CLINICAL CARDIOVASCULAR THERAPEUTICS

Series editors
Henry A. Punzi, M.D.
Walter Flamenbaum, M.D.

Volume 1

Hypertension

editors

Henry A. Punzi, M.D.
Medical Director
Trinity Hypertension and Diagnostic Research Center
Carrollton, Texas

Walter Flamenbaum, M.D.
President
Health and Sciences Research, Inc.
Englewood Cliffs, New Jersey

Futura Publishing
Company, Inc.
Mount Kisco, NY
1989

Copyright 1989
Futura Publishing Company, Inc.

Published by
Futura Publishing Company, Inc.
2 Bedford Ridge Rd., P.O. Box 330
Mount Kisco, New York 10549

Clinical Cardiovascular Therapeutics ISSN# : 1045-8417
ISBN# : 0-87993-372-0

All rights reserved.
No part of this book may be translated or reproduced in any form without the written permission of the publisher.

Printed in the United States of America.

*This volume is dedicated to
Angela Punzi and Judith Flamenbaum
without whose support and efforts
we could not have accomplished so much.*

Contributors

Richard P. Ames, M.D.
Clinical Professor of Medicine, Columbia University, College of Physicians and Surgeons, and Director, Hypertension Service, St. Luke's Roosevelt Hospital, New York, New York

John H. Bauer, M.D.
Professor of Medicine, Hypertension Section, Director, Department of Medicine, Division of Nephrology, University of Missouri, Columbia, Missouri

Sydney H. Croog, Ph.D.
Professor, Department of Behavioral Sciences and Community Health, University of Connecticut Health Center, Farmington, Connecticut

Murray Epstein, M.D.
Professor of Medicine, University of Miami, School of Medicine, Nephrology Section, Miami, Florida

Walter Flamenbaum, M.D.
President, Health and Sciences Research, Inc., Englewood Cliffs, New Jersey

Fetnat M. Fouad-Tarazi, M.D.
Head, Cardial Function Lab, Department of Heart and Hypertension Research, The Cleveland Clinic Foundation, Cleveland, Ohio

William H. Frishman, M.D.
Professor of Medicine, Albert Einstein College of Medicine, Director of Medicine, Hospital of Albert Einstein College of Medicine, Bronx, New York

Ray W. Gifford, Jr., M.D.
Senior Vice Chairman Division of Medicine, Senior Physician, Department of Hypertension and Nephrology, The Cleveland Clinic Foundation, Cleveland, Ohio

Katherine S. Jones
Project Manager, Lewin/ICF, Washington, DC

CONTRIBUTORS • v

Barry J. Materson, M.D.
Associate Chief of Staff, Education, Professor of Medicine, Veterans Administration Medical Center, Miami, Florida

E. Paul MacCarthy, M.D.
Director, Hypertension Program, Cincinnati, Ohio

David A. McCarron, M.D.
Professor of Medicine, Co-Head, Division of Nephrology and Hypertension, Division of Nephrology, Oregon Health Sciences University, Portland, Oregon

Franz H. Messerli, M.D.
Director of Clinical Hypertension Laboratory, Professor of Medicine, Tulane University of Medicine, Ochsner Clinic, New Orleans, Louisiana

Joel M. Neutel, M.D.
Clinical Instructor of Medicine, Veterans Administration Medical Center, Long Beach, California

James R. Oster, M.D.
Professor of Medicine, Associate Chief of Medical Service, University of Miami, School of Medicine, Nephrology Section, Miami, Florida

Mark S. Paller, M.D.
Associate Professor of Medicine, University of Minnesota, Department of Medicine, Minneapolis, Minnesota

H. Mitchell Perry, Jr., M.D.
Professor of Medicine, Director of Hypertension Division, Washington University School of Medicine, St. Louis, Missouri

Thomas G. Pickering, M.D., D.Phil.
Professor of Medicine, Cardiovascular Center, The New York Hospital–Cornell Medical Center, Cornell Medical Center, Hypertension Center, New York, New York

Marc A. Pohl, M.D.
Department of Hypertension and Nephrology, The Cleveland Clinic Foundation, Cleveland, Ohio

Henry A. Punzi, M.D.
Medical Director, Trinity Hypertension and Diagnostic Research Center, Carrollton, Texas

CONTRIBUTORS

Garry P. Reams, M.D.
Associate Professor of Medicine, Department of Medicine, Division of Nephrology, University of Missouri, Columbia, Missouri

Helen C. Redman, M.D.
Professor of Radiology, University of Texas, Southwestern Medical Center, Dallas, Texas

Molly E. Reusser
Research Associate, Division of Nephrology and Hypertension, Oregon Health Sciences University, Portland, Oregon

Robert J. Rubin, M.D.
President, Lewin/ICF, Washington, D.C.

W. Michael Ryan, M.D.
Department of Internal Medicine, Section on Hypertension, Ochsner Clinic and Alton Ochsner Medical Foundation, New Orleans, Louisiana

Ernesto E. Salcedo, M.D.
Department of Cardiology, The Cleveland Clinic Foundation, Cleveland, Ohio

James A. Schoenberger, M.D.
Roberts Professor and Chairman, Department of Preventive Medicine, Rush-Presbyterian-St. Luke's Medicine Center, Chicago, Illinois

David H. G. Smith, M.D.
Clinical Instructor of Medicine, Hypertension Section, Veterans Administration Medical Center, Long Beach, California

Donald G. Vidt, M.D.
Chairman, Department of Hypertension and Nephrology, The Cleveland Clinic Foundation, Cleveland, Ohio

Michael A. Weber, M.D.
Chief, Hypertension Section, Veterans Administration Medical Center, Long Beach, California

Myron H. Weinberger, M.D.
Professor of Medicine, Director, Hypertension Research Center, Specialized Center for Research in Hypertension, Indiana University Medical Center, Indianapolis, Indiana

Foreword

The therapy of hypertension is now the most common indication for patient visits to physicians as well as for the use of legal drugs. Although orally effective therapy has been available for over 30 years and many millions of patients have been effectively treated, the field of antihypertension therapy is now undergoing significant change. Overall precepts, long held and institutionalized, such as the diuretic-first stepcare approach, are being attacked and discarded, to be replaced by significantly different approaches. Drugs such as reserpine and methyldopa, used in millions of patients, are being withdrawn from formularies, being replaced by a mix of new, totally differently acting agents. Concerns about subtle adverse effects, including some such as sleep and sexual function that are difficult to assess, are increasingly being addressed and considered.

At the same time that all of the changes are being made in drug therapy, a continually increasing amount of data about nondrug therapies is being made available. The impetus comes both from concerns about drugs and from the involvement of more and more people with fairly mild hypertension wherein the modest antihypertensive efficacy from nondrug therapies would be expected to provide adequate protection.

With all of these changes, it is obvious that keeping up has become increasingly difficult. Therefore, the availability of a book such as this is welcome. It is composed of separate chapters covering every phase of antihypertensive therapy written by people who are actively involved in clinical investigation about the areas they cover. Special circumstances such as the perioperative period, pregnancy, and old age are given special emphasis. Particular attention is paid to adverse effects of therapy—both overt symptoms and hidden biochemical changes. All of this follows a thorough analysis of the background of hypertension including its natural history and diagnostic evaluation, as well as the burgeoning use of ambulatory blood pressure monitoring. All in all, this book should be useful as an up-to-date, state-of-the-art review of what many of us continue to believe is the most important unsolved problem in clinical medicine—the proper therapy of hypertension.

Norman M. Kaplan, M.D.
Professor of Internal Medicine
The University of Texas
Southwest Medical Center
Dallas, Texas

Introduction

The medical "history" of hypertension—its diagnosis and treatment—to a great degree parallels the overall pattern of the changes in medicine in general. The cycles relative to the varying emphasis on diagnosis and treatment, cause and effect, safety and efficacy, serve to underscore this parallel. Similarly, the cycle of books about hypertension has varied from personal descriptive contributions to large-scale encyclopedic tomes.

The present volume has grown out of the encouragement of our colleagues to provide a current and palatable contribution lending a contemporary perspective for the health care professional. Like other similar efforts, our objectives became more global in order to encompass our desires to attain a broader cardiovascular approach. The current volume, *Clinical Cardiovascular Therapeutics: Hypertension* is the first in a series having the therapy of cardiovascular diseases as the central theme. To those who share our view, the series provides the "bigger picture." To others with a different perspective and different goals, the various volumes should be viewed as an opportunity to choose among the various contributions.

The organization of this volume is neither new nor ideal. To both of us, it represents a bridge similar to our own education and experiences. After a consideration of the background and diagnostic principles, including newer techniques such as ambulatory blood pressure monitoring, we proceed to a review of the end-organ effects of hypertension. The next sections deal with the specifics of both nonpharmacologic and pharmacologic therapy, with the contribution on quality of life linking with reviews related to some specific subsets of hypertensives.

There are a number of people who have made this task both enjoyable and possible. The contributors have offered advice and support and their help is gratefully acknowledged. Similarly, the entire staff at Futura, and Steven Korn in particular, have provided warmth and professionalism allowing us to concentrate on the book. Our own office staffs, despite our promise to the contrary, have been their usual source of expertise and competence, and for this we thank both Marie Ruocco and Janith Mills. This adventure was and remains a very personal undertaking for both editors and we owe an overwhelming debt to our teachers, our patients, and our families.

Henry A. Punzi, M.D.
Walter Flamenbaum, M.D.

Contents

Foreword vii
Introduction ix

Chapter 1. **Pathophysiological and Pathogenic Aspects of Hypertension**
Franz H. Messerli, M.D., and
W. Michael Ryan, M.D. 1

Chapter 2. **The Diagnosis and Evaluation of the Hypertensive Patient**
Richard P. Ames, M.D. 23

Chapter 3. **The Role of Ambulatory Blood Pressure Monitoring**
Joel M. Neutel, M.D., David H. G. Smith, M.D., and Michael A. Weber, M.D. 43

Chapter 4. **Core Organ Effects**

Part I **Uses for Echocardiography in Hypertension**
Fetnat M. Fouad-Tarazi, M.D., and
Ernesto E. Salcedo, M.D. 57

Part II **Cerebral**
Ray W. Gifford, Jr., M.D. 65

Part III **Renal**
John H. Bauer, M.D., and
Garry P. Reams, M.D. 83

Chapter 5. **Nondrug Therapy of Hypertension**
Molly E. Reusser and
David McCarron, M.D. 97

Chapter 6. **Diuretics**
Barry J. Materson, M.D. 117

Chapter 7. **Calcium Antagonists in the Management of Hypertension**
Murray Epstein, M.D., and James R. Oster, M.D. 131

Chapter 8. **Converting Enzyme Inhibitors in the Treatment of Hypertension**
James A. Schoenberger, M.D. 155

CONTENTS

Chapter 9.	Beta-Adrenergic Blockade in Systemic Hypertension William H. Frishman, M.D.	167
Chapter 10.	Vasodilators E. Paul MacCarthy, M.D.	183
Chapter 11.	Centrally Acting Antihypertensive Agents H. Mitchell Perry, Jr., M.D.	207
Chapter 12.	Quality of Life and the Hypertensive Patient: Clinical Aspects Sydney H. Croog, Ph.D.	221
Chapter 13.	Hypertension and Concomitant Disease Henry A. Punzi, M.D.	247
Chapter 14.	Hypertension in the Elderly: Impact, Pathophysiology, and Treatment Myron H. Weinberger, M.D.	269
Chapter 15.	Hypertension in the Perioperative Period Thomas G. Pickering, M.D., D.Phil.	283
Chapter 16.	Hypertension and Pregnancy Mark S. Paller, M.D.	293
Chapter 17.	Urgent, Emergent, and Refractory Hypertension Donald G. Vidt, M.D.	315
Chapter 18.	Lipids and the Cost-Effectiveness of Antihypertensive Therapy Katherine S. Jones and Robert J. Rubin, M.D.	335
Chapter 19.	Renovascular Hypertension: A Radiologist's Point of View Helen C. Redman, M.D.	351
Chapter 20.	Renovascular Hypertension: An Internist's Point of View Marc A. Pohl, M.D.	367
Chapter 21.	The Future Henry A. Punzi, M.D., and Walter Flamenbaum, M.D.	395
Index		399

Chapter 1

Pathophysiological and Pathogenetic Aspects of Essential Hypertension

Franz H. Messerli and W. Michael Ryan

Introduction

Essential or primary hypertension can be defined as a blood pressure elevation, the etiology of which remains unknown. The term "essential" is a misnomer; it was thought that the elevation of blood pressure was "essential" to force blood through an atherosclerotic arterial tree in order to perfuse vital organs—a concept that has been refuted in recent decades. Although the exact etiology of essential hypertension remains unknown, an extensive body of knowledge has been accumulated regarding the pathogenesis and pathophysiology of blood pressure elevation. This chapter reviews some current concepts (and omits others) concerning the pathogenesis and pathophysiology of essential hypertension and provides the practicing physician with a logical framework upon which to build a specific and effective treatment plan.

Cardiovascular Findings

Hypertension is by definition a hemodynamic disorder. The hemodynamic hallmark of essential hypertension is an inappropriate increase in total peripheral resistance (TPR) that is mediated by increases

From Punzi HA, Flamenbaum W (eds): *Hypertension*. Mount Kisco, NY, Futura Publishing Co., Inc., © 1989.

in arterial as well as venous tone. The exact hemodynamic profile found in a given patient is, however, modified by age, body habitus, sex, and race.

Age

Extensive epidemiologic studies by Berenson and others have demonstrated that essential hypertension begins during childhood. Between the ages of 5 and 16 years, blood pressure appears to correlate most directly with body height and less so with weight. Children who consistently "track" above the 75th percentile with respect to blood pressure have a significantly increased risk of becoming hypertensive when adults.

Borderline Hypertension

A variety of studies from all over the globe has documented that young patients with so-called labile, juvenile, or borderline hypertension are hemodynamically characterized by a small but definite increase in cardiac output (Fig. 1) resulting from an increased heart rate and an augmented myocardial contractility. Intravascular volume is distributed centripetally toward the cardiopulmonary circulation and away from the periphery, indicating constriction of the capacitance vessels. Thus, venous constriction is one of the earliest manifestations of blood pressure elevation. The increase in arterial pressure seems to be related to the increase in cardiac output, and TPR remains numerically normal. Clearly, however, this normalcy is not appropriate in the presence of an elevated cardiac output. In a normotensive subject, a similar increase in cardiac output would lead to a fall in TPR. Thus, the term "inappropriately normal TPR" has been used to characterize the hemodynamic abnormality of borderline hypertension. Not surprisingly, with maximal exercise TPR remains distinctly elevated in patients with borderline hypertension when compared to TPR in normotensive subjects.

Concomitantly with the increase in cardiac output, a mild increase in renal blood flow is often seen. Plasma renin activity when related to 24-hour urinary sodium indicates a high-renin state. Similarly, plasma norepinephrine levels have been found to be elevated in patients with borderline hypertension compared to age-matched normotensive subjects. Pharmacological interventions demonstrate that a subset of pa-

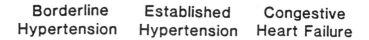

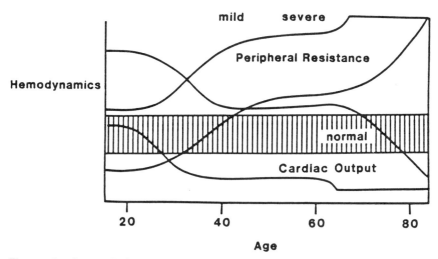

Figure 1. Systemic hemodynamics of essential hypertension change with age and progressive severity of hypertension. The young borderline hypertensive patient is characterized by a high cardiac output and a numerically normal resistance. In established essential hypertension, cardiac output reverts to normal, and resistance becomes distinctly elevated. In the elderly hypertensive patient and in those with congestive heart failure, cardiac output falls and resistance becomes even more elevated. (With permission from Messerli FH: Individualization of antihypertensive therapy: an approach based on hemodynamics and age. J Clin Pharmacol 21:517–528, 1981.)

tients with borderline hypertension exhibit a hyper-beta-adrenergic state, whereas others seem to be characterized by a hypovagotonic state. This would indicate that a net increase in adrenergic activity accompanies or causes the hemodynamic features of borderline hypertension.

Established Essential Hypertension

As hypertensive cardiovascular disease progresses, cardiac output starts falling and TPR becomes more and more elevated. Thus, middle-aged patients with established essential hypertension are hemodynamically characterized by a normal cardiac output and an elevated TPR (Fig. 1). Concomitantly with these hemodynamic changes, intravascular volume becomes progressively contracted. A close inverse correlation between intravascular volume and TPR has been demonstrated in patients with untreated essential hypertension by various investigators. This volume contraction in established essential hypertension further attests to the fact that the capacitance vessels (veins) are actively participating in the pathogenesis of blood pressure elevation.

Renal blood flow falls as hypertensive cardiovascular disease progresses, whereas glomerular filtration rate (GFR) remains relatively well preserved. As a consequence, filtration fraction becomes distinctly elevated. Plasma renin activity has been found to be normal in the majority of patients with essential hypertension, although some have inappropriately low and unresponsive plasma renin activity whereas others display predominantly high-renin values. Plasma catecholamines have been found to be normal or only slightly elevated in patients with established essential hypertension.

Hypertension in the Elderly

With further progression of hypertensive cardiovascular disease, the heart, despite adaptive hypertrophy, can no longer generate the force to maintain arterial pressure at its high preset levels. Cardiac output starts falling, and TPR increases, indicating intensified vasoconstriction (Fig. 1). Thus, an elderly patient with essential hypertension is characterized hemodynamically by a low cardiac output (caused by a small stroke volume and a low heart rate) and a distinctly elevated TPR. Renal blood flow falls further because of nephrosclerosis, and GFR begins to decrease. However, an increase in creatinine and blood urea nitrogen is rare in elderly hypertensive patients because the fall in GFR rarely exceeds 50% and muscle mass (the source of creatinine) diminishes with age.

Plasma renin activity usually is low and unresponsive in elderly patients with essential hypertension. However, with the manifestation of congestive heart failure, an increase in the activity of the renin-angiotensin-aldosterone cascade may occur. In patients with congestive heart failure, plasma renin activity can be greatly stimulated, particularly when there is no peripheral edema. Plasma catecholamines increase with progressive severity of hypertension and age and reach their highest levels in the elderly. In patients with congestive heart failure, a further increase in plasma norepinephrine levels can be observed.

Target Organ Disease

A persistently elevated arterial pressure results in profound effects in the so-called target organs: the brain, heart, and kidneys. While initially these functional and morphological changes appear to be adaptive responses to abnormal hemodynamics, they ultimately contribute to much of the morbidity and mortality from persisting hypertension. Additional discussions of these core organs in hypertension can be found in Chapter 4.

The Heart

The heart plays a dual role in the pathophysiology of essential hypertension. First, it generates the force that is needed to maintain arterial pressure at its elevated levels. Second, as a target organ, it suffers and becomes damaged from long-standing hypertension. The first evidence of cardiac adaptation to an increase in arterial pressure can be found in childhood and adolescence. Studies have shown that children whose blood pressures were above the 90th percentile had higher left ventricular mass and posterior wall thickness than children with normal arterial pressure.

As hypertension progresses, the septal wall, posterior wall, and relative wall thicknesses increase, indicating concentric left ventricular hypertrophy (LVH), an increase in wall thickness at the expense of chamber volume (Fig. 2). Even in this phase, some patients have been reported to have inappropriate septal hypertrophy, suggesting either a different genetic predisposition or a different adaptation to the hemodynamic pattern. We recently documented in two different populations of hypertensive patients in New Orleans and in Bonn (Germany) a close correlation between 24-hour urinary sodium and left ventricular mass (Fig. 3). A high salt intake therefore seems to facilitate the development of LVH, and, conversely, a low-salt diet may prevent or slow down this process. Early in this process, left atrial emptying index decreases, indicating diastolic dysfunction associated later with impaired ventricular compliance. At the same time, manifestations of left atrial enlargement can be found. However, only between 1% and 15% of patients who fulfill echocardiographic criteria of LVH (posterior wall thickness exceeding 11 mm) also have electrocardiographic evidence of LVH. Clearly, the electrocardiogram is a relatively insensitive and late indicator of LVH in hypertension.

The presence of LVH by ECG criteria predisposes the patient to left ventricular ectopic activity and more complicated arrhythmias. We have

6 • HYPERTENSION

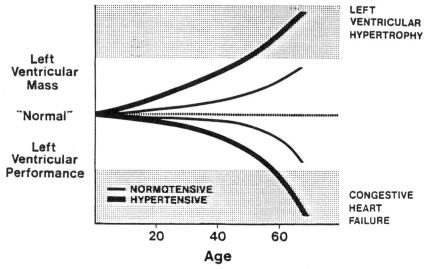

Figure 2. Changes in left ventricular performance with age. (Reproduced from Messerli FH: Clinical determinants and consequences of left ventricular hypertrophy. Am J Med 75:51–63, 1981.)

documented that such patients have a significantly higher prevalence of premature ventricular contractions and score higher with regard to Lown's classifications than patients without electrocardiographic evidence of LVH or normotensive subjects. The Framingham study has shown that the occurrence of both echo- and electrocardiographic LVH puts the patient at risk for sudden death and other cardiovascular mortality, irrespective of levels of arterial pressure. Twenty-four-hour Holter monitoring allows us to identify patients who are at the highest risk and therefore need the most aggressive therapeutic intervention.

Findings from our laboratory have indicated that ventricular ectopic activity occurs not only in concentric LVH but can be found in patients with eccentric LVH as well (an increase in wall thickness and left ventricular mass, with chamber dilatation). A variety of recent studies from the United States and abroad have confirmed and extended our data on the arrhythmogenicity of the hypertrophied left ventricle.

The Kidneys

An abnormality in renal blood flow could also participate in the pathogenesis of essential hypertension, either initiating or sustaining

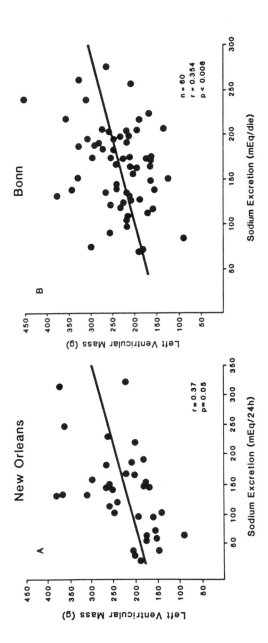

Figure 3. The correlation between 24-hour sodium excretion and left ventricular mass in a homogeneous population of hypertensive patients in Bonn and in a biracial population in New Orleans.

the increase in arterial pressure. Regardless of whether or not the kidney plays a central role in the pathogenesis of essential hypertension, numerous studies document that the kidney suffers as a target organ from long-standing hypertension. In young patients with borderline hypertension who are characterized by an elevated cardiac output, renal blood flow also can be elevated. It has been shown that normotensive offspring of hypertensive parents are also characterized by an increased renal blood flow. As hypertension becomes more established, renal blood flow falls rapidly, mostly because of a reduction in cortical perfusion. A variety of methods has been used to document the reduction in cortical perfusion. Whether the reduction in cortical blood flow is due to arteriosclerosis, vascular constriction, or both remains unknown.

GFR has been shown to remain fairly well preserved despite a decline in renal blood flow in essential hypertension. These findings point to an increased intraglomerular pressure, which mainly determines the GFR. Previously, it was suggested that an increased intraglomerular pressure was the pathogenetic guidepost to the development of nephrosclerosis in various kidney diseases, regardless of their etiology. An increased intraglomerular pressure is mediated either by relatively decreased afferent or increased efferent vascular resistance in the kidney. As a result of a normal GFR and a reduced renal blood flow, filtration fraction increases distinctly. Thus, the classical renal findings in early established essential hypertension consist of a normal GFR, a low renal blood flow (mainly because of a reduction in cortical perfusion), an increase in filtration fraction, and probably an increase in intraglomerular pressure. In later stages of hypertensive disease, the renal vascular bed also exhibits an enhanced response to vasodilators such as phentolamine and angiotensin-converting enzyme inhibitors.

What are the clinical consequences, if any, of these early adaptations in renal function through arterial hypertension? Unfortunately, the kidney is an organ with a function that is difficult to quantitate accurately in clinical practice. Serum creatinine, creatinine clearance, and other semiquantitative function tests usually are normal in mild nephrosclerosis. When challenged with a saline load, most patients with essential hypertension excrete the sodium at a faster rate than normotensives. This so-called exaggerated natriuresis occurs in hypertension that results from a variety of conditions, suggesting that this is a hemodynamic effect caused by the elevated arterial pressure per se. A saline load produces a greater increase in renal blood flow and GFR in hypertensives than it does in normotensive control subjects.

Are there any other means of suspecting a decrease in renal blood flow short of measuring para-aminohippuric acid clearance? We found that serum uric acid correlated inversely with renal blood flow and directly with renal vascular resistance in a population of patients with early essential hypertension and in normotensive subjects who had no evidence of disturbances of uric acid metabolism, such as gout, obesity, alcohol abuse, etc. In contrast to renal blood flow, cardiac output and GFR showed no uric acid-independent pattern. We therefore concluded that unexplained mild hyperuricemia in patients with essential hypertension most likely reflects early vascular involvement, that is, a decrease in renal blood flow and an elevated renal vascular resistance, which are manifestations of early nephrosclerosis.

The Brain

In contrast to the heart and, to a lesser extent, the kidneys, early target organ damage in the brain cannot be measured with diagnostic tools. Unfortunately, all too often the first cerebral manifestation of essential hypertension is a transient ischemic attack or a stroke.

The function of the central nervous system is dependent on a continuous and constant amount of glucose and oxygen. In order to fulfill these requirements, cerebral blood flow has been shown to remain constant despite impressive fluctuations in arterial pressure. Cerebral arterioles dilate when blood pressure falls and constrict when blood pressure rises. These compensatory changes in arterial tone seem to be mediated by intraluminal pressure changes. Sustained increases in arterial blood pressure therefore produce arteriolar vasoconstriction. Arterial changes in brains of patients with long-standing, untreated hypertension include atherosclerosis of large arteries and fibrinoid necrosis of small vessels. These changes are associated with the small aneurysms found classically in the same regions as intracerebral hemorrhages, and the small cystic infarcts (lacunae) that are common autopsy findings in brains of patients suffering from prolonged hypertension. Common long-term complications of untreated hypertension also include intracerebral bleeding, with or without associated subarachnoid bleeding, and occlusive disease of the larger vessels (transient ischemic attack, cerebral infarction) and smaller vessels (lacunae).

Demographic Aspects

Race

Essential hypertension has been found to be a more common and more severe disease in black patients than it is in white patients. Thus, for any given level of arterial pressure, black patients have more severe hypertensive target organ disease in the heart and kidneys than white patients. These epidemiologic differences notwithstanding, we were unable to document a pathophysiological correlate when we examined systemic and regional hemodynamics in black patients and in white patients a few years ago. For any given level of arterial pressure, black patients had blood volumes and levels of TPR similar to those of white patients. In two subsequent studies, however, we found an increase in renal vascular resistance and left ventricular mass in black patients who were matched with white patients with regard to mean arterial pressure. Although systemic hemodynamic findings are similar in the two races, target organ disease is obviously more pronounced in black patients. These pathophysiological observations lend credence to the epidemiologic finding that essential hypertension is a more severe disease among black populations than it is among white populations.

Gender

In 1968, Pickering, after reviewing the epidemiologic evidence, came to the conclusion that for any given level of blood pressure, women fare better than men. We recently examined systemic hemodynamics in 100 women with mildly established essential hypertension and compared them with hemodynamics in an equal number of men who were matched with regard to mean arterial pressure and age. Premenopausal women were characterized hemodynamically by a lower TPR and a higher cardiac output than men of similar age and arterial pressure. With menopause, these hemodynamic differences between the sexes tended to disappear. Vascular resistance, at least to some extent, parallels vascular disease, and the fact that it is lower in women indicates that they are likely to have a lower incidence of vascular disease at any level of arterial pressure. Our pathophysiological observations provide a correlate to half a century of clinical and epidemiologic observation that hypertension is a more benign disorder in women than it is in men.

Aspects of Essential Hypertension • 11

Obesity-Hypertension

Cardiovascular Findings

Any increase in body mass (muscular or adipose tissue) requires a higher cardiac output and expanded intravascular volume to meet the elevated metabolic requirements. Thus, from a hemodynamic standpoint, obesity corresponds with a mild state of volume overload. Provided that arterial pressure remains unchanged, in obese patients an elevated cardiac output will result in a fall in TPR. Therefore, for any level of arterial pressure, cardiac output is higher and systemic vascular resistance is lower in an obese patient than in a lean patient.

Since heart rate remains unchanged when a patient becomes obese, the increase in cardiac output occurs by means of an expanded stroke volume. An elevated left ventricular filling pressure and end-diastolic volume in overweight subjects increases preload, which gives rise to chamber dilatation. According to La Place's law, chamber dilatation increases wall stress, which increases afterload. The dilated left ventricle adapts to these stresses, if they persist, by an increase in muscle mass. Therefore, obesity produces predominantly left ventricular hypertrophy and dilatation, or eccentric hypertrophy, regardless of the level of arterial pressure (Fig. 4). In a study of a heterogeneous population of 171 patients, we recently showed that body weight and body surface area were the most powerful determinants of left ventricle chamber size, wall thickness, and muscle mass (Fig. 5). Indeed, patients who were more than 50% overweight had a 50% prevalence of LVH (defined as posterior wall thickness exceeding 11 mm).

It has been known for many years that obesity takes a toll on the heart. Hippocrates noted that sudden death is more common in the obese than in the lean. We recently demonstrated that obese patients who lacked electrocardiographic evidence of LVH but who had distinct eccentric LVH on the echocardiogram had a markedly increased prevalence and complexity of ventricular ectopy than slender patients or obese patients without LVH (Fig. 6). These observations suggest that an electrophysiological abnormality may be the cause of the epidemiologic findings in the Framingham cohort identifying obesity as an independent risk factor for sudden death and other cardiovascular morbidity and mortality.

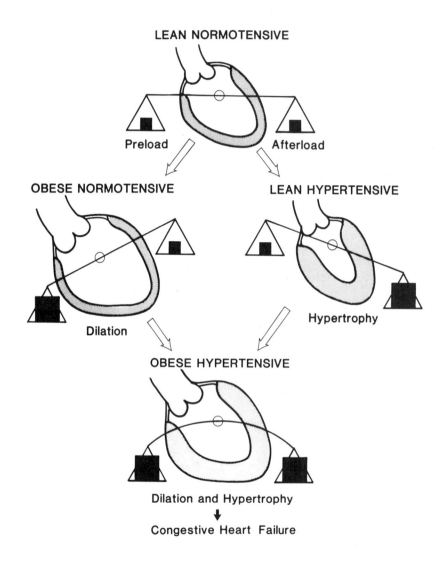

Figure 4. Effects of obesity and hypertension on the left ventricle. (With permission from Messerli FH: Cardiovascular effects of obesity and hypertension. Lancet I:1165–1168, 1982).

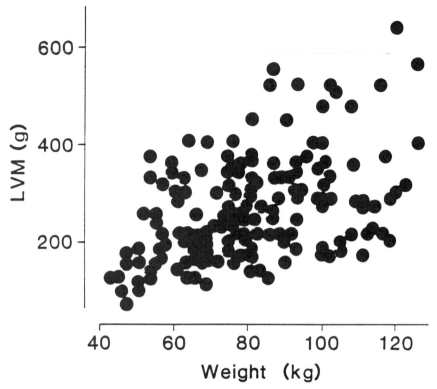

Figure 5. High prevalence of ventricular ectopy in obese patients with eccentric left ventricular hypertrophy when compared to obese patients without left ventricular hypertrophy or lean subjects.

The Obesity-Hypertension Connection

It is postulated that mild obesity may protect a given patient from the deleterious effects of hypertension by reducing systemic vascular resistance and thus decreasing hypertensive target organ damage, and there are data to support this hypothesis. We have shown that systemic vascular resistance and renal vascular resistance are lower in obese patients than in lean subjects with similar arterial pressures. Likewise, there is an inverse correlation between body weight and renal vascular resistance. Investigators have suggested that the lower vascular resistance in obese patients possibly decreases the risk of hypertensive retinopathy, nephrosclerosis, cerebrovascular disease, and other cardio-

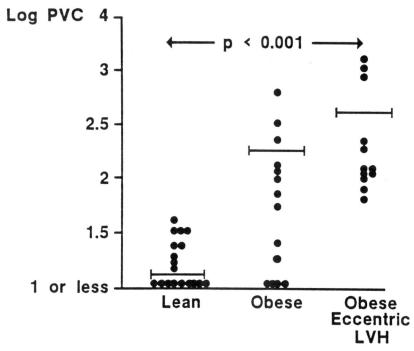

Figure 6. The classic left ventricular response to an increase in afterload, such as occurs in hypertension, is left ventricular hypertrophy. In contrast, the left ventricular response to a volume overload, such as occurs in obesity, is dilatation and eccentric left ventricular hypertrophy. (With permission from Messerli FH, Nunez BD, Ventura HO, et al: Overweight and sudden death: increased ventricular ectopy in cardiopathy of obesity. Arch Int Med 147:1725–1728, 1987.)

vascular morbidity and mortality. However, the increased intravascular volume and preload in obesity should place these patients at high risk for congestive heart failure. These arguments support Volhard's observations—made more than 50 years ago—that pale hypertension predisposes to vascular disease and nephrosclerosis and red hypertension predisposes to heart failure.

Obesity produces eccentric LVH regardless of arterial pressure. In contrast, the cardiac response to arterial hypertension and increased afterload consists of concentric LVH. When obesity and hypertension occur in the same patient, both preload and afterload are elevated, presenting a double burden to the left ventricle. The dual workload imposed on the heart by obesity and hypertension causes severe cardiac hypertrophy. Over 50 years ago, it was demonstrated that, when compared to the normal value of 272 g, heart weight averaged 376 g in obese subjects without known heart disease and 467 g in subjects who were both obese and hypertensive.

Congestive heart failure occurs in a high percentage of morbidly obese patients irrespective of arterial pressure. Investigators have demonstrated impaired left ventricular function and compliance, as well as high end-diastolic pressures, in patients with significant obesity. We recently demonstrated that patients who are more than 50% overweight have normal left ventricular function as measured by velocity of circumferential and fractional fiber shortening. However, the left atrial emptying index, a sensitive indicator of diastolic ventricular emptying compliance, is markedly decreased in obese normotensive and obese hypertensive patients, thus demonstrating diastolic ventricular dysfunction in obesity. Although diastolic ventricular dysfunction occurs early in obesity, we showed that diastolic ventricular compliance is most markedly decreased in obesity-hypertension. In addition, preliminary data from our laboratory indicate that contractility, when measured by a preload-independent index (end-systolic stress/end-systolic volume index), is decreased early in obesity-hypertension. This systolic and diastolic dysfunction and increased preload will tax the heart and, not surprisingly, lead to premature congestive heart failure in obesity, particularly in obesity-hypertension.

Weight Reduction

Weight reduction in obese hypertensive patients is clearly associated with a fall in arterial pressure, but the underlying mechanism remains obscure. The reduction in pressure has been attributed to alterations in body fluid partitions by reduced sodium intake and falls in renin and aldosterone levels. Weight loss reduces the sympathetic drive to the cardiovascular system, allowing a redistribution of the intravascular volume from the cardiopulmonary area to the periphery, thereby reducing venous return (preload), cardiac output, and arterial pressure. As has been shown, weight loss may be associated with a small but significant decrease in left ventricular mass and septal and posterior wall thickness. However, in a recent study of patients who were morbidly obese, a weight loss of 55 kg induced by gastric resection resulted in improved systolic left ventricular performance but did not significantly reduce septal or posterior wall thickness.

Regardless of the mechanism, weight loss clearly reduces the double burden imposed on the heart by obesity and arterial hypertension; decreases preload, afterload, and sympathetic stimulation; and may reverse cardiac hypertrophy. Unloading the heart from this twofold burden should become a major goal in the prevention and treatment of cardiac diseases.

Pathogenetic Aspects of Essential Hypertension

What are the pathogenetic mechanisms leading to the progressive increase in peripheral vascular resistance once essential hypertension becomes established? Why do patients undergo a hemodynamic transition from a "hyperdynamic" hemodynamic phase, with a high cardiac output, to a "vasculogenic" hemodynamic phase, with a high vascular resistance? While no one clear, unifying answer is as yet forthcoming, it appears certain that primary hypertension is the result of the dynamic interplay of several related systems (neuronal, humoral, cellular, etc). We will explore some of these systems both individually and collectively as they interrelate in the pathogenesis and maintenance of primary hypertension.

Sympathetic Nervous System

That the autonomic nervous system is vitally important in blood pressure homeostasis has been known for decades. Evidence for this importance comes partially from experience with patients manifesting genetic or acquired autonomic dysfunction in which normal, posture-related sustenance of arterial pressure is impossible to maintain; these individuals exhibit sometimes profound hypotension. Furthermore, it is clear that pharmacological or surgical blockade of the sympathetic nervous system can effect peripheral vasodilatation, lower arterial pressure, and produce orthostatic hypotension. The "hyperdynamic" hemodynamic profile described above, present in many young patients with borderline hypertension, appears to be mediated largely by increased sympathoadrenal drive. Elevations in plasma catecholamine levels are found occasionally. It is likely that augmented central (i.e., brain stem) sympathetic outflow and increased receptor sensitivity to circulating catecholamines play a role in elevating cardiac output and peripheral vascular resistance. Epinephrine, secreted episodically from the adrenal medulla, appears to be taken up into the presynaptic regions of the peripheral sympathetic nerves, resulting in amplified release of stored norepinephrine into the nerve synapses.

Recent research into the dopaminergic system revealed a decrease in central dopaminergic activity in primary hypertension. Since dopamine is known to elicit natriuresis, is vasodilatory, particularly in the renal vascular bed, and decreases aldosterone secretion from the adrenal cortex, decreased dopamine output by the medullary vasomotor centers could result in chronic sodium retention and excessive peripheral vasoconstriction.

Young patients with borderline hypertension exhibit excessive increases in plasma norepinephrine during stressful mental tasks. Other provocative maneuvers involving the sympathetic nervous system (e.g., cold pressor tests) also reveal abnormal responses in hypertensives and in normotensives from hypertension-prone families. In addition, baroreceptor regulation of increases in mean arterial pressure also appears blunted in these two groups. Thus, a genetic predisposition (through uncertain mechanisms) toward exaggerated adrenergic responses to stressful stimuli, coupled with a blunting of normal baroreceptor suppression of pressure surges may set the stage for the initiation and maintenance of "essential" hypertension.

The Renin-Angiotensin System

The renin-angiotensin system has emerged over the past 15 years as a major hormonal axis involved in both pressure and sodium homeostasis. The juxtaglomerular apparatus of the kidney was thought initially to be the predominant source of renin. However, work in our laboratory and elsewhere provided strongly suggestive evidence of intact renin-angiotensin systems in many other tissue sites throughout the body, such as the brain (neurohypophysis), testes, uterus, salivary glands, and cardiac and vascular myocytes.

Several stimuli result in renin release from the juxtaglomerular cells, such as (1) decreased distal tubular sodium concentration, (2) decreased effective plasma volume and perfusion pressure at the afferent arteriolar level, and (3) increased renal sympathetic nerve activity causing renin release via a beta-receptor. Renin acts upon circulating angiotensinogen to produce the decapeptide, angiotensin I, a hormone with no known biological activity. Upon entering the pulmonary circulation, converting enzyme cleaves off two amino acids, resulting in the octapeptide, angiotensin II, one of the most potent vasoconstrictors known. In addition to its ability to markedly raise peripheral and renal vascular resistances, angiotensin II is a very potent stimulus for aldosterone secretion by the adrenal cortex. Therefore, as a normal adaptive response to a perceived decrease in effective perfusion to one or both kidneys, renin-mediated angiotensin II production can result in elevation of mean arterial pressure by vasoconstriction (directly) and by sodium and water retention (indirectly, through aldosterone).

There is also strong evidence that angiotensin II and the sympathetic nervous system interact synergistically, each system augmenting the activity of the other. For example, presynaptic angiotensin II receptors may increase norepinephrine release from peripheral sympathetic nerves. Central angiotensin II receptors may also facilitate medullary sympathetic nerve outflow. Young hypertensives tend to possess not only enhanced sympathetic drive but also, for the most part, relatively high plasma renin activity when indexed to 24-hour urinary sodium excretion. However, these elevations in plasma renin activity decrease with age, and elderly hypertensives tend to have low and unresponsive renin levels.

Atrial Natriuretic Factor

The pioneering work of de Bold revealed that the heart is an endocrine organ. Crude atrial extracts were found to have natriuretic and vasodilatory activities. It was further discovered that atrial myocytes of mammals manufactured and secreted a circulating 128 amino-acid peptide that possessed several circulatory effects. The release-signal for this atrial natriuretic factor (ANF) was determined to be volume-mediated stretching of the atrial walls. Thus, the heart, in response to volume overload, compensates for this overload by the elaboration of a peptide hormone causing marked natriuresis, increased renal and splanchnic blood flow, and suppression of both renin and aldosterone release. Thus, it effects a reduction in circulating blood volume and restores atrial dimensions to normal.

While it is clear that ANF probably plays an important role in blood volume/pressure homeostasis, its role in the pathogenesis and maintenance of hypertension is controversial. It has been suggested that there is a complimentary interaction between the ANF and the renin-angio-

Aspects of Essential Hypertension • 19

tensin-aldosterone systems, the atrial peptide modulating release of renin (and thus angiotensin II) and aldosterone. A derangement of this interaction could therefore be operative in primary hypertension, resulting in excessive vasoconstriction and relatively expanded intravascular volume. The specific mechanisms whereby ANF effects its vasodilatation/natriuresis have yet to be fully elucidated. Circulating levels of ANF have not been found to correlate with arterial pressure; however, normotensive offspring of hypertensive parents recently have been shown to have a blunted ANF plasma response to sodium loading. This leads to the intriguing hypothesis that prehypertensive individuals have defective release mechanisms for ANF. Conversely, an end-organ insensitivity (renal, adrenal, vascular wall) to the effects of ANF in primary hypertension may also be present. Clearly, much exciting work remains to be done concerning this "cardiac hormone."

Local Vascular Factors

Recent evidence reveals that the blood vessel itself, in addition to its conduit function, is capable of complex metabolic activities including the local release of vasoactive peptides as well as cellular trophic responses to circulating neurohumoral factors. Vascular hypertrophy has been thought of as an adaptive response to elevated arterial pressure in order to reduce wall stress. However, data in certain animal models of hypertension suggest that vascular wall hypertrophy may be a *primary* event. Whatever the stimulus for hypertrophy, the increased wall-to-lumen ratio will result in enhanced vasoconstrictive responses to contractile agonists (Folkow hypothesis). Angiotensin II is an important stimulant for vascular cell hypertrophy, as is mechanical wall stretch due to hypertension itself. Endothelial cells are capable of synthesizing local peptides (such as endothelium-derived relaxation factor) that significantly modulate the vessel wall contractile response. Many other influences on vessel wall hypertrophy and contractile response exist. These include platelet-derived (platelet-derived growth factor [PDGF], prostaglandins, leukotrienes, serotonin, etc.), endothelium-derived (endothelium-derived growth factor, interleukin-I, prostaglandins), and myocyte-derived (PDGF, interleukin-I) substances.

One of the more exciting recent advances in the molecular biology of arterial smooth muscle was the discovery of a 21 amino-acid peptide, endothelin, which is produced and secreted by vascular endothelial cells. Endothelin's importance appears to be related to its potent vasoconstrictor activity, especially in the renal and pulmonary vascular beds. In fact, it seems to be the most potent vasoconstrictor yet discovered. It has been noted that endothelin causes a marked decrease in renal blood flow and glomerular filtration and thereby causes sodium retention. Endothelin also has proven to be a strong stimulus for the release of ANF. Furthermore, it has been postulated that endothelin and ANF may serve as counterregulatory hormones. The extent to which endothelin contributes ultimately to the pathogenesis of hypertension remains conjectural.

Calcium

Probably the most important local vascular factor responsible for vasoconstriction is the calcium ion and its intracellular concentration. Calcium enters smooth muscle cells through "channels," some of which are receptor-mediated while others are voltage-mediated. Calcium then interacts with several cytoplasmic modulatory proteins (e.g., calmodulin). The calcium-protein complex, in turn, activates myosin light-chain kinase (MLCK). It is MLCK that phosphorylates myosin, ultimately resulting in actin-myosin contraction-coupling. This calcium-mediated vasoconstriction is the "final common pathway" whereby circulating vasopressor hormones (such as angiotensin II and norepinephrine) and locally produced peptides (such as endothelin) effect an increase in total and regional vascular resistances. Many investigators feel that excessive accumulation of calcium within the vascular smooth muscle cell is the "essential" cause of the amplified vasoreactivity documented in the resistance vessels of patients with primary hypertension. Intracellular sodium and cyclic adenosine monophosphate levels also correlate positively with intracellular calcium levels. Pathophysiologically, therefore, any cellular defect (e.g., sodium-potassium adenosine triphosphatase inhibition, suppressed sodium-potassium countertransport, etc.) resulting in intracellular sodium accumulation also results in increased calcium availability for the initiation of vascular smooth muscle contraction.

Summary

The hemodynamic hallmark of primary hypertension is an increase in total and regional vascular resistance. This vasospasm is the result of

Aspects of Essential Hypertension • 21

a complex interaction among several distinct biological systems. The intrinsic vasoreactivity of the vascular myocyte is modulated by neuroendocrine vasopressor circulating hormones as well as locally produced vasoactive peptides and growth factors. Vascular hypertrophy, in concert with hyper-reactivity (ultimately mediated via the calcium ion), serves to elevate arterial pressure. Sustained high blood pressure accelerates atherogenesis and thus ultimately induces end-organ dysfunction, accounting for the excess morbidity and mortality seen in hypertensive patients.

Selected References

Berenson GS, Cresanta JL, Webber LS, et al: High blood pressure in the young. Annu Rev Med 35:535–560, 1984.
Caramelo C, Okada K, Tsai P, III, Sodt PC, Messerli FH, et al: Mechanisms of the vascular effect of pressor hormones. Am J Cardiol 62:47G–53G, 1988.
Culpepper WS, et al: Cardiac status in juvenile borderline hypertension. Ann Intern Med 98:1–7, 1983.
Cuneo RC: Effect of physiologic levels of atrial natriuretic peptide on hormone secretion: inhibition of angiotensin-induced aldosterone secretion and renin release in normal man. J Clin Endocrinol Metab 65:765–772, 1987.
Dunn FG, Oigman W, Sundgaard-Riise K, et al: Racial differences in cardiac adaptation to essential hypertension determined by echocardiographic indexes. J Am Coll Cardiol 1:1348–1351, 1983.
Dzau VJ: Cell biology of vascular hypertrophy in systemic hypertension. Am J Cardiol 62:30G–35G, 1988.
Dzau VJ: Significance of vascular renin-angiotensin pathway. Hypertension 8:553, 1986.
Dzau VJ, Re RN: Evidence for the existence of renin in the heart. Circulation 75(Suppl I):I-34, 1987.
Frohlich ED, Messerli FH, Dunn FG, et al: Greater renal vascular involvement in the black patient with essential hypertension: a comparison of systemic and renal hemodynamics in black and white patients. Miner Electrolyte Metab 10:173–177, 1984.
Julius S: Interaction between renin and the autonomic nervous system in hypertension. Am Heart J 116:611–616, 1988.
Julius S: Transition from high cardiac output to elevated vascular resistance in hypertension. Am Heart J 116:600–606, 1988.
Laragh JH: Atrial natriuretic hormone, the renin-aldosterone axis, and blood pressure-electrolyte homeostasis. N Engl J Med 313:1330–1340, 1985.
Masaki T: The discovery, the present state, and the future prospects of endothelin. J Cardiovasc Pharmacol 13(Suppl 5):S1–S4, 1989.
McMurry JJ: Atrial natriuretic factor inhibits isoproteronal and furosemide-stimulated renin release in humans. Hypertension 13:9–14, 1989.
Messerli FH: Cardiopathy of obesity—a not-so-Victorian disease. (editorial) N Engl J Med 314:378–379, 1986.

Messerli FH (ed): The Heart and Hypertension. New York, Yorke Medical Publishers, 1987.
Messerli FH, Sundgaard-Riise K, Ventura HO, et al: Clinical hemodynamic determinants of left ventricular dimensions. Arch Intern Med 144:477–481, 1984.
Messerli FH, Garavaglia GE, Schmieder RE, et al: Disparate cardiovascular findings in men and women with essential hypertension. Ann Int Med 107:158–161, 1987.
Messerli FH, DeCarvalho JGR, Christie B, et al: Essential hypertension in black and white subjects: hemodynamic findings and fluid volume state. Am J Med 67:27–31, 1979.
Messerli FH, Ventura HO, Glade LB, et al: Essential hypertension in the elderly: haemodynamic intra-vascular volume, plasma renin activity, and circulating catecholamine levels. Lancet ii:983–986, 1983.
Messerli FH, Schmieder RE, Nunez BD, et al: Heterogeneous pathophysiology of essential hypertension: implications for therapy. Am Heart J 112:886–893, 1986.
Messerli FH, Ventura HO, Elizardi DJ, et al: Hypertension and sudden death: increased left ventricular ectopic activity in ventricular hypertrophy. Am J Med 77:18–22, 1984.
Messerli FH, Nunez BD, Ventura HO, et al: Overweight and sudden death: increased ventricular ectopy in cardiopathy of obesity. Arch Int Med 147:1725–1728, 1987.
Messerli FH, Frohlich ED, Dreslinski GR, et al: Serum uric acid in essential hypertension: an indicator of renal vascular involvement. Ann Intern Med 93:817–821, 1980.
Needleman P, Adams SP, Cole BR, et al: Atriopeptins as cardiac hormones. Hypertension 7:469–482, 1985.
Pickering GW: High Blood Pressure. London, Churchill-Livingstone, 1955, p 312.
Re RN: Cellular biology of renin-angiotensin systems. Arch Intern Med 144:2037, 1984.
Schmieder RE, Messerli FH: Obesity hypertension. Med Clin North Am 71:991–1001, 1987.
Schmieder RE, Messerli FH, Garavaglia GE, et al: Dietary salt intake: a determinant of cardiac involvement in essential hypertension. Circulation 78:951–956, 1988.
Tuck ML: The sympathetic nervous system in essential hypertension. Am Heart J 112:877–885, 1986.

Chapter 2

The Diagnosis and Evaluation of the Hypertensive Patient

Richard P. Ames

Introduction

Hypertension has become a household word in recent years. Public awareness of the high prevalence of the condition, of its role in cardiovascular morbidity, and of the effectiveness of treatment has created an atmosphere of urgency about therapy. The very simplicity of blood pressure measurement and the widespread availability of blood pressure measuring devices provides a setting at present in which treatment may be instituted too hastily. Proper diagnosis of hypertension is still the basis for good medical care. The diagnosis of hypertension usually requires time and certainly requires an attention to detail. Isolated blood pressure readings may not be representative of the prevailing levels of arterial pressure. General apprehension about the numbers and insufficient appreciation of the indolent nature of the disease put pressure on the doctor to prescribe immediately. Treatment is often the course of least resistance.

It is the purpose of this chapter to outline the most important points in the diagnosis of the hypertensive patient. This chapter draws on the guidelines of the Joint National Committee on Detection, Evaluation, and Treatment of High Blood Pressure. The chapter also incorporates the perspective of the author based on two decades of personal experience with hypertensive patients.

The Detection of Hypertension

The Measurement of Blood Pressure

An accurate recording of the blood pressure is critical to the proper diagnosis of hypertension. Blood pressure fluctuates continuously; this lability is due, in part, to identifiable factors (Table 1). Some of these factors can be controlled by standardizing the circumstances of measurement.

Some practical points in effecting the standardization of the casual (office) measurement need emphasis. Even mild exertion can raise blood pressure acutely in some patients. Thus, even though a patient may have waited 10–15 minutes in a waiting room, a short walk to the examining room may be sufficient exertion to raise blood pressure above basal levels. Another 5 minutes of complete rest is often necessary to allow the pressure to settle back to basal.

Another cause of an acute pressor response, insufficiently appreciated, is talking. A quiet conversation often raises blood pressure by 20/10 mmHg in hypertensive persons. In particularly reactive individ-

Table 1
Tips for Standardizing the Casual Blood Pressure Measurement

1. Patient sitting or supine for at least 5 minutes.
2. When sitting, the patient should be resting against the back of the chair.
3. Arm should be supported at the level of the heart.
4. Proper cuff size, based on measurement of arm circumference.
5. Remove constricting clothing above the cuff.
6. Avoid eating or smoking for 1 hour before the measurement. Avoid coffee for 3 hours.
7. Avoid bladder and bowel distention.
8. Minimize anxiety-provoking circumstances.
9. Avoid talking for 2 minutes before measurement.
10. Allow at least 30 seconds between measurements on the same arm.
11. Be alert to the auscultatory gap.
12. Use fifth phase (disappearance) of Korotkoff sounds.
13. In arrhythmias, record values at which the majority of heart beats are heard as Korotkoff sounds.
14. Record blood pressure at least once after 2 minutes standing.

Diagnosis and Evaluation • 25

uals, the increase can be twice as much. The prohibition from talking during the process of blood pressure measurement is one of most difficult to contend with. A useful routine to cope with these various influences on blood pressure levels is to proceed as follows. First, get the patient comfortably settled in a chair with a back support or supine on an examining table. Apply the cuff to the bared arm, with the arm supported at the level of the heart. Take the interval history, and without further conversation, do an interval physical examination, examine any laboratory data, and record the findings in the chart. *Then* take the blood pressure two or three times. A minute or two should elapse between blood pressure recordings. Although it is reported that readings can be taken as rapidly as every 15 seconds, my own observation suggests that rapidly repeated recordings are lower than the initial measurement. A longer pause between measurements tends to give more reproducible numbers. If successive readings differ by more than 10 mmHg in either systolic or diastolic pressure, additional recordings should be obtained. Use the average of the two closest determinations.

For sitting blood pressure measurements, which are more widely used than supine readings, the patient's chair should have a back-rest. Blood pressure may be raised above basal when the patient's back is unsupported, as when sitting on an examining table.

The ingestion of coffee can raise blood pressure in some circumstances. The degree of blood pressure elevation varies inversely with the regularity of usage. In the habitual nondrinker, coffee may raise blood pressure by an average of 14/10 mmHg for 2 to 3 hours. This effect may abate completely after a week of steady coffee usage. However, abstinence from it for as little as 24 hours following regular usage can partially restore the pressor effect. In view of the varying sensitivity of the individual to the hypertensive action of caffeine, avoidance of it for 3 to 4 hours before blood pressure measurement eliminated another extraneous influence.

Blood pressure should be measured in both arms at the initial visit. If a notable difference is found, the arm with the higher readings should be used in subsequent visits.

Cuff Size

Obtaining an auscultatory blood pressure reading which is close to the true intra-arterial pressure requires a cuff of the appropriate width. More correctly stated, it is the bladder within the cuff that determines the accuracy of the measurement. Readings are most accurate when the bladder width is 40% of the circumference of the upper arm. Stated conversely, the cuff is appropriate if the circumference of the patient's arm is 2.5 times (±10%) the width of the bladder. A narrow cuff will give a reading higher than the true intra-arterial pressure. A wide cuff gives a falsely low reading. Cuffs are available in the United States in sizes termed adult, obese, and thigh cuffs. Standard adult cuffs have bladders that are 12 to 12.5 cm in width depending on the manufacturer. The "obese" cuffs are all 15 cm in width, while thigh cuffs vary from 18 to 20 cm in width. Errors in measurement usually do not exceed 10 mmHg in small arms, even when a thigh cuff is used. The more significant problem comes in using a narrow cuff in the obese or muscular individual. An example of this would be the use of an adult cuff for a person whose upper arm is 50 cm in circumference. This cuff would be too narrow and would give systolic readings of approximately 20 mmHg above the true intra-arterial level. For an arm of 40 cm in circumference, the adult cuff is still too narrow and gives readings of approximately 10 mmHg above the intra-arterial value of systolic blood pressure. Since obese arms represent the most common and most important mismatch problem, it is perhaps simplest to recognize that adult cuffs are satisfactory for upper arms of up to 33 cm in circumference, obese cuffs for arms up to 41 cm in circumference, and thighs cuffs for arms of greater than 41 cm in circumference. For even greater simplicity, it can be stated that obese and thigh cuffs can be used on most arms (26 to 50 cm in circumference) without errors of greater than 10 mmHg in systolic or 5 mmHg in diastolic readings. Measurement errors of greater than 10 mmHg routinely occur only with the use of adult cuffs in large arms that are greater than 40 cm in circumference.

Proper cuff size is readily recognized by vertical lines marked on the cuff. These lines indicate the arm circumference appropriate to the cuff. Specifically, in wrapping the cuff around the arm, the bladder edge of the cuff should fall between the two vertical lines. If large cuffs are not immediately available for individuals with an obese upper arm, a more accurate reading may be obtained by applying the adult cuff to the forearm and listening over the radial artery for the Korotkoff sounds.

Pseudohypertension

Cuff measurements of blood pressure may occasionally be elevated in individuals whose intraarterial pressure is actually normal. This can occur when narrow cuffs are applied on large arms, as noted above. It can also occur when appropriate-sized cuffs are used. Although infrequent, this circumstance has been most often observed in elderly individuals who have rigid, noncompressible arteries. The air pressure in the cuff required to obliterate the Korotkoff sounds is greater than the actual hydraulic pressure exerted by the blood against the walls of the arteries. Thus, the cuff readings overestimate the level of intra-arterial pressure, leading to the hazards of overtreatment. The presence of this condition should be sought in all elderly patients. It is likely to be found more frequently in those with marked elevations in blood pressure (especially systolic blood pressure) and an absence of end-organ damage. Individuals who have symptoms of postural hypotension despite persistent elevations in auscultatory blood pressure readings during treatment should be reassessed for the presence of this condition.

This condition can be detected by Osler's maneuver. This maneuver is carried out by palpating the radial artery before and during inflation of the blood pressure cuff. The radial artery normally collapses and becomes impalpable when cuff pressure is higher than the intra-arterial systolic pressure. Arterial rigidity and pseudohypertension would be suspected when the radial artery is still palpable at a cuff pressure sufficient to obliterate the Korotkoff sounds.

The Osler maneuver is carried out by first ascertaining the systolic pressure by auscultation. Then one palpates the radial artery while inflating the cuff above the level of systolic pressure. If the radial artery remains palpable as a nonpulsating cord, the maneuver is positive. Intra-arterial pressure measurements may be needed to confirm the findings. Direct measurements in these circumstances have revealed intra-arterial readings of systolic pressure as much as 50 mmHg below auscultatory recordings. Diastolic pressure may also be overestimated in pseudohypertension.

Home Blood Pressure Measurements

The problem of blood pressure lability and so-called "white-coat hypertension" is believed to cause false diagnosis in a notable fraction of individuals with a diagnosis of hypertension. In one study, 21% of individuals labeled with hypertension actually had normal blood pressure when measurements were made outside the office. This has led to recommendations for more widespread use of home blood pressure measurements and ambulatory recordings by automated noninvasive devices. Data are now accruing to indicate that such measurements correlate more closely with cardiac hypertrophy and even with cardiovascular morbidity than do office readings. These measurements are considered appropriate for evaluating patients who have anxiety, labile and borderline hypertension, and an unsatisfactory response to therapy. I will confine my comments to home blood pressure measurements because ambulatory recordings are discussed elsewhere in this volume.

It is premature at present to base diagnosis and treatment routinely on home blood pressure measurements. There are a number of reasons for this opinion. First and foremost, virtually all of the epidemiologic information relating blood pressure levels to cardiovascular disease are based on casual or office readings. In addition, the clinical trial data documenting the effectiveness of treatment are based on causal measurements. Similar evidence is not available for home blood pressure recordings. Thus, the scientific foundation of our knowledge concerning prognosis and treatment is based on casual rather then home-based blood pressure measurements. When a more substantial body of such evidence is available for home readings, it will be appropriate to disseminate the practice.

Second, the peaks of blood pressure elevation that are labeled the "white-coat phenomenon" may be due, in many instances, to a failure to observe the details of blood pressure measurement described above. Third, if spikes in blood pressure precipitate strokes and other end-organ damage, rather than average levels of pressure, then the "white-coat" effect may be a useful indicator. The occurrence of cardiovascular events in the morning hours when blood pressure is known to rise may be a manifestation of this phenomenon.

Fourth, many patients are not emotionally suited to unsupervised determinations of blood pressure at home. For them, the measurements create undue anxiety and a fixation on short-term fluctuations in the levels. This apprehension can cause invalidism, absenteeism, excessive telephone calls to doctors, and self-adjustment of medication. This may interfere with the establishment of a stable regimen of treatment.

Finally, there may be substantial divergences between the home readings and the office measurements. What does one do with patients who report home recordings of 120/70 mmHg when office readings are always 170/110 mmHg? Is the office measurement ignorable because it is believed to be simply the white-coat effect? What biases influence the values that patients report? Patients soon learn that they influence therapy with these recordings. There may be numerous motivations for them to want to do this. Thus, home readings may introduce a subjective element that is unsatisfactory for science and unsuitable for certain patients.

Home and ambulatory measurements, nevertheless, represent one of the more promising areas for current and future investigation. The early evidence suggests that these methods will define more clearly the individuals at risk for cardiovascular disease. However, until more extensive documentation is available, the technique of home recordings should be used on a selective basis.

Establishing the Diagnosis of Hypertension

The diagnosis of hypertension is made simply by blood pressure recordings. In fact, the measurement of blood pressure is so easy that there may be a tendency to overdiagnose the condition. The key points are to measure blood pressure properly (Table 1) and to refrain from settling on the diagnosis until elevations in blood pressure have been recorded on three successive visits spaced over a few weeks to a few months. Given the known lability of blood pressure, a single recording of casual levels of pressure is rarely sufficient unless the elevation is severe and the patient symptomatic from it.

The Joint National Committee on the Detection, Evaluation, and Treatment of High Blood Pressure has established criteria for the clas-

Table 2
Classification of Blood Pressure Readings

Range (mmHg)	Category
Diastolic	
<85	Normal blood pressure
85–89	High normal
90–104	Mild hypertension
105–114	Moderate hypertension
≥115	Severe hypertension
Systolic, when diastolic pressure is <90	
<140	Normal blood pressure
140–159	Borderline isolated systolic hypertension
≥160	Isolated systolic hypertension

Reprinted by permission of the Joint National Committee on the Detection, Evaluation, and Treatment of High Blood Pressure. Arch Int Med 148:1023–1038, 1988.

Table 3
Follow-up Criteria for First Blood Pressure Measurement

Blood Pressure Range	Follow-up Interval
Diastolic mmHg	
<85	Recheck within 2 years
85–89	Recheck within 1 year
90–104	Confirm within 2 months
105–114	Evaluate within 2 weeks
≥115	Evaluate immediately
Systolic when diastolic <90 mmHg	
<140	Recheck within 2 years
140–199	Recheck within 2 months
≥200	Evaluate within 2 weeks

Reprinted by permission of the Joint National Committee on the Detection, Evaluation, and Treatment of High Blood Pressure. Arch Int Med 148:1023–1038, 1988.

sification of hypertension. Widely accepted, these criteria adhere to the time-honored tradition of using 140/90 mmHg as the cut-off level between hypertension and normal blood pressure (Table 2). The Committee has also suggested intervals for follow-up visits which set a deliberate place to the diagnostic phase of the encounter (Table 3). Even when elevations in blood pressure are moderately high, measurements should be made over a week or two before the diagnosis is established. In mild hypertension, the tempo is even more unhurried. This cautious pace minimizes overdiagnosis of hypertension by allowing time for short-term and intermediate-term stress reactions to abate. However, once confirmed by repeated elevations, the diagnosis is inescapable and a workup is indicated.

Evaluation of the Hypertensive Patient

The medical history and physical examination have assumed an even greater role in the evaluation of the hypertensive patient than in former times. This is true because the laboratory workup is currently more selective due to cost considerations and the recognized low prevalence of secondary hypertension. The limitations on routine testing means that a heightened alertness to the findings of history and physical is required to identify patients needing a more extensive workup. The objectives of the workup are: (1) to detect the presence of end-organ

Diagnosis and Evaluation • 31

damage; (2) to identify secondary causes of hypertension; (3) to identify other risk factors for cardiovascular disease.

The Medical History

The critical information needed from the medical history is tabulated in Table 4. Positive responses to any of these historical points should serve as the stimulus for additional questioning and specific diagnostic evaluation. Records from other sources of medical care should be re-

Table 4
Key Information in the History

1. Course of the Hypertension
   a. Duration
   b. Usual and highest blood pressure recordings
   c. Drugs taken: effectiveness and side effects
   d. Hospitalization, if any
2. Target Organ Assessment
   a. Headaches, visual symptoms
   b. Dyspnea, ankle edema
   c. Heart attack or angina pectoris
   d. Stroke or motor weakness
   e. Claudication
   f. Prior urinalysis or tests of renal function
3. Family History
   a. Cardiovascular disease before age 55 in parents or siblings
   b. Age and causes of death in parents and siblings
   c. Kidney disease, diabetes mellitus
4. Personal History
   a. Sodium and alcohol use, special diets
   b. Other medications:
      Nonsteroidal anti-inflammatory drugs
      Oral contraceptives
      Adrenocorticosteroids
      Sympathomimetic amines as in nasal decongestants and appetite suppressants
      Psychotropic drugs:
         monoamine oxidase inhibitors
         Tricyclics
5. Symptoms of secondary causes
   a. Episodes of sweating, palpitations, anxiety
   b. Muscle weakness
   c. Flank pain and hematuria
6. Other cardiovascular risk factors
   a. Pack-years of smoking
   b. Prior cholesterol measurements
   c. Weight at the age of 21, and subsequent changes
   c. Diabetes mellitus

32 • HYPERTENSION

quested, if available. Specific historical points regarding the presence of renovascular hypertension are detailed in a chapter elsewhere in the volume, therefore, they are not repeated here.

The Physical Examination

The important points of the physical examination are listed in Table 5. Often omitted, determination of body weight is essential to establishing the ideal weight limits for the individual. A specific weight goal should be set for each patient who is outside the ideal range. It is generally not appreciated that an individual's weight in adulthood should not exceed that reached at age 21. The weight at age 21 may serve as a goal for obese individuals in whom the standard weight tables may seem unrealistic.

Weight should be measured at each visit, not at widely spaced intervals. Changes in weight as small as 1–2 pounds can be clues to the reason for failure to achieve or maintain blood pressure control during treatment. For convenience, weight can be recorded with the patient

Table 5
Focus of the Physical Examination

a. Height and weight
b. Vital signs
c. Body habitus and fat distribution
d. Funduscopic findings:*
   anteriolar narrowing (grade 1)
   arteriovenous nicking (grade 2)
   hemorrhages, exudates (grade 3)
   papilledema (grade 4)
e. Neck vein distention, carotid pulsation and bruits, thyroid gland size
f. Pulmonary rales, dullness to percussion
g. Precordial pulsatons, heart rhythm, gallop, loudness and splitting of second heart sound
h. Abdominal striae, organomegaly, masses, bruit, aortic pulsations
i. Leg edema, cyanosis, femoral pulsations and bruit, pedal and posterior tibial pulses
j. Focal neurological deficits and abnormal reflexes

* Grades of funduscopic findings correspond to the Keith-Wagener classification

Diagnosis and Evaluation • 33

clothed but with shoes and outer garments, i.e., jackets and coats, removed. The same balance-arm scale should be used at each visit to keep technical variables to a minimum.

The distribution of fat on the body also assumes importance. Central obesity has been identified as a risk factor for cardiovascular morbidity. A waist-to-hip circumference ratio of greater than 1:1 portends excess cardiovascular disease. Also, fat pads located in the supraclavicular region and the back of the neck typify Cushing's syndrome, a rare secondary cause of hypertension.

In the asymptomatic hypertensive, the funduscopic examination is the area most likely to reveal an abnormality. Arteriovenous nicking, the most common abnormality found, is most meaningful when observed in vascular crossings at a distance from the optic disc. The crossing defects are considered a sign of atherosclerosis rather than hypertension per se. It is important to assess the caliber of the arterioles of the fundus. The normal ratio of the diameter of artery to vein is 2:3. The comparison of artery and vein must be made at a similar distance from the optic disc. The arteriolar narrowing of hypertension usually becomes visually detectable at a ratio of 1:2. Hemorrhages and exudates are seen in severe and accelerated hypertension. Papilledema is the hallmark of malignant hypertension. There should be a rough correspondence between the eye findings and the height of the blood pressure. When hemorrhages, exudates, or papilledema are observed in individuals with mild and asymptomatic hypertension, a cause other than blood pressure elevation should be considered. On the other hand, a severe elevation of blood pressure in the presence of normal fundi and organ function suggests that the hypertension is a nonsustained spike.

Evaluation of the neck veins often poses difficulties. Pulsation of the internal jugular vein is the most tell-tale sign of congestive heart failure, yet it is a subtle pulsation to observe because it is a broader, more diffuse wave movement in the neck. The external jugular vein is more readily apparent, but engorgement of it does not immediately indicate congestive failure. Filling of the external jugular vein from above must be interrupted by compressing the vein at the mandible with the thumb. The vein normally collapses with this maneuver. If the vein remains distended or shows a filling wave above the clavicle when the patient is resting at 30° or more from the horizontal, then venous pressure is elevated.

Pulmonary rales suggest congestive heart failure but can be confounded by the presence of concomitant pulmonary disease. Simple but important signs that often precede the development of rales are a rapid respiratory rate or a prolonged expiratory phase of respiration. Diminished or absent breath sounds and dullness to percussion suggest advanced heart failure and the presence of pleural effusion, which typically appears first in the right pleural cavity.

The cardiac examination can give clues to hypertrophy, enlargement, and organ failure. A sustained and forceful apical impuse suggests hypertrophy. Displacement of the apical impuse to the left and a parasternal lift indicate chamber enlargement. A fourth heart (S_4 gallop) foretells a loss of compliance of the left ventricle. A third heart sound together with a rapid rate may indicate incipient heart failure. A reversal of the physiological splitting of the second heart sound, best heard at the base, occurs when the left ventricular systolic ejection time is prolonged, a finding in long-standing severe hypertension. Normally, the second heart sound becomes split at the end of inspiration due to a delay in closure of the pulmonic valve. In reversed splitting, the split disappears at the end of inspiration as the pulmonic valve closure moves into synchrony with the late closing of the aortic valve. The sign also occurs in left bundle branch block and is difficult to detect when the heart rate is rapid.

On the abdominal examination, organomegaly and an epigastric bruit are the most important signs. Clinically significant stenosis of the renal arteries often causes a bruit with both systolic and diastolic components. Palpable aortic pulsations may indicate the presence of an aneurysm. On the other hand, pulsations of a normal aorta may be palpable in a thin individual with relaxed abdominal musculature. In the elderly individual, the palpable aorta may be tortuous but not dilated. Ultrasonography is needed to make the distinction.

In bed-ridden patients with hypertension and congestive heart failure, edema is often missed because it is redistributed from the lower portions of the legs to the flanks, thighs, and presacral regions. The detection of the edema in these locations is crucial to the proper management of these patients. These patients usually need the addition of a diuretic to their therapeutic regimen, or an increase in the dose of a diuretic, to control both the hypertension and the heart failure.

The physical examination may also give clues to secondary forms of hypertension. Kidney enlargement and abdominal bruits have already been mentioned. Tenderness over the lower abdomen combined with dullness to percussion in the suprapubic area may indicate bladder distention and urinary obstruction. This may cause a volume-expansion form of hypertension.

Coarctation of the aorta may be suspected from a variety of physical

Diagnosis and Evaluation • 35

findings. Most prominent of these is a delay in the femoral pulse wave. This sign is elicited by palpating the radial and femoral pulse simultaneously. Normally, the femoral pulsation precedes the radial pulse; in coarctation, this is reversed. The femoral pulsation may or may not be faint. The key physical finding in the coarctation is a normal or low blood pressure in the leg and an elevated pressure in the arm. There may be a discrepancy of blood pressure between the right and left arm if the coarctation occurs above the origin of the left subclavian artery. Coarctation may cause a bruit audible in the posterior chest region. There may be enlargement and tortuosity of intercostal arteries on the chest wall.

Primary aldosteronism has few physical signs. Generalized muscle weakness and latent tetany may be found. Tetany may be elicited by Chvostek's or Trousseau's signs.

Pheochromocytoma is characterized by lability of blood pressure yet fully half of patients have sustained hypertension. Postural hypotension occurs in some patients. Tachycardia, a coarse resting tremor, pallor, and sweating are other clues to excessive circulating catecholamines.

Cushing's syndrome may be recognizable by the truncal obesity, florid "moon facies," posterior cervical and supraclavicular fat pads, and violaceous strial of abdomen and thighs.

Laboratory Tests

The minimum labortory workup needed in asymptomatic hypertension is listed in Table 6. A microscopic examination of the urine sediment is usually not helpful even when the dipstick part of a routine urinalysis is normal. The blood workup is best accomplished by a complete blood count and automated battery of 20–26 biochemical tests. In

Table 6
Minimum Laboratory Workup

Dipstick urinalysis (microscopic also if dipstick is abnormal)
Hemoglobin or hematocrit
Creatinine, potassium, fasting glucose concentrations
Total cholesterol, high density lipoprotein cholesterol, fasting triglycerides
Electrocardiogram

36 • HYPERTENSION

this way, the clinician gets a comprehensive assessment of the patient's body chemistry and is prepared to evaluate changes in the event of intercurrent illness or side effects of treatment. When finances are a constraint, the blood testing could be limited to the items in Table 6. With the three lipid measurements, low density lipoprotein cholesterol (LDL) can be calculated according to the formula: LDL cholesterol = total cholesterol − (high density lipoprotein cholesterol + triglycerides 6). This formula is valid for triglycerides at least up to 400 mg/dL, and perhaps as high as 1,000 mg/dL. If total cholesterol exceeds 200 mg/dL, or LDL cholesterol exceeds 130 mg/dL, the lipid profile should be repeated at least once to verify the presence of hyperlipidemia. Bear in mind that all male hypertensives automatically have two risk factors (i.e., their sex and elevated blood pressure) for coronary heart disease; therefore, the cut-off levels specified above represent their goal levels for cholesterol-lowering, according to the guidelines of the National Cholesterol Education Program.

The only other test essential in the initial examination is the electrocardiogram (ECG). Left ventricular hypertrophy detected by ECG is a recognized additional risk factor for cardiovascular disease. The presence of ventricular hypertrophy calls for an early start of treatment. The echocardiogram is actually more sensitive in identifying hypertrophy of the ventricle. There is accumulating evidence that cardiac hypertrophy identified in this way presages cardiovascular disease. However, the prognostic advantage of this early detection requires further clarification. Until this clarification is available and the cost of the test declines, the echocardiogram should be used selectively and electively. The workup is detailed in Table 7.

When aldosteronism is suspected, urinary potassium excretion should be measured at a time when hypokalemia is present. High urinary potassium (>40 mEq per day) is consistent with aldosteronism; urinary potassium of less than 20 mEq per day suggests that the hypokalemia is due to extra-renal losses, not to aldosteronism. If the patient is taking diuretics, they should be stopped and urinary potassium measured after an interval of 2 or more weeks. If high urinary potassium is found, urinary aldosterone should be measured after 3 days of high sodium intake. The sodium loading should be at least 12 grams of sodium chloride supplement per day. Sodium excretion should be measured in the urine collection for aldosterone in order to document compliance with the high sodium intake. Urinary aldosterone of 8 μg/day or more is diagnostic of aldosteronism in the presence of urinary sodium of 250 mEq or more per day. Plasma renin should be measured at the

Table 7
Laboratory Investigation of Primary Aldosteronism

A. Document urinary potassium wasting
   1. Preparation: no diuretic for 2 weeks
   2. Tests: 24 hour urinary K^+, serum K^+
   3. Result and interpretation:
      a. Urinary K <20 meq = aldosteronism absent
      b. Urinary K >40 meq = aldosteronism present
         Serum K <3.5 mEq/L
B. Confirm presence of aldosteronism
   1. Preparation: no diuretic, 12 grams of sodium chloride supplement per day for 3 days
   2. Tests: 24-hour urinary aldosterone and sodium concentrations, plasma renin activity
   3. Results and interpretation
      a. Aldosterone <4 µg/day = aldosteronism/absent
      b. Aldosterone >8 µg/day = aldosteronism/present
      c. Renin < 2 ng/mL/hr = aldosteronism is primary
      d. Renin >2 ng/mL/hr = aldosteronism is secondary
   (Interpretations appropriate if urinary sodium >250 meq/day)
C. Locate tumor
   1. Preparation: hydration
   2. Test: computerized tomography (CT) of adrenal glands
   3. Result and interpretation
      a. Unilateral enlargement = solitary adenoma
      b. Bilateral enlargement = nodular hyperplasia
      c. Normal adrenal size = adenoma is small or absent
D. Further localization (for individuals with normal adrenal glands by CT scan)
   1. Preparation: hydration
   2. Test: adrenal vein catheterization for aldosterone concentration
   3. Result and interpretation
      a. Tenfold difference in aldosterone concentration between sides = solitary adenoma
      b. Concentrations high but less than two-fold difference between sides = bilateral hyperplasia

This workup is indicated for unprovoked serum potassium <3.5 mEq/L or for K 2.5 mEq/L during diuretic therapy.
Surgery is indicated for solitary adenoma; medical therapy is indicated for bilateral hyperplasia.

same time to rule out secondary aldosteronism. In primary aldosteronism, plasma renin should suppress to less than 2 ng/mL/hr.

The next step is to distinguish solitary adenoma from bilateral nodular hyperplasia of the adrenal cortex. Computerized tomography (CT) scanning can localize adrenal tumors as small as 1 cm in diameter. If a solitary tumor is identified, no further testing is needed before surgery. If the CT scan is negative, an adenoma of less than 1 cm diameter may be present. Adrenal vein sampling by percutaneous catheterization may be needed. In solitary adenoma, there is typically a tenfold difference in aldosterone concentration between the two sides. In bilateral hyperplasia, aldosterone levels are high on both sides and the difference between sides is less than twofold. It is often helpful to measure plasma cortisol in adrenal vein samples to assure proper catheter placement. Cortisol should be similarly elevated on both sides.

Pheochromocytoma

Pheochromocytoma needs be evaluated only in individuals with suggestive symptoms and signs. Refractoriness to therapy and pressor responses to anesthesia or antihypertensive drugs are additional indications for workup (Table 8). The simplest of the screening tests is the 24-hour urinary metanephrine assay. It is superior to urinary catecholamines or vanillylmandelic acid. Plasma catecholamines are more specific than urinary testing but are technically more difficult. To avoid spurious elevation, which can be evoked by stimuli as minor as venipuncture, an indwelling needle or catheter must be inserted a half hour before blood sampling. The patient should also remain recumbent during this time. In pheochromocytoma, plasma calecholamines are usually greater than 2,000 ng/L. If catecholamines are in the gray zone of 500–2,000 ng/L, the clonidine suppression test can aid in the diagnosis. In this test 0.3 mg of clonidine is given orally and should suppress catecholamines, measured 3 hours later, by 50% or more. Failure to suppress indicates the presence of pheochromocytoma.

The next step is to localize the tumor. CT scan of the adrenal accomplishes this in 90% of cases. In the other 10% of cases, adrenal vein and regional venous sampling are needed. The risk of pressor responses is ever-present; a syringe loaded with phentolamine should be kept at hand during abdominal venous sampling.

Diagnosis and Evaluation • 39

Table 8
Laboratory Investigation for Pheochromocytoma

A. Screening test for suspected tumor
 1. Preparation: none
 2. Test: urinary metanephrines
 3. Result and interpretation: greater than 1.0 mg/24 hours or 1.0 mcg/mg creatinine = tumor is possible
B. Confirm catecholamine excess
 1. Preparation: indwelling needle; patient supine for 30 minutes
 2. Test: plasma catecholamines
 3. Result and interpretation
  a. Catecholamines >2000 ng/L = tumor present
  b. Catecholamines 500–2000 ng/L = tumor possible; suppression test needed
C. Differential diagnosis of borderline catecholamine excess (clonidine suppression test)
 1. Preparation: same as B1; 0.3 mg clonidine
 2. Test: plasma catecholamines before and 3 hours after oral clonidine
 3. Result and interpretation: failure of plasma catecholamines to decrease by 50% from baseline 3 hours after clonidine = tumor present
D. Locate tumor
 1. Preparation: hydration
 2. Test: computerized tomography (CT) of adrenal glands
 3. Result and interpretation
  a. Tumor demonstrable if >1 cm diameter
  b. Scan normal = tumor <1 cm or extra-adrenal location
E. Further localization if CT scan normal
 1. Preparation: hydration; intravenous phentolamine available in syringe
 2. Tests: abdominal and pelvic CT scan; selective arteriography of adrenals and suspected sites catheterization of adrenal veins and inferior vena cava for regional catecholamine assay
 3. Results and interpretation: Identification of tumor by CT scan or arteriography requires confirmation by venous catecholamine assay

Tips for Special Situations

Monitoring Hypertension in the Hospitalized Patient

Several important points can be made about evaluating blood pressure levels of the hypertensive patient in the hospital. First, physicians should take their own readings of the patient's blood pressure each day. Blood pressure measurements by others are not always made with the same care and accuracy as those by the physician. While the appearance of the physician may cause a temporary spike in blood pressure, measurements taken near the end of the visit have satisfactory reliability.

Blood pressure measurements should be taken with the patient standing as well as supine or in a sitting position. Hospitalized patients tend to stay in bed much of the time even if not acutely ill. Because of this, it is often quickest to record pressure only with the patient supine. This is unsatisfactory practice because orthostatic effects are easily missed, especially in the elderly and atherosclerotic patient who is likely to have sluggish baroreceptor reflexes. Certain classes of antihypertensive drugs impair these reflexes further. Such painstaking evaluation may seem unduly time-consuming, but it can forestall the problem of patients collapsing.

Blood pressure decreases spontaneously in some hypertensives during a hospital stay. This phenomenon has been attributed to a number of factors, such as reduced mental stress, improved control of dietary sodium, and more reliable intake of medication. Previously established drug regimens may prove excessive in the hospital and require tapering. It must be remembered that blood pressure will rise again after discharge. Therefore, patients need to be followed up periodically with this in mind. This is one of several reasons why the antihypertensive drug regimen is best established in the outpatient setting.

The New Patient Currently Receiving Treatment

In this era of the widespread awareness of the hazards of untreated hypertension, the physician often encounters a new patient who is already receiving treatment. These patients deserve the same evaluation as described in this chapter for the untreated new patient. However, an additional consideration is appropriate. A trial of step-down therapy is indicated if blood pressure is less than 140/90 mmHg after the first few visits. This is important because the care with which the original diagnosis was made is usually unknown. Even if the steps described in the preceding sections were meticulously followed, other circumstances that can affect the blood pressure may have changed. For example, folowing the original diagnosis, the patient may have made substantial life style changes, such as losing weight, reducing dietary sodium intake, eliminating alcohol use, changing jobs, or stabilizing his personal life. In mild hypertension, one or more of these changes might drop the blood pressure back into the normal range. While it has been accepted dogma that the therapy of hypertension, once started, is life-long, this belief is a carry-over from experience with moderate and severe hypertension. Mild hypertension is different. In the Australian trial, 30% of the placebo group was normotensive at each annual visit. A somewhat smaller percentage of patients in the Hypertension Detection and follow-

Diagnosis and Evaluation • 41

up Program and the Multiple Risk Factor Intervention Trial had the same experience. Bear in mind that in these trials the hypertension was diagnosed by strict criteria; yet the hypertension did not persist. In a controlled study of step-down therapy, 25%–35% of patients have remained off drug therapy in follow-up of 3 to 4 years. Of course, these patients need to be followed for years because relapse of hypertension can occur at any time.

Selected References

Bravo EL, Gifford RW Jr: Pheochromocytoma: Diagnosis, localization and management. N Engl J Med 311:1298–1303, 1984.
Bravo EL, Tarazi RC, Dustan HP, et al: The changing clinical spectrum of primary aldosteronism. Am J Med 74:641–651, 1983.
Frohlich ED, Grim C, Labarthe DR, et al: Recommendations for human blood pressure measurements by sphygmomanometers. Circulation 77:502A–514A, 1988.
Gifford RW Jr, Kirkendall W, O'Connor DT, et al: Office evaluation of hypertension. Hypertension 12:283–293, 1989.
Joint National Committee. The 1988 Report of the Joint National Committee On Detection, Evaluation, and Treatment of High Blood Pressure. Arch Int Med 148:1023–1038, 1988.
Messerli FH, Ventura HO, Amodeo C: Osler's maneuver and pseudohypertension. N Engl J Med 312:1548–1551, 1985.

Chapter 3

The Role of Ambulatory Blood Pressure Monitoring

Joel M. Neutel, David H.G. Smith, Michael A. Weber

Introduction

The epidemiologic evidence that defines the risks associated with hypertension and the benefits to be expected from treatment is nearly all based on readings of blood pressure (BP) made in the clinical setting. However, several hypertension treatment trials conducted over the past few years have raised serious concern regarding the accuracy of blood pressure measurements obtained in a conventional manner. It has been observed that over 30% of placebo-treated patients in such studies have been found to have normal blood pressures at the end of the trials despite the application of rigorous diagnostic criteria at the beginning of the study. Other trials have described some patients who, after having been discontinued from antihypertensive medication, have remained normotensive on an indefinite basis. The most likely basis for these findings is that many of the patients entering the study were in fact normotensive at the outset but had transiently elevated blood pressures in the clinical setting which resulted in overestimation of blood pressure and diagnosis of hypertension.

A major contributor to the marked inaccuracy of standard clinical methods for measuring blood pressure is the pressor response triggered by an alerting reaction in a subject undergoing a medical examination.

From Punzi HA, Flamenbaum W (eds): *Hypertension*. Mount Kisco, NY, Futura Publishing Co., Inc., © 1989.

Frequently, this response is sufficient to elevate the blood pressure of normotensive subjects well into the hypertensive range, the so-called "white-coat hypertension." Furthermore, the magnitude of the response will differ among individuals and under different circumstances, making it difficult or impossible to establish a baseline blood pressure. Since the decision to treat hypertension depends largely on the level of the pressure, it becomes critical to obtain data from the patient that are truly representative of the average arterial pressure, which, given our currently accepted methods for BP determination, may be an extremely difficult task.

However, recent advances in medical technology have resulted in the development of fully automatic, lightweight, portable, noninvasive BP recorders that are capable of accurately monitoring changes in BP over periods of 24-hours or more. The commercial availability of such recorders raises the question of their relevance to the practical management of hypertensive patients.

This chapter has three purposes: (1) to examine the available instrumentation for continuous blood pressure monitoring; (2) to investigate the use of these techniques for better understanding the physiology and characteristics of blood pressure; and (3) to outline its potential value in the management of hypertensive patients.

Instrumentation

Most of the early work done on continuous BP monitoring utilized portable intra-arterial equipment which required cannulation of a brachial artery and a miniaturized perfusion pump to preserve the patency of the intra-arterial cannula. Although it is generally accepted that this method is a desirable means of measuring BP because it is capable of measuring every systolic and diastolic pressure during the period of monitoring, it is invasive and associated with potential morbidity and is therefore generally only used for research purposes. Nonetheless, because of its accuracy, this method is still regarded as a gold standard against which the accuracy of other methods can be measured.

Today, almost all of the work done on ambulatory BP monitoring, particularly in the United States, utilizes noninvasive techniques. The currently available ambulatory monitors, now made by several manufacturers, are small easily portable devices that allow the patients reasonable flexibility in following their day-to-day activities. The systems consist of a standard arm cuff that is inflated at predetermined intervals by a small battery powered pump unit carried on a shoulder strap or attached to the patient's belt. The modern systems are capable of measuring blood pressure using two separate methods: auscultatory and oscillometric. The auscultatory method employs a small microphone placed over the brachial artery that listens to the Korotkoff sounds in the same fashion as a human observer with a stethoscope. Because these machines can make erroneous readings based on external artifactual sounds, some of the available devices also use chest leads that provide electrocardiographic R-wave gating to ensure that the sounds heard by the microphone are true Korotkoff sounds rather than artifact. The oscillometric method works by perceiving subtle changes in air pressure within the cuff systems caused by fluctuations of the brachial artery. It is able to discriminate the systolic BP from the mean BP (taken to be the lowest pressure at which the maximum pulse amplitude is maintained); and from these two measurements, using an algorithm, it calculates the diastolic BP. All blood pressures measured throughout the monitoring period are stored in a memory system contained within the unit and can be extracted on completion of monitoring. Most of the available blood pressure monitoring systems can be interfaced with personal computers to provide printouts of the whole-day blood pressure readings together with some preliminary analysis and statistics. The data can be saved for future reference and comparison.

Semiautomatic systems that require the patient to inflate the cuff are also available. However, they are obviously unable to measure blood pressure when the patient is sleeping. Also in our experience, it is unusual for patients to obtain frequent regular recording with these systems, and thus they are less useful to clinicians and researchers.

More recently there have been preliminary evaluations of noninvasive devices that measure blood pressures in the circulation of the finger or the earlobe, but these methods are not yet generally available.

Accuracy

In order to establish a role for ambulatory BP monitors in hypertension, it became critical to demonstrate the accuracy or reproducibility of these systems when comparing them to the current accepted gold standards. Graettinger and his colleagues compared BP readings obtained on the two different types of ambulatory monitors, auscultatory and oscillometric, to those obtained intra-arterially. They demonstrated that there were significant correlations ($p<0.001$) between each non-

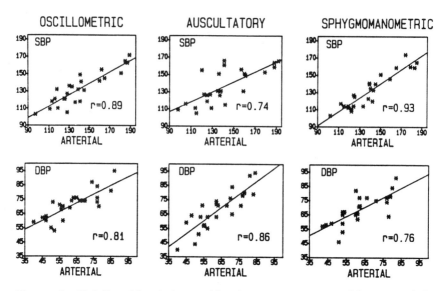

Figure 1. Relationships between blood pressure measured intra-arterially and by oscillometric or auscultatory portable devices or by a mercury sphygmomanometer in 25 hospitalized patients. Data shown are for systolic blood pressure (SBP) and diastolic blood pressure (DBP). All correlations are significant (p<0.001 in each case). With permission from Graettinger WF, Lipson JL, Cheung DG, et al: Validation of portable noninvasive blood pressure monitoring: Comparisons with intra-arterial and sphygmomanometer measurements. Ann Heart J 116:1155–1160, 1988.

invasive method and the intra-arterial method for systolic and diastolic BP (Fig. 1). Further, they demonstrated a significant correlation (p<0.001) between each of the noninvasive methods and a standard mercury sphygmomanometer for both systolic and diastolic BPs (Fig. 2). Similar findings have been reported by other authors using different systems. It is important to emphasize that these studies of accuracy have been carried out in patients or volunteers in a relatively quiet setting. It has not been established whether the portable equipment provides accurate readings during vigorous motion.

It must be accepted that with any system, whether intra-arterial or noninvasive, the recordings obtained will include some readings that are artifactual (usually as a result of excessive movement) that must be edited out. But given these provisos, it is generally accepted that the noninvasive systems are accurate and provide clinically relevant data.

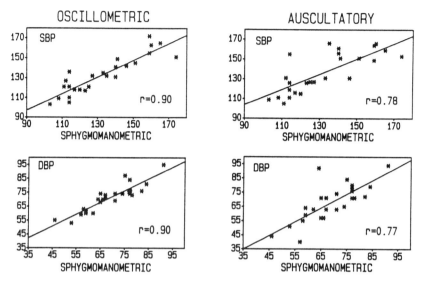

Figure 2. Relationships between blood pressure measured by a mercury sphygmomanometer and oscillometric or auscultatory devices in 25 hospitalized patients. Data shown are for systolic blood pressure (SBP) and diastolic blood pressure (DBP). All correlations are significant ($p<0.001$ in each case). With permission from Graettinger WF, Lipson JL, Cheung DG, et al: Validation of portable noninvasive blood pressure monitoring: Comparisons with intra-arterial and sphygmomanometer measurements. Ann Heart J 116:1155–1160, 1988.

Physiological Relevance

The principal evidence supporting the physiological relevance of whole-day blood pressure monitoring has been the demonstration of a definite and reproducible circadian pattern of blood pressure. Blood pressures are at their highest levels during the daytime hours, forming a plateau between 8 am and 6 pm. The blood pressure then falls steadily until it reaches a nadir at about midnight. It then slowly rises until 5 am, after which it abruptly increases to the daytime levels (Fig. 3). Studies comparing normal volunteers with hypertensive patients have shown that both groups have almost identical circadian patterns, with the hypertensive patients consistently at a higher level than the normal subjects (Fig. 4).

It seems likely that this pattern of blood pressure is determined to some extent by activity of the sympathetic nervous system, for it has

48 • HYPERTENSION

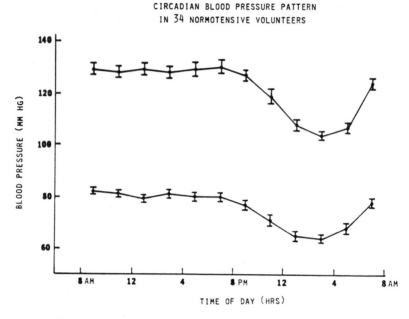

Figure 3. Typical circadian pattern of blood pressure. With permission from Drayer JIM, Weber MA, Hoeger WJ: Whole-day blood pressure monitoring in ambulatory normotensive men. Arch Intern Med 145:271–274, 1985.

been shown that plasma concentrations of the neurotransmitter neurophrine have a circadian pattern similar to that of blood pressure. The increase in sympathetic activity which occurs during arousal may be an important factor in producing the sharp rapid early morning increase in blood pressure.

Of further physiological relevance is the reproducibility of the circadian pattern from one day of monitoring to another. Early studies with intra-arterial devices established that the 24-hour blood pressure is repeatable when studied on consecutive days and also when studied on separate days several weeks apart. Similar findings have been obtained with noninvasive techniques both in hospitalized subjects and in ambulatory subjects undergoing their routine daily activity (Fig. 5). It should be remembered, however, that there can be variations within individual patients from one day of monitoring to another, especially if there are differences in the type of activity undertaken during those days.

Further evidence for physiological relevance is the relationship be-

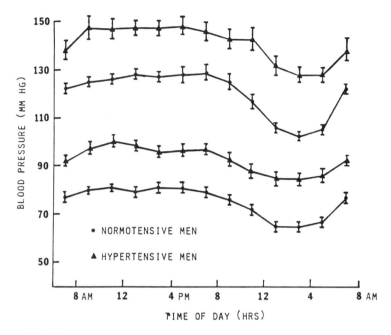

Figure 4. Whole-day systolic and diastolic blood pressure averages in 29 age-matched pairs of hypertensive and normotensive men.

tween blood pressure and left ventricular muscle mass. This relationship is based on the assumption that the mass of the left ventricle should be proportional to the blood pressure, either as a reflection of the workload of the heart required to sustain a given level of blood pressure or, possibly, because blood pressure and heart size are each dependent on a third factor, such as activity of the sympathetic nervous system. Correlations between left ventricular muscle mass and conventionally measured blood pressures have been comparatively weak, but several studies have demonstrated that average whole-day blood pressures (mean of all readings obtained during the 24-hour monitoring period) have a far closer relationship with heart size. Apart from changes occurring in the myocardium, changes as a result of hypertension occurring in the fundi and the kidney were found to be more closely related to the mean pressure obtained over 24-hours than to conventional readings (three or more) obtained in the office setting.

It could thus be argued that the whole-day blood pressure may have prognostic importance to the individual patient. Indeed, an earlier study that used a form of ambulatory blood pressure monitoring indicated that

50 • HYPERTENSION

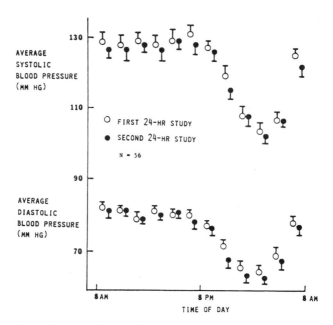

Figure 5. Systolic and diastolic blood pressures during automated ambulatory blood pressure monitoring in 56 normal volunteers. Values shown are averages for the 12 2-hour periods comprising the full day. Data are given for two separate days of monitoring, 2–6 weeks apart. None of the differences between the values on the two days of monitoring are significant. (With permission from Weber MA, Drayer JIM, Brewer DD: Repetitive blood pressure measurements: Clinical issues, techniques, and data analysis. In: Scheving LE, et al (eds). Chronobiotechnology and Chronobiological Engineering, Martinue Nijhoff, The Netherlands, 1987, pp 270–277.)

this technique is probably superior to measurements of conventional blood pressure in predicting major cardiovascular events. In patients followed for 5 years, cardiovascular death and mortality rates were found to be highest in patients with mild hypertension whose ambulatory blood pressure values exceeded their office measurements.

Data Analysis

There is as yet no clear agreement among users and investigators on the optimal approach for interpreting data from 24-hour monitoring. The average of all blood pressures obtained during the day (provided that they are obtained uniformly throughout the entire 24-hour period) is a reproducible value and has the virtue of being simple to calculate. It has been shown that whole-day systolic and diastolic blood pressure

Ambulatory Blood Pressure Monitoring • 51

averages were lower than corresponding casual (office) values by mean values of 10 and 5 mmHg, respectively. Thus, for example, the recommended diagnostic criterion (by the Joint National Committee) of 140/90 mmHg based on casual blood pressure averages would correspond to whole-day values of 130/85 mmHg. A further advantage of using the average of multiple readings during a full 24-hour period helps compensate for inaccuracies produced by acute fluctuations in BP and the variations associated with its circadian pattern.

An alternative way of analyzing the data is by dividing the 24-hour period into diurnal (6 am–10 pm) and nocturnal (10 pm–6 am) periods which would negate the effect of the lower blood pressures that occur during the hours of sleep on the daytime mean. However, it has been demonstrated that the blood pressure and heart rate averages during each of these periods correlated closely with those for the full 24-hours. Moreover, there was a strong correlation between the diurnal and nocturnal averages even though the absolute values during the night were substantially lower than those during the day.

Other authors have described a context called the "blood pressure load," which quantifies the percentage of readings throughout the day that exceed established criteria (90 mmHg for diastolic and 140 mmHg for systolic blood pressures). All persons including those who are truly "normotensive," may have some readings throughout the day that exceed these arbitrary levels. Therefore, the important secondary objective is to determine the point at which the diastolic and systolic load is clearly excessive and indicative of a diagnosis of hypertension.

The interested clinician will, of course, scrutinize all of the individual readings and trends throughout the 24-hour period to determine whether any additional useful clinical insights can be obtained.

The approach for the analysis of 24-hour monitoring which we have found most useful is based on the division of the 24-hour period into 12 consecutive 2-hour periods. We then obtain averages for each of these periods (average of all readings taken during that 2-hour period). Occasionally a 2-hour period is composed entirely or predominantly of antifactual, erroneous, or omitted readings and thus cannot be used in obtaining the whole-day average. One approach to this problem is deriving an interpolated reading statistically to provide a value for the missing 2-hour period.

Ultimately, as with all clinical tests, the interpretation and therapeutic consequences arising from blood pressure monitoring data must be based at least in part, on experience and judgment. More research will be required with greater numbers of patients and longer periods of follow-up before the definitive method will be described.

Indications for Continuous BP Monitoring Use in Diagnosis of Hypertension

Making a diagnosis of hypertension in usual clinical practice appears to be a simple task. With the use of criteria established by the Joint National Committee on the Detection, Evaluation, and Treatment of High Blood Pressure, it seems necessary only to carefully measure the BP by conventional means on two or three occasions before deciding that a patient's BP is normal or that a diagnosis of hypertension should be made. However, this approach may not be accurate. In the Australian Therapeutic Trial of Mild Hypertension, approximately 2000 patients with conventionally measured diastolic BP in the range of 95 to 110 mmHg were treated with placebo for 3 years so as to provide a control group for patients receiving active medication. By the end of the study, approximately 40% had BPs in the normotensive range. Almost certainly the majority of patients whose BPs became normal during the study were normotensive individuals who had been erroneously diagnosed at the start of the study. Similar results have been described by other authors. Other evidence for misdiagnosis comes from studies of the effects of discontinuing antihypertensive therapy in hypertensive patients. A sizable percentage of patients who discontinued their antihypertensive treatment remained normotensive indefinitely, once again placing doubt over the assigned diagnosis.

Studies with continuous intra-arterial measurements have revealed a marked rise in blood pressure during the performance of the conventional measurement procedure. When performed by a physician, this may result in increases of the resting BP by as much as 27/15 mmHg. Studies with noninvasive monitoring techniques have also explored this issue and have shown that blood pressure in most participants is lower for the day as a whole than when measured conventionally in a clinical setting.

Because BPs obtained from continuous monitoring correlates more closely with target organ damage, are better predictors of cardiovascular prognosis, and are diagnostically accurate, this technique would appear to be the method of choice in the clinical setting. However, the prevalence of hypertension is so high that it would be impractical to carry out prolonged blood pressure measurements in all patients. Thus, patient selection for this procedure becomes an important issue.

For the purposes of diagnosis of hypertension, patients with blood pressures in the moderate to severe range, specifically diastolic blood pressure values exceeding 110 mmHg, are unlikely to be normotensive during long-term monitoring. It is also unnecessary to undertake this additional diagnostic procedure in patients who already have evidence of target organ damage such as left ventricular hypertrophy, hypertensive fundal changes, abnormal renal function, or proteinuria. A strong family history of hypertension or premature cardiovascular disease can support the office diagnosis of hypertension. Similarly, patients with clearly normal blood pressure on casual office readings would not benefit from 24-hour monitoring.

Thus, automated blood pressure monitoring appears most appropriate for patients with an office diagnosis of mild to moderate hypertension, as well as the group of so-called borderline or labile hypertensives. This applies more particularly to patients who claim to be normotensive at home but have elevated pressures in the clinic or the hypertensive patient who has occasional but inconsistent normal readings in the office (white-coat hypertension).

Other groups of patients who may benefit from 24-hour monitoring are (1) patients whose BP is inappropriately high for their degree of target organ damage, suggesting a large "white-coat" component; (2) normotensive patients who are at high risk of developing hypertension because of their race or family history, who may benefit from early detection and treatment of hypertension, or from the reassurance that they do not have clinical hypertension; (3) those subjects who are extremely likely to develop "white-coat hypertension" will clearly benefit from continuous monitoring. It should be appreciated that the reaction responsible for causing an elevated casual blood pressure will be more marked in a patient in whom the outcome of the medical examination has importance on their lives and careers. Such may be the case during the annual flight medical examination of a pilot or at an insurance physical. Differentiating between true hypertension and examination-induced hypertension in these patients may be difficult or impossible. Yet this is the group in which a correct diagnosis is critical. It has been demonstrated that many of the methods used by cautious physicians to standardize the measurement environment in an attempt to alleviate the BP response may be of little or no benefit. Under these circumstances, 24-hour monitoring is extremely useful.

Use in Treatment

Apart from playing an important role in diagnosing hypertension, 24-hour monitoring is extremely useful in the treatment of hypertension.

First, it allows clear quantification of treatment effects over the entire 24-hour period. This is important as there can be little argument that a smooth sustained reduction of blood pressure throughout the day and night should be the accepted criterion for successful treatment of hypertension. Furthermore, monitoring a hypertensive patient outside of the clinical environment will frequently avoid overtreatment of patients whose treated blood pressure level is higher in the clinic because of a pressor response occurring in the presence of a doctor giving the physician a false indication of inadequate treatment.

When considering the treatment of hypertension, another aspect that has recently been the focus of increasing attention has been the early morning rapid rise in blood pressure. Epidemiologic studies have clearly demonstrated that this period corresponds very closely with the maximal incidence of nonembolic strokes and myocardial infarction. Clearly for this reason it becomes crucial to obtain good therapeutic blood pressure control during these hours. Of further importance is the fact that it is frequently this time just prior to the next day's dose that one would expect a downward trend in the antihypertensive effect of agents given once daily. With the convenience of these once-a-day compounds gaining increasing popularity among both physician and patients in the treatment of mild to moderate hypertension, it becomes critical to assess the duration of efficacy of a long-acting antihypertensive agent. Treating a hypertensive patient with a single dose of a drug which loses its protective value towards the end of the 24-hour period, frequently the very time that the patient is at the greatest risk of sustaining target organ damage, is certainly not optimal. Previously, it was practically and logistically almost impossible to assess blood pressure during this crucial early morning period of patient arousal from sleep; however, these anbulatory devices provide a convenient means of assessing efficacy over the entire 24-hour period.

Use in Research

Ambulatory blood pressure monitoring should probably be a standard part of clinical trials assessing antihypertensive efficacy. There are three advantages to this technique. First, since whole-day blood pressure monitoring is more reliable than conventional methods for diagnosing hypertension, it would restrict entry into trials of those patients whose hypertension is established and who are more likely to respond to treatment and include patients who are not truly hypertensive but have elevated blood pressure levels on casual blood pressure monitoring. A second benefit is that long-term automated blood pressure monitoring provides reproducible values from one day of monitoring to another thereby providing a more reliable index of treatment responses than by conventional methods. The third benefit of this approach is that the duration of action of antihypertensive effect persists throughout the entire day whether it provides shorter term efficacy and peaks and troughs of the study medications.

The Future

Although continuous ambulatory blood pressure monitoring is a fairly new technique, the major technological advances in this field continue to make the procedure more convenient and reliable, adding to the temptation of using these systems more frequently in clinical practice. As more 24-hour blood pressure data are accumulated, the values of these machines in both the diagnosis and the treatment of hypertension is becoming increasingly evident. However, a major obstacle to the routine use of continuous blood pressure monitoring is in the legitimate concerns that this methodology could add considerably to the already extremely high cost of treating hypertension. However, these concerns may be unfounded since the results of ambulatory blood pressure monitoring may have an impact on cost in several ways. If the information obtained was not used in the decision to treat patients, then cost would invariably increase by the price for the procedure. However, using the results as a basis of whom to treat might eventually lead to a substantial reduction in cost for treatment. It has been demonstrated that if in the region of 38% of patients initially labeled as hypertensive had average ambulatory pressures low enough to permit observation without drug treatment, then the cost of ambulatory monitoring would be offset by the lack of cost for treatment of those subjects having lower blood pressures, and over the long term may eventually reduce the cost by preventing unnecessary treatment. Furthermore, it will save many patients an unnecessary financial burden as well as the many potential problems associated with being labeled as hypertensive and being treated for hypertension.

Much more work still needs to be done in this field, particulary in better defining criteria for its interpretation, but there is little doubt that used thoughtfully, these systems will become a valuable, cost-effective tool with an important role to play in the overall management of hypertensive patients.

Selected References

Ambulatory Blood Pressure Monitoring. Weber MA, Drayer JIM (eds). New York, Springer-Verlag, 1984.
Clinical Application of Automated Whole-day Blood Pressure Monitoring. Am Heart J 116:4, 1988.
Drayer JIM, Gardin JM, Brewer DD, et al: Disparate relationships between blood pressure and left ventricular mass in patients with and without left ventricular hypertrophy. Hypertension 9(suppl II):II-61–II-64, 1987.
Drayer JIM, Weber MA, Nakamura DK: Automated ambulatory blood pressure monitoring: A study in age-matched normotensive and hypertensive men. Am Heart J 109:1334–1338, 1985.
Graettinger WF, Lipson JL, Cheung DG, et al: Validation of portable noninvasive blood pressure monitoring: Comparisons with intra-arterial and sphygmomanometer measurements. Am Heart J 116:1155–1160, 1988.
Hypertension Detection and Follow-Up Program Cooperation Group. Five year findings of the hypertension and detection follow-up program: (I) reduction: In mortality of persons with high blood pressure including mild hypertension. JAMA 262:2562–2571, 1979.
Krakoff LR, Eison IT, Philips RH, et al: Effect of ambulatory blood pressure monitoring on the diagnosis and cost treatment for mild hypertension. Am Heart J 116:1152–1154, 1988.
Management Committee of the Australian Therapeutic Trial in Mild Hypertension: Untreated mild hypertension. Lancet 1: 1:185–191, 1982.
Mancia G, Bertinieri G, Grassi G: Effects of blood pressure measurement by the doctors on patients' blood pressure and heart rate. Lancet 2;695–697, 1983.
Modern Approaches to Blood Pressure Measurements: Patient Education. J Hypertension 7 (suppl 3) May 1989.
Neutel JM, Beritz H, Sindelman C, et al: Flight medical: a common cause of "reactive hypertension" in pilots. Aviation Medicine Quarterly 1:117–124, 1987.
Perloff D, Sokolow M, Cowan R: The prognostic value of ambulatory blood pressure. JAMA 249:2793–2793, 1983.
Weber MA: Automatic BP recorders and 24-hour monitoring. Current Opinion in Cardiol 2:748–757, 1987.
Weber MA: Whole-day blood pressure. Hypertension 11:288–298, 1988.
Weber MA, Cheung DE, Graettinger WF, et al: Characterization of antihypertensive therapy by whole-day BP monitoring. JAMA 259(22):3281–3285, 1988.
Weber MA, Drayer JIM: Role of blood pressure monitoring in the diagnosis of hypertension. J Hypertension 4(Suppl 5):S325–S327, 1986.
Weber MA, Drayer JIM, Baird WM: Echocardiographic evaluations of left ventricular hypertrophy. J Cardiovasc Pharmacol S61-S69, 1986.
Weber MA, Drayer JIM, Nakamura DK, et al: The circadian BP pattern in ambulatory normal subjects. Am J Cardiol 54:115–119, 1984.
Weber MA, Drayer JIM, Wyle FA, et al: Reproducibility of whole-day blood pressure pattern in essential hypertension. Clin Exp Hypertension A4:1377–1390, 1982.

Chapter 4

Core Organ Effects: Part I Uses for Echocardiography in Hypertension

Fetnat M. Fouad-Tarazi and
Ernesto E. Salcedo

Introduction

The heart is a primary end-organ in terms of the systemic effects of hypertension. Echocardiography may help in the identification of structural and functional cardiac changes, in the establishment of the diagnosis of significant hypertension, in determining the prognosis of hypertensive heart disease, in the choice of first line of therapy, as well as in the recognition of some complications related to hypertension. There is increasing experimental and clinical data supporting the important role echocardiography plays in the cardiac management and follow-up of hypertensive patients. Thus, practically, echocardiography frequently proves cost-effective in the management of clinical hypertension.

Structural Changes in Hypertensive Heart Disease

Our previous experience in the evaluation of untreated hypertensive patients has shown that 42% of these patients had normal left ventricles by echocardiography, whereas 22% had asymmetric septal hypertrophy, 20% had concentric left ventricular hypertrophy, and 16%

From Punzi HA, Flamenbaum W (eds): *Hypertension*. Mount Kisco, NY, Futura Publishing Co., Inc., © 1989.

had evidence of left ventricular dilation. Similar experience has been published by others showing that cardiovascular disease developing in hypertensive patients can be detected by echocardiography even prior to ECG or x-ray abnormalities become apparent. These experiences and many others have revealed that these structural cardiac changes are not strongly correlated with blood pressure levels. In our experience, the correlation between systolic blood pressure and left ventricular mass index, although significant, did not exceed 0.5 with an index of determination of 25% whether the correlation was performed in untreated hypertensives, treated hypertensives, or in the hypertensive population as a whole. Other centers have also reported analogous experience using casual measurements of either systolic blood pressure, diastolic blood pressure, or mean arterial pressure as the independent variable.

These findings may represent another indication that blood pressure, per se, is not an adequate index of afterload. Indeed, a more adequate definition of afterload includes the combination of pressure, left ventricular radius, and left ventricular wall thickness. According to such relationship between left ventricular stress and left ventricular mass, ventricular hypertrophy was classified as appropriate (with normalized wall stress) or inappropriate (low stress type or high stress type). The correlation between end-systolic stress and left ventricular mass index, however, was not much better than the correlation between blood pressure, per se, and left ventricular mass, suggesting that nonvascular factors play an important role in the development of left ventricular hypertrophy in hypertension. Many such factors have been identified and/or suggested, including: adrenergic activity and catecholamines, angiotensins, the newly reported myocardial hypertrophy factor, and possibly other genetic disturbances. In this respect, the Framingham study has revealed the occurrence of various patterns of left ventricular hypertrophy (asymmetric, concentric, or eccentric) in the normotensive offspring of hypertensive patients. Moreover, previous reports in the spontaneously hypertensive rat have demonstrated that left ventricular hypertrophy precedes the occurrence of hypertension in the young animals.

In the evaluation of left ventricular hypertrophy in hypertensive patients, one has to be cautious in the use of echocardiography because of the possible occurrence of technical pitfalls. M-mode echocardiography has been shown to be of higher resolution than 2D-echocardiography in the calculation of ventricular wall thickness and left ventricular mass; the method is also simpler and requires less sophisticated computer programing. However, unless performed under two-dimensional echocardiographic guidance, M-mode echocardiography may give erroneous results. Left ventricular M-mode echocardiography should always be recorded at the same site (level of tip of the mitral valves) in order to allow comparison of data acquired at different time intervals and comparison of data obtained from different patients. Despite this cautious approach, the angulation between the anterior wall of the aorta and the axis of the interventricular septum may introduce important artifactual changes in the septal thickness recorded in the M-mode format. Moreover, age has been shown to influence left ventricular wall thickness and left ventricular mass/volume ratio, indicating that controls for hypertensive patients should be age-matched.

Functional Changes in the Hypertensive Heart

Early on in our experience with hypertensive heart disease, we realized that the use of average values of left ventricular systolic functional indices—such as left ventricular percent fractional shortening—and velocity of fiber shortening may hide important information in individual patients. Therefore, evaluation of left ventricular systolic functional indices in relation to afterload—defined as LV end-systolic stress—became a valuable practice as illustrated in Figure 1.

In recent years, noninvasive procedures have allowed the assessment of left ventricular diastolic function in hypertension using radionuclide ventriculography and M-mode echocardiography. Echocardiography has offered many indices for noninvasive evaluation of left ventricular diastolic function. The rate of change of left ventricular internal diameter in diastole and the rate of posterior wall thinning have been well recognized in recent years. Moreover, combined with noninvasive phonocardiography, ECG, and carotid pulse tracing, M-mode echocardiography can be utilized successfully in the determination of diastolic time intervals; A_2O, the time between closure of the aortic valve and opening of the mitral valve is a good measure of left ventricular relaxation time. Finally, the combination of left ventricular pressure and M-mode echocardiography allows the determination of left ventricular pressure-volume loops and the calculation of left ventricular compliance characteristics.

In our experience as well as in the reports by others, left ventricular filling rate was found to be reduced in a large proportion of hypertensive patients at a time when left ventricular systolic function was still within normal limits. The causes of these early diastolic functional changes have

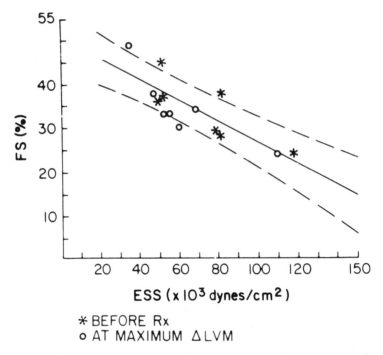

Figure 1. Effect of regression of left ventricular hypertrophy on cardiac performance expressed as the relationship between left ventricular percent fractional shortening (FS%) and left ventricular end-systolic stress (ESS). All points after therapy remained within the 95% confidence limits of the correlation obtained before treatment. * = hypertensive patients before and ° after treatment with enalapril. (With permission from Nakashima Y, Fouad FM, Tarazi RC: Regression of left ventricular hypertrophy from systemic hypertension by enalapril. Am J Cardiol, 1984.)

not been determined yet, but their clinical importance in cardiovascular regulation is just becoming recognized. In this respect, we have reported a reduced ability to vasoconstrict in response to head-up posture or peripheral venous pooling in hypertensive patients with reduced left ventricular filling rate as compared to normal volunteers and to hypertensives with normal left ventricular filling rate.

Role of Echocardiography in the Diagnosis of Unrecognized Hypertension

On many occasions, hypertension is not stable. The fluctuating nature of hypertension in some patients may be confusing to the physician and to the patient. Moreover, the cardiovascular impact of office hypertension, orthostatic hypertension, and exercise hypertension that may occur in some otherwise normotensive individuals is not yet clear. As previously shown by 24-hour ambulatory blood pressure recording, blood pressure fluctuation during the day may be of major importance in the determination of cardiac changes. Thus, better correlations have been reported with 24-hour ambulatory blood pressure averages and left ventricular mass as compared to correlations obtained by using casual blood pressure measurements. Also, work blood pressure had proven to be more strongly related to left ventricular mass than casual blood pressure determinations. Such findings have gained other practical importances. For example, the presence of left ventricular hypertrophy in a patient with occasional hypertension might indicate that blood pressure or hypertensive factors are present more often than detected during office visits in such a patient. Such diagnoses are of importance since left ventricular hypertrophy in hypertension has been reported by the Framingham group to be of major prognostic value as far as survival and occurrence of arrhythmias.

Echocardiography in the Choice of First-Line Therapy in Hypertensive Patients

Left ventricular echocardiography may be used in various ways to either choose or monitor treatment of hypertension. Left ventricular dilation, for example, suggests the need for diuretic use. In this respect, we have observed in seven normal volunteers and nine hypertensive patients that intravenous furosemide (40 mg) induces echocardiographic left ventricular diameter changes within 30 minutes. All subjects lost weight and increased their hematocrit in response to this diuretic administration, whereas blood pressure did not change significantly (Table 1). M-mode echocardiography revealed a reduction of left ventricular end-diastolic volume by 8.9 ± 6 mL in normal individuals and 7.9 ± 6 mL in hypertensive patients. These findings indicate that furosemide therapy results in a reduction of left ventricular preload even without changes of afterload. This might be one of the most important mechanisms by which diuretics improve left ventricular congestive symptoms in heart failure.

Another therapeutic aspect relates to the recent acknowledgement of regression of left ventricular hypertrophy in hypertension. This alteration in left ventricular mass in hypertension received attention after

Table 1
Response to IV Furosemide (40 mg) in normal volunteers and hypertensive patients

	Normals	Hypertensives
n	7	9
ΔB·wt (kg)	−1.2 ± 0.2**	−1.1 ± 0.4**
ΔHct (%)	+2.5 ± 1.0*	+2.5 ± 2.0*
ΔSBP (mmHg)	−0.1 ± 4	+4 ± 14
ΔLVEDV (ml)	−8.9 ± 6*	−7.9 ± 6*
ΔLV FS (%)	−0.001 ± 0.03	0.002 ± 0.03

* p<0.01 vs. baseline; ** p<0.0001.
Abbreviations: B·wt = body weight; Hct = hematocrit; SBP = systolic blood pressure; EDV = end diastolic volume; FS = fractional shortening; LV = left ventricle.

the widespread recognition that the hypertensive "adaptive" left ventricular hypertrophy may not be necessarily beneficial to the function of the hypertensive heart in the long-term follow-up. Clinically, the Framingham study has shown that 45% of hypertensive patients with left ventricular hypertrophy, in hypertension is associated with reduced adrenergic responsiveness, the reduced left ventricular coronary flow reserved, and is eventually complicated by left ventricular dilation and failure. Thus, the initial adaptive mechanisms in the hypertensive hypertrophied heart may lead to cardiac decompensation. Regression of ventricular hypertrophy became, therefore, a goal of antihypertensive therapy. Proven successful in the animal model, it was tried afterward in hypertensive patients. Since then, several studies have revealed the successful induction of ventricular hypertrophy by medical therapy in hypertensive patients; in this respect, not all antihypertensive therapy was shown to produce regression of ventricular hypertrophy. The most successful agents were sympatholytics, converting enzyme inhibitors, and calcium entry blockers. Diuretics and beta-blockers have been rather disputed as far as their effectiveness in reducing left ventricular mass. On the other hand, vasodilators of the pure arteriolar variety, were either unsuccessful in reducing left ventricular mass or have even led to an increase in left ventricular mass in some instances (such as minoxidil) probably due to the associated reflex adrenergic stimulation. In this context, it is of importance to note that clinical studies did not show deterioration of cardiac performance in association with reduction of left ventricular mass, at least under resting conditions.

Therefore, assessment of left ventricular dimensions by echocardiography has the potential of facilitating decision-making regarding the choice of first line of antihypertensive therapy.

Summary

The heart is a primary end-organ in terms of the systemic effects of hypertension. In recent years, echocardiography allowed the noninvasive assessment of cardiac structural and functional changes in hypertension. Moreover, echocardiography could be helpful in determining the prognosis of hypertensive heart disease in the choice of first-line therapy as well as in the recognition of some complications related to hypertension. The clinical relevance of the gained observations make the test cost-effective in the management of hypertensive patients.

Selected References

Devereux RB, Pickering TG, Alderman MH, et al: Left ventricular hypertrophy in hypertension. Prevalence and relationship to pathophysiologic variables. Hypertension 9(Suppl II):II-53–II-60, 1987.
Dreslinski GR, Frohlich ED, Dunn FG, et al: Echocardiographic diastolic ventricular abnormality in hypertensive heart disease: atrial emptying index. Am J Cardiol 47:1087–1090, 1981.
Fouad-Tarazi FM: Left ventricular diastolic function in hypertension. Circulation 75 (Suppl I):I-48–I-55, 1987.
Fouad-Tarazi FM, Liebson PR: Echocardiographic studies of regression of left ventricular hypertrophy in hypertension. Hypertension 9(Suppl II):II-65–II-68, 1987.
Leenen FHH, Reeves RA: Role of echocardiography in managing the hypertensive patient. Drug Therapy November:53–65, 1984.
Grossman W: Cardiac hypertrophy: Useful adaptation or pathologic process? Am J Med 69:576–584, 1980.
Marcus ML, Mueller TM, Gascho JA, et al: Effects of cardiac hypertrophy secondary to hypertension on the coronary circulation. Am J Cardiol 44:1023–1028, 1979.
Pfeffer JM, Pfeffer MA, Fishbein MC, et al: Cardiac function and morphology with aging in the spontaneously hypertensive rat. Am J Physiol 237(4):H461–H468, 1979.
Savage DD, Abbott RD, Padgett S, et al: Epidemiologic features of left ventricular hypertrophy in normotensive and hypertensive subjects. In: ter Keurs HEDJ, Schipperheyn JJ (eds), Cardiac Left Ventricular Hypertrophy, Boston, Martinus Nijhoff Publishers, 1983, pp 3–16.
Sen S, Petscher C, Ratliff N: A factor that may initiate myocardial hypertrophy in hypertension. Hypertension 9:261–267, 1987.

Smith VE, Katz AM: Relaxation abnormalities part II: clinical aspects. Hosp Prac 19:149–172, 1984.
Strauer BE: Functional dynamics of the left ventricle in hypertensive hypertrophy and failure. Hypertension 6(Suppl III):III-4–III-12, 1984.
Tarazi RC, Levy MN: Cardiac responses to increased afterload: state of the art review. Hypertension 4:II8–II18, 1982.
Tarazi RC, Sen S, Fouad FM, et al: Regression of myocardial hypertrophy: conditions and sequelae of reversal in hypertensive heart disease. In: Alpert NR (ed), Perspective in Cardiovascular Research, Vol. 7: Myocardial Hypertrophy and Failure. New York, Raven Press, 1983, pp 637–652.

Chapter 4

Core Organ Effects: Part II Cerebral

Ray W. Gifford, Jr.

Introduction

The brain is one of the major target organs for the development of sequelae in patients with hypertension. Conversely, hypertension is a major risk factor for cerebrovascular disease and its complications, including cerebral infarction and hemorrhage, transient ischemic attacks, multi-infarct dementia, and Binswanger's disease. Compared to cigarette smoking and hypercholesterolemia, hypertension is a more important risk factor for ischemic brain disease than it is for ischemic heart disease.

This chapter addresses the immediate effects of blood pressure reduction on cerebral blood flow as well as the long-term effects on preventing or reducing the risk of ischemic, hemorrhagic, and embolic stroke. To understand the consequences of blood pressure reduction on cerebral blood flow, it is important to describe the concept of cerebral autoregulation of blood flow, as well as the protective effect of the baroreceptor reflexes.

Cerebral Autoregulation

Cerebral blood flow is not primarily under the influence of the autonomic nervous system. Cerebral blood flow is maintained within re-

From Punzi HA, Flamenbaum W (eds): *Hypertension*. Mount Kisco, NY, Futura Publishing Co., Inc., © 1989.

Table 1
Autoregulation of Cerebral Blood Flow in Normotensive and Hypertensive Subjects

	Mean Arterial Blood Pressure (mmHg)			% of Rest MABP	
Group	Control	Lower Limit of Autoregulation	Lowest Tolerated	Lower Limit of Autoregulation	Lowest Tolerated
Normotensive (n = 10)	98 ± 10	73 ± 9	43 ± 8	74 ± 12	45 ± 12
Hypertensives (n = 13)	145 ± 17	113 ± 17*†	65 ± 10*	79 ± 10	45 ± 6
Controlled hypertensives (n = 9)	116 ± 18	96 ± 17	53 ± 17	72 ± 29	46 ± 16

Values given as means ± SD. MABP = mean arterial blood pressure.
* p <0.01 for difference between normotensives and hypertensives.
† p <0.01 for difference between controlled and uncontrolled hypertensives.
(Adapted from Strandgaard S: Autoregulation of cerebral blood flow in hypertensive patients. The modifying influence of prolonged antihypertensive treatment on the tolerance to acute, drug-induced hypotension. Circulation 53:720–727, 1976, with permission.)

markably narrow limits over a wide range of systemic arterial pressure. When blood pressure rises, cerebral vasoconstriction increases cerebral vascular resistance and prevents a commensurate rise in cerebral blood flow; when blood pressure falls, vasodilatation prevents a decrease in cerebral blood flow. In young healthy normotensive subjects, cerebral blood flow remains relatively constant between systemic mean arterial pressures of 70 to 150 mmHg. The lower limit of cerebral autoregulation is the mean arterial pressure below which cerebral blood flow begins to fall (Fig. 1). Symptoms of cerebral ischemia do not develop at this point because the brain can compensate for the reduced blood flow by extracting more oxygen from the blood. When this compensatory mechanism finally fails, symptoms, such as lightheadedness, clamminess, yawning, nausea, and restlessness appear before the subject faints. The mean arterial pressure at which symptoms of cerebral ischemia appear is the "lowest tolerated pressure," and is usually 30–40 mmHg lower than the lower limit of cerebral autoregulation (Table 1). When blood pressure exceeds the upper limit of cerebral autoregulation, hyperperfusion of the brain occurs, which many authorities believe is the genesis

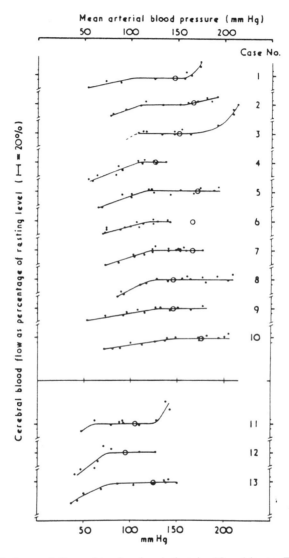

Figure 1. Autoregulation of brain circulation in 13 subjects. The ordinate shows cerebral blood flow as a percentage of the resting level. For each curve cerebral blood flow ± 10% is marked. The curves were drawn by simple visual interpolation of the points. An estimate of the patients' habitual mean arterial pressure is indicated by an open circle. It is clearly seen how the autoregulation curves of the hypertensive patients (cases 1–10) are shifted upwards when compared with the controls (cases 11–13). In addition, some of the patients show an upper limit of autoregulation beyond which cerebral blood flow increases. (With permission from Strandgaard S, Olesen J, Skinhoj E, et al: Autoregulation of brain circulation in severe arterial hypertension. Br Med J 1:507–510, 1973.)

of hypertensive encephalopathy. This is known as the "breakthrough" phenomenon.

It is the current consensus that cerebral autoregulation is mediated by a myogenic reflex in the wall of the arterioles and/or by a metabolite such as adenosine so that a fall in mean arterial pressure causes relaxation of the resistance vessels, and a rise in mean arterial pressure triggers vasoconstriction to protect the brain from excessive pressure and flow. In normotensive healthy individuals, blood pressure can be reduced abruptly with little or no adverse effect on cerebral blood flow until mean arterial pressure of approximately 70 mmHg is reached (Table 1) and mean arterial blood pressure can rise abruptly to approximately 150 mmHg without a consequent change in cerebral blood flow.

Effect of Hypertension on Cerebral Autoregulation

The curve of autoregulation is shifted to the right in chronically hypertensive patients so that the lower limit of autoregulation is in the range of 100 to 115 mmHg and the lowest tolerated mean arterial pressure at which anoxic symptoms occur is 55–75 mmHg (Table 1). Presumably the upper limit of cerebral autoregulation is also shifted to the right (a higher level of mean arterial pressure) but this hasn't been studied adequately. The clinical lesson is that blood pressure should not be reduced rapidly or excessively for chronically hypertensive patients to avoid undesirable reduction in cerebral blood flow. The mean arterial pressure that represents the lower limit of autoregulation for a normotensive subject approximates the lowest tolerated mean arterial pressure for a hypertensive patient (Table 1).

Treatment of hypertension tends to shift the autoregulatory curve back toward normal (or to the left) such that hypertensive patients can tolerate lower blood pressures without jeopardizing cerebral blood flow after they have been on treatment for several weeks compared to when treatment was first started (Table 1; Fig. 2). A rule of thumb for the clinician to gauge safe levels of mean arterial pressure is that the lower limit of autoregulation is approximately 75% of resting mean arterial pressure, and the lowest tolerated mean arterial pressure is about 45% of resting mean arterial pressure, whether patients are normotensive, untreated hypertensives, or treated hypertensives (Table 1).

Baroreceptor Reflexes

Autoregulation protects the brain from all but the most severe decreases in blood pressure. In addition, the baroreceptor reflexes prevent

Core Organ Effects: Cerebral • 69

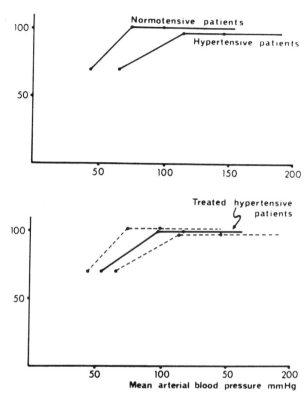

Figure 2. (Top panel) Mean curves of autoregulation of cerebral blood flow (CBF) in normotensive and severely hypertensive human subjects. Each curve is defined by the mean values of resting blood pressure, the lower limit of CBF autoregulation, and the lowest tolerated blood pressure. The curve from the hypertensive patients is shifted to the right on the blood pressure axis. (Bottom panel) Mean curve of CBF autoregulation in patients with a formerly severe hypertension, which at the time of the study was effectively controlled by antihypertensive treatment. The curve falls between the two curves above, which are shown by dotted lines. (With permission from Strandgaard S: Autoregulation of cerebral blood flow in hypertensive patients. The modifying influence of prolonged antihypertensive treatment on the tolerance to acute, drug-induced hypotension. Circulation 53:720–727, 1976.)

70 • HYPERTENSION

Table 2
Antihypertensive Drugs That Can Cause Orthostatic Hypotension

Bethanidine
Guanadrel
Guanethidine
Pargyline
Prazosin
Terazosin

systemic hypotension. Baroreceptor reflex activity tends to be less effective in the elderly and in hypertensives than in younger or normotensive individuals. Cerebral acute and chronic vascular disease also diminishes baroreflex sensitivity, making those patients more susceptible to hypotension.

Perhaps related to this phenomenon is the observation by Caird and co-workers that 24% of 494 people aged 65 years or more living at home had an orthostatic decrease of at least 20 mmHg in systolic blood pressure that was unassociated with symptoms. This underscores the importance of measuring blood pressure in the standing position as well as the seated or supine position *before* and during antihypertensive therapy and also militates against the use of antihypertensive agents that have a propensity to cause or aggravate orthostatic decreases in blood pressure (Table 2), especially in elderly patients.

Effect of Antihypertensive Drugs on Cerebral Blood Flow

Drugs that have no direct effect on cerebral vasculature will decrease cerebral blood flow only when blood pressure has been reduced below the lower limit of autoregulation. An example is diazoxide, which has no direct vasodilating effect on cerebral vasculature, although it is a potent vasodilator of other vascular beds.

Dihydralazine is a cerebral vasodilator and therefore will maintain cerebral blood flow below the lower limit of autoregulation but may increase intracranial pressure, which is undesirable, especially for patients with acute stroke or head trauma and cerebral edema because it will reduce cerebral blood flow. Dihydralazine can also interfere with autoregulation. Sodium nitroprusside has an effect similar to dihydralazine, although it is less likely than dihydralazine to increase intracranial pressure at low levels of blood pressure. Dihydralazine can produce a "patchy," uneven perfusion where areas of high and low flow coexist. Sodium nitroprusside is less likely to do this.

Ganglionic blockers and alpha-adrenergic blockers abolish the weak alpha-adrenergic constriction of the larger cerebral resistance vessels that occurs during experimental hemorrhagic hypotension. Trimethaphan does not increase intracranial pressure.

Unlike dihydralazine and sodium nitroprusside, ganglion blockers, adrenergic blockers, and angiotensin-converting enzyme (ACE) inhibitors actually shift the lower limit of autoregulation of cerebral blood flow toward the left (toward lower pressures). Calcium channel blocking agents such as nifedipine, nitrendipine, and verapamil are cerebral vasodilators that increase cerebral blood flow acutely and maintain cerebral blood flow in spite of blood pressure reduction during chronic therapy.

One of the calcium channel blocking drugs, nimodipine, has been used extensively in the treatment of acute subarachnoid hemorrhage with encouraging results with respect to mortality and morbidity. The effect of nimodipine on cerebral blood flow has been disputed. Some studies showed an increase while others showed no effect. Vasospasm around the bleeding site was reduced but not abolished by nimodipine, and there was no difference in continuous electrocardiographic recordings between the placebo and actively treated groups. It has been suggested that nimodipine may protect the neurons from ischemic damage, perhaps by preventing calcium influx.

Treatment of Hypertension for Patients with Cerebral Vascular Disease

Most of the results referred to in the previous section have come from acute short-term studies and may not be pertinent for chronic therapy of hypertension. Treatment of hypertensive emergencies including acute hypertensive encephalopathy is discussed in a separate chapter.

Acute Ischemic Stroke

Unless hypertension is severe (e.g., >180/110 mmHg) treatment should be withheld following an acute ischemic infarct because autoregulation is lost or severely impaired during an acute insult and flow will passively follow blood pressure. If systolic blood pressure is ≥180 mmHg and/or the diastolic blood pressure is ≥110 mmHg or if the patient has impending heart failure, blood pressure should be reduced gradually to levels no lower than 160/100 mmHg. Theoretically, an ACE inhibitor (captopril, enalapril, or lisinopril) is the drug of choice because these agents tend to shift the autoregulatory curve toward lower levels. Agents that tend to cause unpredictable orthostatic hypotension (Table 2) should be avoided, as should beta-blockers, which can reduce cardiac output and hence decrease cerebral blood flow. Calcium channel blocking drugs can be used cautiously in small doses because most have been shown to have a vasodilating effect on the cerebral circulation.

Transient Ischemic Attacks

Hypertension should be treated in patients with transient ischemic attacks. Blood pressure should be reduced gradually and orthostatic hypotension should be avoided if at all possible (Table 2). Drugs of choice include ACE inhibitors, calcium channel blockers, low-dose diuretic and centrally acting adrenergic inhibiting agents. Once hypertension is controlled, aspirin should be prescribed in a dose of 0.3 g daily or every other day.

There is no doubt that transient ischemic attacks are harbingers of stroke, and control of hypertension lessens this risk. A Doppler/ultrasound scan of the extracranial arteries in the neck is usually advisable, looking for a significant stenosis or ulcerated atheromata that might be treated surgically. The concern that reduction of blood pressure for hypertensive patients with transient ischemic attacks might precipitate a stroke has not been substantiated by clinical experience. Indeed, control of blood pressure is usually accompanied by a diminution in frequency of the transient ischemic attacks.

Lacunar Infarcts

This syndrome of "little strokes" leading eventually to bilateral neurological signs, gait disturbances, sensory changes, pseudobulbar palsy, and dementia is almost always accompanied by hypertension. The symptoms are due to multiple tiny infarcts (lacunae) in the white matter of the hemispheres, brain stem, and cerebellum.

Control of blood pressure is the only hope of retarding the progress of this syndrome, but patients often do not tolerate blood pressure medications well. The goal should be to keep the blood pressure as nearly normal as the patient can tolerate, using regimens similar to those recommended for patients with transient ischemic attacks (see above).

Binswanger's Disease

While dementia of the Binswanger's type has been attributed to hypertension, there is no evidence that treating hypertension is beneficial in this condition, although there is no harm in making the attempt. If reducing blood pressure seems to worsen the dementia, treatment should be discontinued.

Postcerebral Infarction

Once a patient has recovered from the acute phase of cerebral infarction, the neurological deficit has stabilized, and the patient is ambulatory (usually three or four weeks after the stroke), hypertension should be treated with the same regimens that would be used for hypertensive patients who have never had a stroke. The goal should be to normalize blood pressure (< 140/90 mmHg).

Surprisingly, these patients tolerate blood pressure reduction quite well, including inadvertent orthostatic hypotension. If it becomes necessary to use orthostatic agents to control blood pressure, patients should be warned about rising from the seated or recumbent positions rapidly.

Methyldopa has been used to treat hypertensive patients with cerebral vascular disease (cerebral infarction and/or transient ischemic attacks). Average cerebral blood flow was low initially (Table 3). After two weeks of treatment, mean arterial pressure and cerebral vascular resistance were significantly reduced and cerebral blood flow was significantly increased. Since methyldopa is an inhibitor of the sympathetic nervous system, it is unlikely that it had a direct effect to reduce cerebrovascular resistance, hence the reduction in cerebrovascular resistance must be related to autoregulation.

If reduction of blood pressure is poorly tolerated and produces symptoms of cerebral ischemia unrelated to measurable hypotension, the clinician should suspect that the patient has severe bilateral carotid

Table 3
Effect of Antihypertensive Therapy on Cerebral Hemodynamics in 13 Patients With Cerebrovascular Disease

MAP		CBF		CVR	
C	Rx	C	Rx	C	Rx
125.2 ± 16.6	105.9 ± 14.6	44.5 ± 11.0	48.9 ± 10.6	2.97 ± 0.76	2.27 ± 0.58
p <0.01		p <0.05		p <0.001	

MAP = mean arterial pressure (mmHg); CBF = cerebral blood flow (mL/100 g brain/min); CVR = cerebral vascular resistance (mmHg/mL/100 g brain min); C = before treatment; Rx = at end of 2 weeks treatment with methyldopa. (Adapted from Meyer JS, Sawada T, Kitamura A, et al: Cerebral blood flow after control of hypertension in stroke. Neurology 18:772–781, 1968, with permission.)

and/or vertebral basilar occlusive disease or drug-induced orthostatic hypotension. Doppler/sonographic scans will help rule out disease in the neck, but intracranial lesions can also cause this syndrome and may require angiography for diagnosis. Another possibility is pseudohypertension due to severe medial sclerosis of the brachial arteries and their branches, yielding spuriously high blood pressure readings by indirect sphygmomanometry. This diagnosis can be suspected when the radial artery is easily palpable and can be rolled under the examiner's fingers after the pulse has been obliterated by occluding the brachial artery with the blood pressure cuff.

Prevention of Stroke

Primary Prevention

Many of the large prospective controlled clinical trials have shown that treatment of hypertension reduces the incidence of fatal and nonfatal stroke. The Australian National Trial and the European Working Party on Hypertension in the Elderly (EWPHE) Trial showed impressive, although not statistically significant reductions in stroke rate.

By analyzing pooled data from nine of the largest clinical trials, a statistically significant reduction in both fatal and nonfatal strokes has been shown (Fig. 3). Data were derived from approximately 43,000 patients with an average follow-up of 5.6 years. Mortality from stroke was significantly reduced by 38% in subjects from the study treatment groups

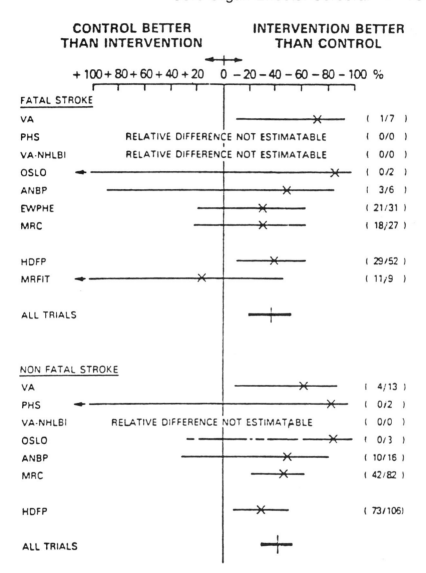

Figure 3. Estimates with approximate 9% confidence intervals of the relative difference in fatal and nonfatal stroke between study intervention and control groups. Number of events (intervention/control) given on right. (With permission from MacMahon SW, Cutler JA, Furberg CD, et al: The effects of drug treatment of hypertension on morbidity and mortality from cardiovascular disease: a review of randomized controlled trials. Prog Cardiovasc Dis 29(Suppl 1):99–118, 1986.)

(95% confidence interval: −53% to −19%). There was also a significant reduction in the incidence of nonfatal stroke by 43% (95% confidence interval: −54% to −29%). The incidence of fatal and nonfatal stroke combined was reduced by 39% (95% confidence interval: −48% to −28%). In a VA placebo-controlled trial there were five subjects in the placebo group who had cerebral or subarachnoid hemorrhage compared to none in the group on active treatment. In other studies no attempt was made to distinguish between hemorrhagic and nonhemorrhagic stroke.

With the exception of the MRC trial all of these clinical trials used a diuretic as initial treatment. In the MRC trial, bendrofluazide was strikingly and significantly more effective in reducing strokes for smokers than propranolol. Whether calcium channel blocking agents and converting enzyme inhibitors will be as effective as diuretics in reducing stroke remains to be determined by future controlled clinical trials using these agents as initial therapy.

Secondary Prevention

Several small trials have shown that control of blood pressure for patients who have already had one stroke will reduce the risk of recurrent stroke, including fatal ones. One large multicenter trial failed to corroborate this.

One study compared a group of 39 hypertensive patients who had one stroke and whose hypertension was treated, with a group of 42 stroke survivors whose hypertension was not treated. During a follow-up period that averaged 3 years, 22 nonfatal and 5 fatal cerebrovascular events occurred in the latter group compared to eight nonfatal and two fatal cerebrovascular events in the treated group.

In a randomized trial in 97 stroke survivors whose diastolic blood pressure was 110 mmHg or greater, antihypertensive medications were given to half of the patients with a goal diastolic blood pressure of 90–100 mmHg. During 5 years of follow-up, 10 untreated and 3 treated patients had fatal cerebral infarction or hemorrhage.

A third study followed 162 hypertensive stroke survivors for periods up to 12 years with an average of 48 months. Antihypertensive medication was given to all patients, and the adequacy of blood pressure control was compared to the frequency of recurrent strokes retrospectively. Blood pressure control was "good" if standing diastolic blood pressure was less than 100 mmHg, "fair" if between 100 and 109 mmHg, and "poor" if greater than 109 mmHg. Patients with good control had a 16% incidence rate of recurrent stroke compared with 32% for patients with fair control and 55% when hypertension was poorly controlled.

A placebo-controlled double-blind multicenter study of the relationship between blood pressure control and recurrent stroke was sponsored by the National Institute of Neurological Diseases and Stroke. Pretreatment blood pressure range was 140–220 mmHg systolic and 90–115 mmHg diastolic. Active drug therapy consisted of a combination of 10 mg of methyclothiazide and 1 mg of deserpidine in 233 patients, while 219 received placebo. Average blood pressure fell from 167/100 mmHg by 26.3/13.3 mmHg in the drug-treated group. There was a small, but statistically insignificant reduction in fatal and nonfatal strokes in the drug-treated group, with 37 strokes occurring in the treated group and 42 in the placebo group. There was a statistically significant reduction in the occurrence of congestive heart failure in the drug-treated group. The conclusion was that hypertension should be treated for stroke victims because treatment did not increase the risk of subsequent strokes and did decrease the incidence of congestive heart failure.

The Chicago Stroke Study found that systolic blood pressure was a more important risk factor for stroke than was diastolic blood pressure and that isolated systolic hypertension (systolic blood pressure ≥160 mmHg and diastolic blood pressure <80 mmHg) increased the risk of stroke by 2.5 times compared to normotensive subjects (Table 4). There

Table 4
Three-Year Incidence of Stroke and of Class 1 Nonembolic Brain Infarction By Level of Sytolic Pressure in Persons With Diastolic Pressure ≤ 79 mmHg, Age 65 to 74: Chicago Stroke Study

Systolic Blood Pressure (mmHg)	No. of Subjects	All Stroke			Class 1 NBI		
		No.	Rate/1,000*	SE	No.	Rate/1,000*	SE
≤ 139	687	26	42	8	14	22	6
140–159	332	17	55	13	7	26	10
≥ 160	204	20	110	27	8	57	23

* Each rate is the mean of eight age-specific, sex-specific, and race-specific rates computed for the category by life table procedure. (With permission from Shekelle RB, Ostfeld AM, Klawans HL: Hypertension and the risk of stroke in an elderly population. Stroke 5:71–75, 1974.)

is no evidence from clinical trials that treatment of isolated systolic hypertension will lessen the risk. The Systolic Hypertension in the Elderly Program (SHEP) is a multicenter trial now in progress to address this issue.

In the analysis of the major clinical trials of antihypertensive therapy, the marked benefit in preventing stroke was clearly contrasted with the failure to demonstrate significant reductions in coronary events. The reason for this difference is not apparent but may relate to the epidemiologic observations that hypertension is the single most important risk factor for stroke but is only one of three major risk factors for coronary disease.

Major differences in the cerebral and coronary circulations play an important role in these observed differences in end-organ sequelae. In the brain, oxygen extraction from the blood can be increased if blood pressure falls below the lower limit of autoregulation, while in the coronary circulation, oxygen extraction is virtually maximal in the resting state, and therefore, this compensatory mechanism is not available when coronary flow is reduced below the level of coronary autoregulation. This is particularly true in the subendocardial areas of the hypertrophied left ventricle where myocardial contraction compromises the vasculature to a greater degree than in more superficial layers and where the lower limit of autoregulation is higher than in more superficial layers, thus making it vulnerable to reductions in blood pressure especially when atherosclerosis of major coronary arteries impairs flow proximally. In my opinion, these authors do not give enough consideration to the demand side of the equation. When blood pressure, especially systolic, is reduced, there is little if any change in the oxygen consumption of the brain, but there is a dramatic decrease in the oxygen requirement of the left ventricle, which could offset the decrease in coronary blood flow.

Summary

Hypertension is the major correctable risk factor in the development of stroke, and there is convincing evidence from large prospective clinical trials that treatment of hypertension has benefit in preventing primary and perhaps secondary stroke. Although hypertensive patients have impaired cerebral autoregulation and baroreflex function, these improve with reduction in blood pressure, the lower limit of autoregulation being approximately 75% of the resting mean arterial pressure.

Unless the hypertension is severe, antihypertensive medication

Core Organ Effects: Cerebral • 79

should be withheld during an acute ischemic stroke until the patient's neurological deficit has stabilized and the patient can ambulate. Thereafter, blood pressure should be reduced gradually to normal levels. Hypertension should be treated in patients with transient ischemic attacks or lacunar infarcts. Drugs that do not interfere with cerebral circulation are preferable to those that cause orthostatic hypotension.

Selected References

Hypertension as a Risk Factor for Stroke

Kannel WB, Dawber TR, Sorlie P, et al: Components of blood pressure and risk of atheroembolic brain infarction: The Framingham Study. Stroke 7:327–333, 1976.
Kannel WB, Wolf PA, Verter MS, et al: Epidemiologic assessment of the role of blood pressure in stroke: The Framingham Study. JAMA 214:301–310, 1970.
Kannel WB: Role of blood pressure in cardiovascular morbidity and mortality. Prog Cardiovasc Dis 17:5–24, 1974.
Shekelle RB, Ostfeld AM, Klawans HL: Hypertension and risk of stroke in an elderly population. Stroke 5:71–75, 1974.

Cerebral Autoregulation

Finnerty FA Jr, Witkin L, Fazekas JF, et al: Cerebral hemodynamics during cerebral ischemia induced by acute hypotension. J Clin Invest 33:1227–1232, 1954.
Kontos HA: Regulation of the cerebral circulation. Ann Rev Physiol 43:397–407, 1981.
Lassen NA, Agnoli A: The upper limit of autoregulation of cerebral blood flow on the pathogenesis of hypertensive encephalopathy. Scand J Clin Lab Invest 30:113–116, 1972.
Skinhoj E, Strandgaard S: Pathogenesis of hypertensive encephalopathy. Lancet 1:461–462, 1973.
Skinhoj E: The sympathetic nervous system and the regulation of cerebral blood flow in man. Stroke 3:711–716, 1972.
Strandgaard S, Olesen J, Skinhoj E, et al: Autoregulation of brain circulation in severe arterial hypertension. Br Med J 1:507–510, 1973.
Strandgaard S: Autoregulation of cerebral blood flow in hypertensive patients. The modifying influence of prolonged antihypertensive treatment on the tolerance to acute, drug-induced hypotension. Circulation 53:720–727, 1976.
Strandgaard S, Paulson OB: Cerebral autoregulation. Stroke 15:413–416, 1984.
Symon L, Held K, Dorsch NWC: On the myogenic nature of the autoregulatory mechanism in the cerebral circulation. Europ Neurol 6:11–18, 1971.
Vinall PE, Simeone FA: Cerebral autoregulation: an in vitro study. Stroke 12:640–642, 1981.

Winn HR, Welsch JE, Rubio R, et al: Brain adenosine production in rat during sustained alteration in systemic blood pressure. Am J Physiol 239:H636-H641, 1980.

Baroreceptor Reflexes

Appenzeller O, Descarries L: Circulatory reflexes in patients with cerebrovascular disease. N Engl J Med 271:820-823, 1964.
Caird FI, Andrews GR, Kennedy RD: Effect of posture on blood pressure in the elderly. Br Heart J 35:527-530, 1973.
Gribbin B, Pickering TG, Sleight P, et al: Effect of age and high blood pressure on baroreflex sensitivity in man. Circ Res 29:424-431, 1971.

Effect of Antihypertensive Drugs on Cerebral Blood Flow

Conen D, Bertel O, Dubach UC: Cerebral blood flow and calcium antagonists in hypertension. J Hypertens 5(Suppl 4):S75-S80, 1987.
Meyer JS, Sawada T, Kitamura A, et al: Cerebral blood flow after control of hypertension in stroke. Neurology 18:772-781, 1968.
Miyamori I, Yasuhara S, Matsubara T, et al: Effects of a calcium entry blocker on cerebral circulation in essential hypertension. J Clin Hypertens 3:528-535, 1987.
Paulson OB, Waldemar G, Andersen AR, et al: Role of angiotensin in autoregulation of cerebral blood flow. Circulation 77(Suppl I):I-55-I-58, 1988.

Nimodipine and Subarachnoid Hemorrhage

Mee E, Dorrance D, Lowe D, et al: Controlled study of nomidipine in aneurysm patients treated early after subarachnoid hemorrhage. J Neurosurg 22:484-491, 1988.
Neil-Dwyer G, Mee E, Dorrance D, Lowe D: Early intervention with nimodipine in subarachnoid haemorrhage. Eur Heart J 8(Suppl K):41-47, 1987.
Scriabine A, Van den Kerckhoff W: Pharmacology of nimodipine. A review. Ann NY Acad Sci 522:698-706, 1988.
Seiler RW, Grolimund P, Zurbruegg HR: Evaluation of the calcium antagonist nimodipine for the prevention of vasospasm after aneurysmal subarachnoid haemorrhage. Acta Neurochir 85:7-16, 1987.
Tettenborn D, Porto L, Ryman T, et al: Survey of clinical experience with nimodipine in patients with subarachnoid hemorrhage. Neurosurg Rev 10:77-84, 1987.

Treatment of Hypertension for Patients with Cerebral Vascular Disease

Hankey GJ, Gubbay SS: Focal cerebral ischaemia and infarction due to antihypertensive therapy. Med J Aust 146:412-414, 1987.

Core Organ Effects: Cerebral • 81

McLaren GD, Danta G: Cerebral infarction due to presumed haemodynamic factors in ambulant hypertensive patients. Clin Exp Neurol 23:55–66, 1987.

Paulson OB, Andersen AR, Vorstrup S: Drugs in acute ischemic cerebrovascular lesion evaluated by regional blood flow measurements in the brain. Agressologie 28:367–371, 1987.

Whisnant JP, Cartlidge NEF, Elveback LR: Carotid and vertebral-basilar transient ischemic attacks: effect of anticoagulants, hypertension, and cardiac disorders on survival and stroke occurrence—A population study. Ann Neurol 3:107–115, 1978.

Prevention of Stroke

Amery A, Brixko P, Clement D, et al: Mortality and morbidity results from the European Working Party on High Blood Pressure in the Elderly Trial. Lancet 1:1349–1354, 1985.

Beevers DG, Fairman MJ, Hamilton M, et al: Antihypertensive treatment and the course of established cerebral vascular disease. Lancet 1:1407–1409, 1973.

Carter AB: Hypotensive therapy in stroke survivors. Lancet 1:485–489, 1970.

Freis ED: The Veterans Administration Cooperative Study on Antihypertensive Agents. Implications for stroke prevention. Stroke 5:76–77, 1974.

Hypertension Detection and Follow-up Program Cooperative Group: Five-year findings of the Hypertension Detection and Follow-up Program. III, Reduction in stroke incidence among persons with high blood pressure. JAMA 247:633–638, 1982.

Hypertension-Stroke Cooperative Study Group: Effect of antihypertensive treatment on stroke recurrence. JAMA 229:409–418, 1974.

MacMahon SW, Cutler JA, Furberg CD, et al: The effects of drug treatment of hypertension on morbidity and mortality from cardiovascular disease: a review of randomized controlled trials. Prog Cardiovasc Dis 29(Suppl 1):99–118, 1986.

Marshall J: A trial of long-term hypotensive therapy in cerebrovascular disease. Lancet 1:10–12, 1964.

Medical Research Council Working Party: MRC trial of treatment of mild hypertension: principal results. Br Med J 291:97–104, 1985.

Strandgaard S, Haunso S: Why does antihypertensive treatment prevent stroke but not myocardial infarction? Lancet 2:658–661, 1987.

The Australian Therapeutic Trial in Mild Hypertension. Lancet 1:1261–1267, 1980.

Miscellaneous

Messerli FH, Ventura HO, Amodeo C: Osler's maneuver and pseudohypertension. N Engl J Med 312:1548–1551, 1985.

Roman GC: Senile dementia of the Binswanger type: A vascular form of dementia in the elderly. JAMA 258:1782–1788, 1987.

Chapter 4

Core Organ Effects: Part III Renal

John H. Bauer and Garry P. Reams

The Pathophysiology of the Essential Hypertensive Kidney

The natural course of essential hypertensive renal disease is characterized by a slowly progressive impairment of renal function. Specifically, there is a progressive rise in renal vascular resistance (RVR), and a progressive fall in effective renal plasma flow (ERPF)/ renal blood flow (RBF). The glomerular filtration rate (GFR) is relatively maintained, although serious renal impairment may occur in up to 20% of essential hypertensive patients (Fig. 1, phases I-V). The initial changes are functional and reversible, presumably mediated by neurohumoral mechanisms, including enhanced renal vascular response to circulating or endogenous norepinephrine and angiotensin II. Subsequently, structural changes occur related to the severity of the hypertension and to the aging process.

Two vascular lesions are observed in the essential hypertensive kidney: hyperplastic elastic arteriosclerosis, most marked in the interlobular arteries, and hyaline arteriolosclerosis, primarily involving the afferent arterioles. Ultimately, as a result of reduced blood flow, the glomeruli undergo ischemic changes. The process begins with wrinkling of the capillary basement membrane followed by its thickening, simplification, and collapse. The initial ischemic glomerular changes are potentially reversible; however, with the appearance of hyaline in the capsular

---

From Punzi HA, Flamenbaum W (eds): *Hypertension*. Mount Kisco, NY, Futura Publishing Co., Inc., © 1989.

PATHOPHYSIOLOGY OF ESSENTIAL HYPERTENSIVE RENAL DISEASE

Time (age-years)

(20-30) PHASE I:
Rise in renal vascular resistance due to functional disturbance of renal vasculature: ? active vasoresponse to endogenous angiotensin II, norepinephrine

(30-40) PHASE II:
Further rise in renal vascular resistance; both functional and structural disturbances in renal vasculature; preservation of glomerular filtration rate (although glomeruli may be ischemic); rise in filtration fraction; microalbuminuria

(40-50) PHASE III:
Further rise in renal vascular resistance; structural disturbances involving both renal vasculature and glomeruli (arteriolar nephrosclerosis); reduction in perfusion disproportionately greater than filtration; sustained rise in filtration fraction; proteinuria.

(50-) PHASE IV:
critical reduction in renal mass: fall in renal vascular resistance (reduction in afferent arteriolar resistance); rise in glomerular capillary hydraulic pressure; progressive fall in GFR; nephrosclerosis, glomerulosclerosis

PHASE V
Chronic renal insufficiency -> ESRD

Figure 1. Pathophysiology of essential hypertensive renal disease. ESRD = end-stage renal disease.

space, the process proceeds to complete obsolescence. Secondary tubular atrophy, thickening of tubular basement membranes, and interstitial fibrosis occurs. Because the vascular lesions are usually distributed in a focal, irregular fashion throughout the renal cortex, the secondary ischemic changes assume a similar pattern of distribution. However, when the vascular lesions are severe and generalized, the entire kidney undergoes ischemic atrophy. Data derived from studies in an animal analogue of essential hypertension, the spontaneous hypertensive rat, provide insight into the intrarenal hemodynamic changes occurring during the progressive phases of essential hypertensive renal disease. There is an initial increase in preglomerular capillary (afferent arteriolar) resistance, which protects the kidney from exposure to an elevated systemic pressure (Figs. 2, 3); although systemic pressure is elevated, the glomerular capillary pressure (P_{GC}) is normal. The normal P_{GC} is a consequence of a physiological, autoregulatory response of the afferent arteriolar resistance to the elevated systemic pressure. These early func-

NORMAL MICROCIRCULATION

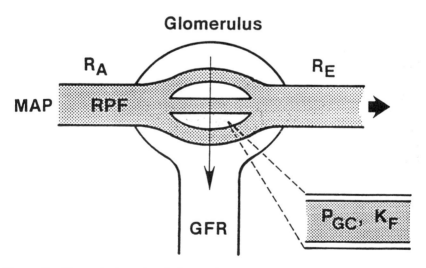

Figure 2. Normal microcirculation—glomerulus. MAP = mean arterial pressure (systemic); RPF = renal plasma flow; GFR = glomerular filtration rate; R_A = afferent arteriolar resistance; R_E = efferent arteriolar resistance; P_{GC} = glomerular capillary pressure; K_f = ultrafiltration coefficient.

ESSENTIAL HYPERTENSION

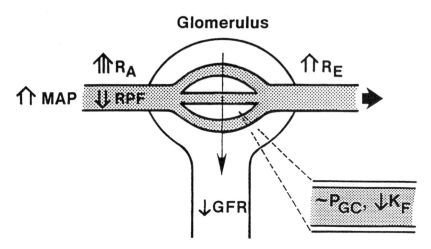

Figure 3. Microcirculation—glomerulus—essential hypertensive kidney (adapted from spontaneously hypertensive rat model; see text).

tional alterations, if extrapolated to the human essential hypertensive kidneys, would be clinically manifested (using renal clearance techniques) by an increase in RVR, and a decrease in ERPF/RBF (see Fig. 1, phase I-II). The filtration fraction (ratio of GFR to ERPF) is increased, due to the relative preservation of GFR. Microalbuminuria may be observed. With the development of irreversible vascular disease (see Fig. 1, phase III-IV), renal mass is gradually lost due to glomerular ischemia. Clinically (using renal clearance techniques), there is a further rise in the RVR, and there is a further decrease in ERPF/RBF. There is a decrease in GFR (now manifested by a rise in the serum creatinine and/or a fall in the creatinine clearance), which is proportionally less than the decrease in ERPF/RBF, sustaining the rise in filtration fraction. Overt proteinuria may be observed. Hypertensive nephrosclerosis is pathologically present. Such a process may require decades to occur, presumably due to the initial protection of the glomerular capillary bed from hemodynamically mediated injury afforded by the increase in preglomerular capillary (afferent arteriolar) resistance, and the slow development of arteriosclerosis and arteriolosclerosis. This process, however, may be accentuated by severe hypertension, or exaggerated by metabolic disorders such as diabetes mellitus.

LOSS OF RENAL MASS/HIGH PROTEIN DIET

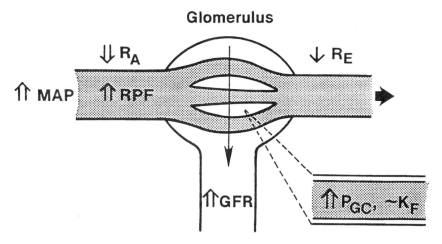

Figure 4. Microcirculation—glomerulus—response to loss of renal mass—high protein diet (adapted from uninephrectomized spontaneously hypertensive rat model; see text).

Once there has been a critical loss of renal mass (greater than 50%), there is a rapid loss of residual renal function (see Fig. 1, phase IV-V). Spontaneously hypertensive rats, undergoing uninephrectomy, experience a significant increase in their P_{GC}. This results from the transmission of systemic pressure to the unprotected glomerular capillary bed, due to a marked reduction in preglomerular capillary (afferent arteriolar) resistance (Fig. 4). The biological stimulus modulating this renal vasodilated state is unknown, but the elevated P_{GC} mediating the glomerular injury is clearly precipitated/aggravated by protein loading. Such functional alterations, if extrapolated to the human, could occur in residual, intact nephrons of the hypertensive nephrosclerotic kidney. Pathologically, mesangial expansion and glomerular sclerosis would occur. Clinically, the GFR would rapidly decrease to end-stage renal disease values.

Therapeutic Considerations

It is generally accepted that treatment of systemic hypertension protects the kidney from hemodynamically mediated injury. However, there are no prospective studies that have systemically examined the relationship between hypertension and the status of renal function in patients with essential hypertension. It is equally clear that renal function may deteriorate during traditional (i.e., stepped-care) antihypertensive therapy. Currently, hypertensive nephrosclerosis accounts for approximately 15%–25% of all end-stage renal disease in the United States.

Furthermore, blacks experience a disproportionate risk of hypertensive end-stage renal disease. There is, at the present, no evidence of a reduction in the incidence of hypertensive nephrosclerosis as a cause of end-stage renal disease.

Recent experimental studies suggest that the resistance state of the preglomerular and postglomerular capillary arterioles may determine if a particular form of antihypertensive therapy will protect the kidney from hemodynamically mediated glomerular injury. In essential hypertension, the initial increase in preglomerular capillary resistance protects the glomerular capillary bed from the transmission of systemic pressure. If preglomerular capillary resistance declines significantly in response to drug therapy, without a concurrent decrease in postglomerular capillary resistance, the glomerular capillary bed could be exposed to a rise in pressure. If preglomerular capillary resistance is already maximally dilated prior to drug therapy (e.g., residual intact nephrons of a nephrosclerotic kidney), drug therapy that reduced systemic pressure would also reduce P_{GC}, provided postglomerular capillary resistance was not increased. Experimentally, drugs that reduce systemic and P_{GC} have protective advantages (i.e., reduce proteinuria, prevent glomerular sclerosis), compared to drugs that reduce only systemic pressure.

Intrarenal Effects of Angiotensin II

During the phases of functional and reversible hemodynamic changes, many similarities exist between the pathophysiological changes occurring in the essential hypertensive kidney and the physiological changes effected by angiotensin II in the normal kidney. All the components of the renin-angiotensin system are present within the kidney (angiotensinogen and angiotensinogen mRNA, renin and renin mRNA, angiotensin-converting enzyme). The generation of angiotensin II from blood-borne and/or intrarenally generated angiotensinogen/angiotensin I should occur. Receptors for angiotensin II have been demonstrated in glomeruli, and glomerular contractile responses have been

MICROCIRCULATION RESPONSE TO ANGIOTENSIN II

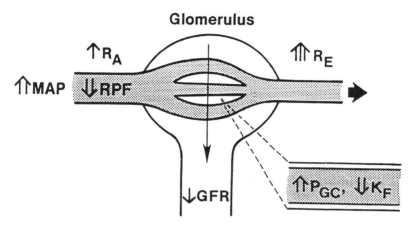

Figure 5. Microcirculation—glomerulus—response to angiotensin II (adapted from euvolemic Munich Wister rat model-exogenous infusion angiotensin II; see text).

observed with low concentrations of angiotensin II. Furthermore, angiotensin II receptors occur in brush-border and basolateral membranes of the proximal tubule, and in longitudinal bands in the inner zone of the outer medulla in association with vasa recta bundles. Experimentally, the exogenous infusion of angiotensin II, which may reflect the intrarenal action of angiotensin II, preferentially constricts the postglomerular capillary (efferent) arterioles, diminishing ERPF/RBF (Fig. 5). The preglomerular capillary (afferent) arterioles are also constricted, either as a direct effect of angiotensin II or as a myogenic response to the increase in systemic pressure. Although the P_{GC} is increased, GFR is unchanged due to a decrease in the ultrafiltration coefficient (K_f) (see below). Thus, there is a characteristic rise in the filtration fraction.

As a consequence of the increase in filtration fraction, there is a decrease in the excretion of sodium and water, physically resulting from the decrease in hydrostatic pressure and the increase in colloid osmotic pressure of the peritubular capillary circulation. In addition to its effect on renal hemodynamics, angiotensin II directly stimulates proximal tubular sodium reabsorption. Angiotensin II may also increase tubular sodium reabsorption by decreasing renal medullary blood flow. Constriction of efferent arterioles of juxtamedullary nephrons or a direct vasoconstrictor action on the vasa recta would lower renal medullary blood flow, increasing medullary interstitial fluid osmolality. Increased medullary osmolality would raise urine concentrating ability, enhancing passive sodium chloride reabsorption in the thin ascending limb of the loop of Henle.

Angiotensin II plays an important role in controlling GFR through two opposing mechanisms: (1) constriction of the efferent arteriole, increasing P_{GC}, and (2) constriction of the glomerular capillary mesangial bed, decreasing the ultrafiltration coefficient (K_f) (see Fig. 5). The K_f is the product of the total glomerular capillary filtering surface area, and the local capillary hydraulic conductance or permeability. Reductions in the K_f value can result from either declines in capillary surface area available for filtration, hydraulic conductance, or both. Angiotensin II reduces the K_f by decreasing the glomerular capillary surface area by promoting mesangial cell contraction. Net GFR will thus depend on the relative effects angiotensin II has on the filtration pressure (P_{GC}) and the K_f.

Angiotensin II also enhances the transglomerular passage of macromolecules (e.g., albumin). Angiotensin II causes an impairment in the size-selective permeability property of the glomerular capillary wall, increasing mesangial traffic and/or trapping of macromolecules. This process may be mediated by angiotensin II's capacity to modulate transmural pressure, via its regulatory effect on efferent arteriolar vasomotor tone. Angiotensin II may also increase transglomerular diffusion and convection of macromolecules, due to increases in the local intraglomerular capillary albumin concentration (a result of the increase in filtration fraction). The increased movement or entrapment of macromolecules within the glomerular mesangium, maintained over a period of time, may be a contributing factor to the development of proteinuria and mesangial sclerosis.

The Renal Effects Of ACE Inhibitors

To the degree that the essential hypertensive kidney is under the tonic influence of angiotensin II, the use of ACE inhibitors, by interrupting the integrity of the systemic and intrarenal renin-angiotensin system could be expected to mitigate the effects of angiotensin II on the glomerular mesangium (normalizing and/or increasing K_f) and on the postglomerular (efferent) arteriolar resistance (decreasing RVR and normalizing P_{GC}) (Figs. 6 and 7). In addition, inhibition of the intrarenal

ESSENTIAL HYPERTENSION / ACEI

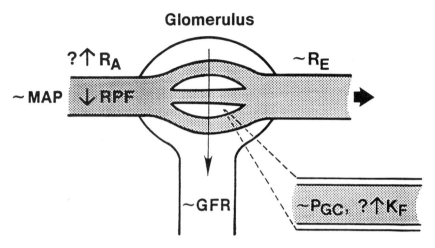

Figure 6. Microcirculation—glomerulus—essential hypertensive kidney response to ACE inhibition (ACEI) therapy (hypothesized response).

effects of angiotensin II on renal tubular epithelium and/or medullary blood flow could result in a natriuresis and diuresis. Angiotensin-converting enzyme inhibition therapy could also be expected to potentiate the vasodepressor kallikrein-kinin tissue system and to stimulate intrarenal production of vasodepressor prostaglandins. Finally, ACE inhibitor therapy could be expected to inhibit norepinephrine release and/or to inhibit post-junctional pressor responses to angiotensin II and/or norepinephrine.

Numerous investigators have demonstrated that ACE inhibitors do have salutary effects on the essential hypertensive kidney, presumably related to drug interruption of the integrity of the intrarenal renin-angiotensin system or to potentiation of the intrarenal vasodilatory systems. In general, RVR is reduced, ERPF/RBF is preserved or improved, and GFR is preserved or improved. There is an initial diuresis and antikaliuresis; there may be a sustained diuresis. Urinary protein excretion is unchanged or decreased. Improvement in renal perfusion and glomerular filtration, observed in essential hypertensive patients with impaired renal function receiving ACE inhibition therapy has not been observed with other classes of antihypertensive drugs (with the possible exception of calcium antagonists).

LOSS OF RENAL MASS/ACEI

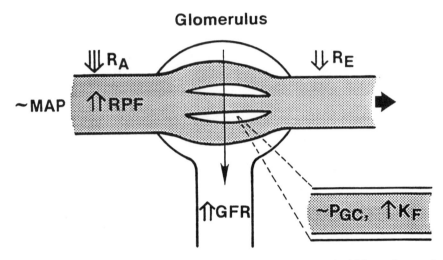

Figure 7. Microcirculation—glomerulus—nephrosclerotic kidney (loss of renal mass) response to ACE inhibition (ACEI) therapy (adapted from remnant kidney—high protein diet—ACEI rat model; see text).

Forty to 50% of patients with essential hypertension fail to increase their ERPF, or fail to enhance their renal vascular responsiveness to an exogenous infusion of angiotensin II, when shifted from a low to a high sodium diet; such patients have been termed "non-modulators." In these patients, the administration of an ACE inhibitor restores their ERPF, and their renal vascular responsiveness, to normal. All of these observations suggest that ACE inhibitor therapy may not only reverse the initial functional pathophysiological changes encountered in the essential hypertensive kidney, but may also attenuate the progression of essential hypertensive renal disease. These effects are presumably mediated by drug attenuation of the intrarenal effects of angiotensin II, with normalization of P_{GC}. Since ACE inhibition therapy largely reverses the pathophysiological changes encountered in the essential hypertensive kidney, one may speculate that the functional and reversible hemodynamic changes observed in the essential hypertensive kidney are the result of excessive endogenous renal tissue production of angiotensin II.

Selected Bibliography

Anderson S, Meyer TH, Rennke HG, et al: Control of glomerular hypertension limits glomerular injury in rats with reduced renal mass. J Clin Invest 76:612–619, 1985.

Anderson S, Rennke HG, Brenner BM: Therapeutic advantage of converting enzyme inhibitors in arresting progressive renal disease associated with systemic hypertension in the rat. J Clin Invest 77:1993–2000, 1986.

Ando K, Fujita T, Ito Y, et al: The role of renal hemodynamics in the antihypertensive effect of captopril. Am Heart J 111:347–352, 1986.

Ardaillou R, Sraer J, Chansel D, et al: The effects of angiotensin II on isolated glomeruli and cultured glomerular cells. Kidney Internat 31 (suppl 20) S74–S80, 1987.

Arendshorst WJ, Beierwalters WH: Renal and nephron hemodynamics in spontaneously hypertensive rats. Am J Physiol 236:F246–F251, 1979.

Bauer JH, Brooks CS, Burch RN: Renal function and hemodynamic studies in low- and normal-renin essential hypertension. Arch Intern Med 142:1317–1323, 1982.

Bauer JH, Gaddy P: Effects of enalapril alone, and in combination with hydrochlorothiazide, on renin-angiotensin-aldosterone, renal function, salt and water excretion, and body fluid composition. Am J Kidney Dis 6:222–232, 1985.

Bauer JH, Jones LB: Comparative studies: Enalapril vs hydrochlorothiazide as first-step therapy for the treatment of primary hypertension. Am J Kidney Dis 4:55–62, 1984.

Bauer JH, Reams GP, Lal SM: Renal protective effect of strict blood pressure control with enalapril therapy. Arch Intern Med 147:1397–1400, 1987.

Birkenhager WH, Schalekamp MADH, Krauss XH, et al: Systemic and renal hemodynamics, body fluids and renin in benign essential hypertension with special reference to natural history. Eur J Clin Invest 2:115–122, 1972.

Blantz RC, Konnen KS, Tucker BJ: Angiotensin II effects upon the glomerular microcirculation and ultrafiltration coefficient of the rat. J Clin Invest 57:419–434, 1976.

Blantz RC, Pelayo JC: In vivo actions of angiotensin II on glomerular function. Fed Proc 42:3071–3074, 1983.

Brazy PC, Stead WW, Fitzwilliam JF: Progression of renal insufficiency: Role of blood pressure. Kidney Int 35:670–674, 1989.

Campbell DJ: Circulating and tissue angiotensin systems. J Clin Invest 79:1–6, 1987.

Castleman B, Smithwick RH: The relationship of vascular disease to the hypertensive state. N Engl J Med 239:729–732, 1948.

Chou SY, Allen AM, Adam WR, et al: Local actions of angiotensin II: Quantitative in vitro autoradiographic localization of angiotensin II receptor binding and angiotensin converting enzyme in target tissues. J Cardiovasc Pharmacol 8 (suppl 10):S35–S39, 1986.

Cohen ML, Kurz KD: Angiotensin converting enzyme inhibition in tissues from spontaneously hypertensive rats after treatment with captopril or MK421. J Pharmacol Exp Ther 220:63–69, 1982.

Cushman DW, Wang FL, Fung WC, et al: Differentiation of angiotensin-converting enzyme (ACE) inhibitors by their selective inhibition of ACE in physiologically important target organs. Am J Hypertension 2:294–306, 1989.

Dworkin LD, Feiner HD: Glomerular injury in unnephrectomized spontaneously hypertensive rats: A consequence of glomerular capillary hypertension. J Clin Invest 77:797–809, 1986.

Dworkin LD, Feiner HD, Randazzo J: Glomerular hypertension and injury in deoxycorticosterone-salt rats on antihypertensive therapy. Kidney Int 31:718–724, 1987.

Dzau VJ: Significance of the vascular renin-angiotensin pathway. Hypertension 8:553–559, 1986.

Faubert PF, Chou SY, Porush JG: Regulation of papillary plasma flow by angiotensin II. Kidney Int 32:472–478, 1987.

Giaconi S, Levanti C, Fommei E, et al: Microalbuminuria and casual and ambulatory blood pressure monitoring in normotensives and in patients with borderline and mild essential hypertension. Am J Hypertension 2:259–261, 1989.

Goldring W, Chasis H, Ranges HA, et al: Effective renal blood flow in subjects with essential hypertension. J Clin Invest 20:637–653, 1941.

Gomez RA, Lynch KR, Chevalier RL, et al: Renin and angiotensinogen gene expression and intrarenal renin distribution during ACE inhibition. Am J Physiol 254:F900–F906, 1988.

Hall JE: Control of sodium excretion by angiotensin II: Intrarenal mechanisms and blood pressure regulation. Am J Physiol 250:R960–R972, 1986.

Hall JE, Guyton AC, Jackson TE, et al: Control of glomerular filtration rate by renin-angiotensin system. Am J Physiol 233:F366–F372, 1977.

Heptinstall RH: Hypertension: II. Essential hypertension. In: Pathology of The Kidney. Vol. I, Third Edition, Little, Brown and Company, Boston, 1983, pp 181–246.

Hollenberg NK, Adams DF, Solomon H, et al: Renal vascular tone in essential and secondary hypertension. Medicine 54:29–44, 1975.

Hollenberg NK, Epstein M, Basch RI, et al: "No man's land" of the renal vasculature. Am J Med 47:845–854, 1969.

Hollenberg NK, Meggs LG, Williams GH, et al: Sodium intake and renal responses to captopril in normal man and in essential hypertension. Kidney Int 20:240–245, 1981.

Hollenberg NK, Swartz SL, Passan DR, et al: Increased glomerular filtration rate after converting enzyme inhibition in essential hypertension. N Engl J Med 301:9–12, 1979.

Huang WC, Ploth DW, Navar LG: Angiotensin-mediated alterations in nephron function in Goldblatt hypertensive rats. Am J Physiol 243:F553–F560, 1982.

Imai Y, Abe K, Seino M, et al: Captopril attenuates pressor responses to norepinephrine and vasopressin through depletion of endogenous angiotensin II. Am J Cardiol 49:1537–1539, 1982.

Keane WF, Raij L: Relationship among altered glomerular barrier permselectivity, angiotensin II, and mesangial uptake of macromolecules. Lab Invest 52:599–604, 1985.

Larochelle P, Gutkowska J, Schiffrin E, et al: Effect of enalapril on renin angio-

Core Organ Effects: Renal • 95

tensin converting enzyme, aldosterone and prostaglandins in patients with hypertension. Clin Invest Med 8:197–201, 1985.

Lindeman RD, Tobin JD, Shock NW: Association between blood pressure and the rate of decline in renal function with age. Kidney Int 26:861–868, 1984.

London GM, Safar ME, Sassard JE, et al: Renal and systemic hemodynamics in sustained essential hypertension. Hypertension 6:743–754, 1984.

Magee JH, Unger AM, Richardson DW: Changes in renal function associated with drug or placebo therapy of human hypertension. Am J Med 36:795–804, 1964.

McClellan W, Tuttle E, Issa A: Racial differences in the incidence of hypertensive end-stage renal disease (ESRD) are not entirely explained by differences in the prevalence of hypertension. Am J Kidney Dis 12:285–290, 1988.

McGee WG, Ashworth CT: Fine structure of chronic hypertensive arteriopathy in the human kidney. Am J Pathol 43:273–299, 1963.

McManus JFA, Lupton CH: Ischemic obsolescence of renal glomeruli. Lab Invest 9:413–434, 1960.

Mimran A, Targhetta R, Laroche B: The antihypertensive effect of captopril. Hypertension 2:732–737, 1980.

Morduchowicz G, Boner G, Ben-Bassat N, et al: Proteinuria in benign nephrosclerosis. Arch Intern Med 146:1513–1516, 1986.

Mujais SK, Kauffman S, Katz AL: Angiotensin II binding sites in individual segments of the rat nephron. J Clin Invest 77:315–318, 1986.

Myers BD, Dean WM, Brenner BM: Effects of norepinephrine and angiotensin II as the determinants of glomerular ultrafiltration and proximal tubule fluid reabsorption in the rat. Circ Res 1975;37:101–110, 1975.

Oliver JA, Sciacca RR, Cannon PJ: Renal vasodilation by converting enzyme inhibition: Role of renal prostaglandins. Hypertension 5:166–171, 1983.

Pedersen EB, Mogensen CF: Effect of antihypertensive treatment on urinary albumin excretion, glomerular filtration rate and renal plasma flow rate in patients with essential hypertension. Scand J Clin Lab Invest 36:231–237, 1976.

Perera GA: Hypertensive vascular disease: Description and natural history. J Chron Dis 1:33–42, 1955.

Raij L, Keane WF: Glomerular mesangium: Its function and relationship to angiotensin II. Am J Med 79 (suppl 3C):24–30, 1985.

Redgrave J, Rabinowe S, Hollenberg NK, et al: Correction of abnormal renal blood flow response to angiotensin II by converting enzyme inhibition in essential hypertension. J Clin Invest 75:1285–1290, 1985.

Reubi FC, Weidmann P, Hodler J, et al: Changes in renal function in essential hypertension. Am J Med 64:556–563, 1978.

Romero JC, Knox FG: Mechanisms underlying pressure-related natriuresis: The role of the renin-angiotensin and prostaglandin systems. Hypertension 11:724–738, 1988.

Rosivall L, Narkates AJ, Oparil S, et al: De novo intrarenal formation of angiotensin II during control and enhanced renin secretion. Am J Physiol 252:F1118–F1123, 1987.

Rostand SG, Brown G, Kirk K, et al: Renal insufficiency in treated essential hypertension. N Engl J Med 320:684–688, 1989.

Samani NJ, Godfrey NP, Major JS, et al: Kidney renin mRNA levels in the early and chronic phases of two-kidney, one-clip hypertension in the rat. J Hypertension 7:105–112, 1989.

Swartz SL, Williams GH, Hollenberg NK, et al: Captopril-induced changes in prostaglandin production. J Clin Invest 65:1257–1264, 1980.

Tracy RE, Marcos-Velez-Duran, Heigle T, et al: Two variants of nephrosclerosis separately related to age and blood pressure. Am J Pathol 131:270–282, 1988.

Unger T, Ganten D, Lang RE, et al: Is tissue converting enzyme inhibition a determinant of the antihypertensive efficacy of converting enzyme inhibitors? Studies with the two different compounds, Hoe498 and MK421, in spontaneously hypertensive rats. J Cardiovasc Pharmacol 6:872–880, 1984.

Unger T, Schull B, Rascher W, et al: Selective activation of the converting enzyme inhibitor MK421 and comparison of its active diacid form with captopril in different tissues of the rat. Biochem Pharmacol 31:3063–3070, 1982.

Velletri P, Bean BL: Comparison of the time course of action of captopril on angiotensin-converting enzyme with the time cause of its antihypertensive effect. J Cardiovasc Pharmacol 3:1068–1081, 1981.

Veterans Administration Cooperative Study Group on Antihypertensive Agents: Effects of treatment on morbidity in hypertension II. Results in patients with diastolic blood pressures averaging 90 through 114 mmHg. JAMA 213:1143–1152, 1970.

Wilkes BM, Pion I, Sollott S, et al: Intrarenal renin-angiotensin system modulates glomerular angiotensin receptors in the rat. Am J Physiol 254:F345–F350, 1988.

Williams GF, Hollenberg NK: Accentuated vascular and endocrine response to SQ 20881 in hypertension. N Engl J Med 297:184–188, 1977.

Wilson SK, Lynch DR, Snyder SH: Angiotensin-converting enzyme labeled with [^{3}H] captopril. J Clin Invest 80:841–851, 1987.

Yoshioka T, Mitarai T, Kon V, et al: Role for angiotensin II in an overt functional proteinuria. Kid Internat 30:538–545, 1986.

Yoshioka T, Shiraga H, Yoshida Y, et al: "Intact nephrons" as the primary origin of proteinuria in chronic renal disease. J Clin Invest 82:1614–1623, 1988.

Chapter 5

Nondrug Therapy of Hypertension

Molly E. Reusser and
David A. McCarron

Introduction

While hypertension is clearly a major health problem in this country, estimated to affect nearly 58 million Americans, the appropriate means of its management in the individual patient is much less certain. Despite advances in recent years in our understanding and utilization of pharmacological agents to control blood pressure, many patients cannot tolerate or do not benefit from the use of antihypertensive drugs. Further, there is the concern, particularly in borderline and mild hypertension, that the risks of pharmacological treatment may outweigh the benefits. Thus, the high prevalence of hypertension and its long-term effects, combined with the personal and economic costs and unresolved questions regarding drug therapy, have resulted in strong interest in identifying nonpharmacological approaches to the treatment of high blood pressure.

Nondrug management of hypertension is not limited to the specific application of a single agent targeted to a single disorder. Unlike drugs, the incorporation of nonpharmacological strategies into an individual's life style may provide a means of preventing high blood pressure. Patients in whom one or more nondrug regimens are effective have the additional benefits of reduced risks of adverse side effects and reduced

From Punzi HA, Flamenbaum W (eds): *Hypertension*. Mount Kisco, NY, Futura Publishing Co., Inc., © 1989.

costs of treatment. Where nonpharmacological approaches alone are inadequate in controlling blood pressure, their use in conjunction with drug treatment can reduce medication requirements, again resulting in lower risks and costs to the patient.

The behavioral and nutritional factors that have been recommended for the management of hypertension have the concomitant advantage of being generally conducive to good health. Life style factors include obesity, alcohol intake, tobacco use, physical exercise, and stress. Dietary components that have been examined in terms of their roles in blood pressure regulation include sodium, calcium, potassium, magnesium, chloride, phosphorus, fat, fiber, protein, and carbohydrates. This chapter focuses on each of these with the caveat that while each dietary factor is presented separately, there are complex nutrient interactions among them that must be considered in assessing their effects. Changes in life style as well as the presence of multiple naturally occurring nutrients in the diet can influence the effects of separate and combined nutritional factors used for the purpose of controlling blood pressure.

Life Style Interventions

Obesity

The direct association between body weight and blood pressure is well established in epidemiologic studies. Similarly, a strong correlation has been demonstrated between body weight and blood pressure and between increases in body weight and the ensuing development of hypertension. Among obese adult Americans between the ages of 20 and 45 years, the relative risk of developing high blood pressure is five to six times that of lean individuals. This link between obesity and blood pressure has been observed in virtually all socioeconomic, age, and ethnic groups and in both male and female subjects.

In obese hypertensive subjects, small reductions in body weight are associated with decreases in blood volume, cardiac output, and mean arterial pressure without changes in total peripheral resistance. A blood pressure-lowering effect of modest weight reduction has been noted in both lean and obese hypertensive subjects, with greater blood pressure reductions in the significantly overweight. Reduced blood pressure occurs with as little as 2–4 kg of weight loss, indicating that the mechanisms invoked by the initial weight loss contribute to the chronic reduction in blood pressure. However, there appears to be a "floor effect"

Nondrug Therapy of Hypertension • 99

of weight loss, beyond which further blood pressure reductions will not occur.

Weight loss programs that lower blood pressure in obese hypertensive subjects generally involve either reduced total caloric intake or decreased intake of fat, carbohydrates, or protein. There is a greater proportional fall in blood pressure with initial caloric restriction than that which follows continuous weight reduction with long-term caloric restriction. Several studies have demonstrated that the antihypertensive effect of weight loss is independent of sodium chloride intake. Individuals who maintain their normal sodium chloride intake may experience greater blood pressure reductions than those who simultaneously restrict sodium chloride and calories. In nearly all subjects, blood pressure remains lowered as long as the weight loss is maintained.

For overweight hypertensive patients whose arterial pressure cannot be sufficiently controlled with weight loss alone, weight loss in conjunction with pharmacological therapy has been shown to decrease blood pressure in treated as well as untreated hypertensive patients. The number and amount of antihypertensive drugs required for blood pressure control may be lessened by weight reduction in obese hypertensive persons. In a study in normal weight hypertensive patients receiving pharmacological treatment, drug requirements were decreased with weight loss.

While nonadherence and recidivism rates are high with this approach, weight loss is the single most effective, safe, and relatively inexpensive means of reducing blood pressure as yet identified and is an optimal first-line approach to blood pressure control in overweight hypertensive patients. Beyond prescribing weight reduction for overweight hypertensive patients, support and reinforcement, such as recommendations for weight loss programs and continuing patient follow-up, may be necessary to achieve and sustain success with this intervention strategy.

Alcohol

One of the major preventable causes of hypertension is alcohol abuse. A number of studies have shown a highly significant correlation within populations among regular alcohol consumption, blood pressure levels, and hypertension. In the Framingham Study, the frequency of hypertension was positively correlated with the consumption of alcohol, although nondrinkers had higher pressures than light drinkers. The prevalence of hypertension has been reported to be three to four times greater in persons consuming more than 30 g of ethanol a day than in abstainers or light drinkers.

Clinical studies have also demonstrated a relationship between alcohol and blood pressure. In some studies, alcohol consumption caused increases in blood pressure in nondrinking normotensive subjects. Even in the studies that reported no change in blood pressure, alcohol reduced systemic vascular resistance and increased cardiac output in this population. Several groups have reported the pressor effect of alcohol in normotensive drinkers. In a randomized, controlled, cross-over trial in 46 healthy male drinkers reduced alcohol intake resulted in modest decreases in blood pressure, most apparent with systolic pressure. In another study, when alcohol consumption was decreased in hypertensive subjects decreases in both systolic and diastolic blood pressure were observed; the reinstitution of alcohol resulted in increased blood pressure. This pressor effect of alcohol is also seen in hypertensive nondrinkers.

While there appears to be a protective effect of ethanol in small amounts (10–30 g/day) against the development of coronary heart disease, the effect on blood pressure is unclear. Of 30 cross-sectional studies of the relationship between alcohol and blood pressure reviewed, seven reported higher blood pressures in subjects consuming less than 30 g of ethanol per day compared to nondrinkers, 11 noted no difference, and 12 reported lower pressures in subjects with ethanol intakes below 30 g a day.

As well as the pressor effect of alcohol, its consumption may interfere with the efficacy of antihypertensive medications. A randomized, cross-over trial in hypertensive subjects was conducted to examine the effect of alcohol on blood pressure. It was observed that pressures were greater during periods of alcohol consumption than during periods when alcohol consumption was markedly decreased and that the pressor effect of ethanol is reversible over two-six weeks in treated hypertensive subjects. Thus, it appears that a general reduction in alcohol consumption levels could substantially reduce the prevalence of hypertension. Further, in hypertensive patients, limiting or eliminating alcohol intake could improve the efficacy of drug therapy, and in cases of mild hypertension even alleviate medications altogether.

Tobacco

Although cigarette smoking results in an acute increase in arterial pressure, prolonged use is not associated with an increased prevalence of hypertension. There is, however, a clear association between smoking and a substantial excess mortality rate at any level of blood pressure. Death due to hypertension is more common in smokers, and they have a higher frequency of malignant hypertension and subarachnoid hemorrhage.

Furthermore, smoking has been shown to attenuate the beneficial effect of antihypertensive therapy. In the Australian Therapeutic Trial in Mild Hypertension, trial endpoints (TEP) of morbidity and mortality were greater in smokers than nonsmokers on placebo therapy. The TEP in women smokers on active therapy was reduced to that of women nonsmokers. In men, the number of TEP in smokers on active therapy was reduced, but clearly not to the level of nonsmokers.

The adverse effect of smoking on the incidence of stroke and coronary events in hypertensive individuals was dramatically demonstrated in the recent Medical Research Council (MRC) Trial. There was a marked increase in stroke rate in smokers versus nonsmokers taking placebo therapy. This increase in stroke rate was also seen in patients taking beta-blockers for treatment of hypertension. In contrast, the increased risk of stroke in smokers was reduced in subjects receiving diuretics. There was also an increase in coronary events in smokers compared to nonsmokers taking placebo therapy. In contrast to the beneficial effect of diuretics on stroke incidence in smokers, neither beta-blocker nor diuretic therapy reduced the increased coronary incidence in smokers.

In the recent Metoprolol Atherosclerosis Prevention in Hypertension (MAPHY) Study, a beneficial effect of beta blockers over diuretics was observed. Cumulative mortality was reduced in smokers receiving beta-blockers compared to smokers given diuretics. The reduction in mortality was caused by a reduction in coronary events. Why these studies produced divergent results is not known.

Thus, while there is no evidence that cigarette smoking increases blood pressure, there is overwhelming evidence that smoking increases the risk of coronary and stroke events in hypertensive persons. There is also strong evidence that cigarette smoking interferes with some forms of antihypertensive therapy. The benefits of tobacco avoidance have been proven conclusively and smoking cessation cannot be too strongly recommended.

Exercise

Evidence from a number of areas suggests a beneficial role for exercise training in lowering blood pressure in hypertensive patients. Epidemiologic studies indicate that active persons have significantly lower at-rest systolic and diastolic blood pressures than their less active counterparts. Some cross-sectional studies have found lower blood pressures among athletes compared to the general population, although in some population studies, including Framingham, physical activity status did not correlate with blood pressure levels.

In a review of six prospective, randomized, controlled clinical trials on the effect of aerobic exercise on blood pressure, five reported a significant reduction in blood pressure. The most impressive and consistent results were observed in a 1986 study by Nelson and co-workers in which subjects with essential hypertension were subjected to a variety of exercise regimens for four-week periods in random order. These investigators found a dose-related effect of exercise on blood pressure, heart rate, peripheral resistance, and cardiac index. In addition, they reported dose-related plasma norepinephrine level decreases with exercise. These studies suggest that chronic isotonic exercise may decrease sympathetic tone in hypertensive persons.

Physical training in persons with mild to moderate hypertension results in blood pressure reductions, independent of weight loss, and smaller, less consistent blood pressure changes in normotensive individuals. In examining metabolic variables affected by physical training, blood pressure reductions appear to be related not as much to changes in body fat as to changes in plasma insulin, blood glucose, and plasma triglycerides. Thus, the blood pressure-lowering effect of training may be a decrease in plasma insulin concentration, possibly associated with reductions in sodium reabsorption and sympathetic activity. Physical exercise, therefore, may facilitate blood pressure control both directly through metabolic changes and indirectly through weight loss.

Exercise may be an effective adjunct to pharmacological as well as other nonpharmacological interventions for the management of high blood pressure. A randomized, double-blind, placebo-controlled trial was conducted to examine the relationships between exercise, hypertension, and beta-adrenergic blockade. It was found that resting blood pressure measured without drug therapy was significantly lowered after exercise conditioning on placebo and on metoprolol, but not on propranolol.

Some antihypertensive drugs have been reported to present problems for persons who exercise. Muscle blood flow may be decreased by diuretic-induced hypokalemia, and exercise-induced increases in heart rate and cardiac output can be inhibited by beta-blockers, which may impair performance. Nevertheless, the hemodynamic response to both aerobic and anaerobic exercise can break through beta-blockade, and an effect of physical training can be realized.

In addition to its hypotensive effects, regular exercise, like most nonpharmacological approaches to the management of high blood pressure, has a favorable influence on other cardiovascular risk factors, including weight loss, smoking cessation, and decreased total cholesterol and increased high density lipids, independent of hypertension. Clearly, as concluded by the Third International Congress on Obesity, regular physical exercise should be among recommendations given for the initial management of mild and moderate hypertension in overweight, inactive patients.

Stress

While it is commonly assumed that "stress" is a key factor in the lives of individuals with high blood pressure, evidence to support the control of hypertension by relieving stress is sparse and inconclusive. The most common behavioral approaches that have been used to lower blood pressure are relaxation techniques (including muscle relaxation, meditation, and yoga), biofeedback, and psychotherapy.

While most studies of stress and hypertension have been poorly controlled, an impressive effect was observed in a well-controlled study by Patel and co-workers in which 204 newly identified hypertensive subjects were randomly allocated to either a biofeedback group receiving training in relaxation and stress management or a control group. After eight weeks of training and again six months later, the biofeedback group showed a significantly greater fall in systolic and diastolic blood pressures than the control group. These observations are consistent with the putative role for the renin-angiotensin system in the production of chronic, stress-induced blood pressure changes. Further, the sustained lower blood pressures suggest that relaxation-based behavioral methods may hold promise as a means of managing hypertension.

One study of hypertension in pregnancy utilized relaxation and biofeedback in 60 subjects. Of these, 18 received relaxation therapy alone, 18 received relaxation therapy and biofeedback, and 24 served as controls. The experimental groups had significantly lower systolic and diastolic blood pressures than the control group. Whereas less than a third of the women in each relaxation group had to be admitted to the hospital during their pregnancies, two thirds of the control group were admitted. There were no significant differences in hospital admissions or blood pressure measurements between the relaxation groups. In pregnant hypertensive patients, in whom every effort should be made to avoid pharmacological treatment, relaxation training may be a useful approach to blood pressure control.

In a study of group therapy in essential hypertension aimed at altering the patients' coping mechanisms, patients continued on their current antihypertensive medications during the study. The group receiving therapy showed impressive decreases in blood pressure compared to controls at the end of active study. Follow-up at three months and one year showed that the positive effect on blood pressure persisted in most patients. Although the results were positive, adherence was a negative factor in the study due to the time involved and the cost of therapy.

In summary, while most forms of relaxation therapy have been found to be at least transiently effective, the number of prospective, randomized, controlled studies is small, and none have conclusively shown relaxation therapy to be practical for long-term management of hypertension. In certain subgroups such as pregnant women, however, behavioral intervention may be an effective adjunctive approach.

Dietary Interventions

Sodium

The role of sodium in the diet has been a subject of controversy for centuries. Epidemiologic data has shown that in primitive societies where intake of sodium is extremely low, hypertension is virtually nonexistent and blood pressure does not increase with age. Industrialized societies, having high intakes of sodium, have a high prevalence of hypertension that does increase with age. On this basis, aside from the multitude of other differences between these two types of populations, high blood pressure is commonly attributed to high salt intake.

An international epidemiologic study entitled "Intersalt," which included more than 10,000 subjects in 52 centers from 32 countries, recently has been completed and may shed definitive light on the questions surrounding the role of dietary sodium in the population. Sodium excretion determined by 24-hour urine collections ranged from 0.2 to 242 mmol/day across the 52 centers. In the 48 centers representing the greatest majority of subjects, the range was only 100 to 242 mmol/day. Sodium excretion was related to blood pressure in individuals, but the relationship was not robust. When the four centers with the lowest sodium intakes were deleted, no relationship could be identified.

There was an identifiable relationship between the slope of blood pressure with age within centers and median sodium excretion. However, sodium excretion was not related to median blood pressure or to the prevalence of hypertension. The inclusion of potassium excretion in the analysis did not alter the relationships. Body mass index and alcohol consumption were shown to have strong, independent effects. The results of the Intersalt study, although undergoing continuing analysis, indicate that the relationship between blood pressure, the prevalence of hypertension, and dietary salt intake is not as strong as has been generally assumed.

A number of clinical intervention trials of sodium restriction in the treatment of hypertension were reviewed, and of 13 prospective, randomized, controlled trials, significant reductions in blood pressure were observed in only three. It was also noted that the fall in blood pressure was related to the height of the initial blood pressure and that there is a clear association between age and blood pressure decreases with dietary salt restriction.

Similar findings regarding initial blood pressure and response to decreased sodium have been found after plotting the relationship between blood pressure and the logarithm of sodium excretion in more than 40 dietary salt restriction trials. The most dramatic results of dietary salt restriction have been reported by MacGregor and colleagues. They performed a randomized, cross-over, placebo-controlled study in which sodium intake was reduced from approximately 150 mmol/day to 90 mmol/day and observed an 8-mmHg decrease in mean blood pressure in the hypertensive subjects.

The heterogeneous results of dietary salt restriction trials may be largely attributable to "salt-sensitivity." It appears that some individuals with high blood pressure are sensitive to the hypertensive effects of sodium chloride, whereas the majority may have hypertension related to other mechanisms. A definition of salt-sensitivity on the basis of responses to either acute salt loading and depletion or to dietary intervention has been formulated by Weinberger and associates. By their definition, one third of normal individuals and approximately one half of hypertensive subjects were salt-sensitive. These numbers were increased for blacks and older subjects. An influence of genetic variance on salt-sensitivity of blood pressure was also reported by these investigators, and they propose a possible genetic marker for the condition.

Recently a new factor has emerged that should be considered in the selection of sodium restriction for the management of blood pressure in hypertensive patients. Studies have now identified an interaction between sodium chloride intake and calcium channel blockers. It appears that the efficacy of these agents is dependent on the ingestion of a higher sodium chloride intake than is currently recommended for hypertensive persons.

While dietary sodium restriction has not been shown to preclude the development of hypertension, it may be ineffective in reducing blood pressure in some patients, and in some cases may actually complicate blood pressure control. There are no known harmful effects of moderate sodium restriction to a level of about 100 mmol/day. Until more reliable means of identifying those patients who will benefit from sodium restriction are available, recommendation of reduced levels of dietary sodium intake is a reasonable approach to the nonpharmacological management of hypertension.

Calcium

Although the potential beneficial impact of increasing dietary calcium intake on the blood pressure of humans remains controversial, low dietary calcium intake and alterations in calcium metabolism have been found in a number of areas to have a remarkably consistent relationship with increased blood pressure in humans. More than 20 independent reports of epidemiologic studies have identified a statistically significant association between the level of dietary calcium intake and either blood pressure or the risk of hypertension. The reports encompass a broad age range, diverse geographic areas, and various ethnic and racial groups. The first National Health and Nutrition Examination Survey is one of the largest data bases that has been used to evaluate this relationship. This data base has been assessed by several groups, and the association between calcium intake and blood pressure has been reported either in the entire population sampled or in specific subgroups.

These studies suggest that the protective effect of adequate dietary calcium against the development of high blood pressure is relatively independent of factors generally associated with hypertension such as age, sex, race, exercise, and weight. However, several studies have indicated partial interactions among dietary calcium, other dietary components, and blood pressure, perhaps the most important being dietary sodium. In addition, it appears that there may be a threshold of approximately 400–600 mg/day of dietary calcium. Below this level, the risk of elevated blood pressure increases sharply; above it, the effect of increasing calcium intake is modest.

A number of calcium intervention trials have been conducted in which dietary calcium has been increased to various levels of supplementation, ranging from 0.4 to 2 g/day in the form of a calcium salt (citrate, gluconate, or lactogluconate) or dietary calcium. A modest antihypertensive effect of calcium was detected in approximately two thirds of these trials, with average decreases of 4- to 7-mmHg systolic and 2- to 4-mmHg diastolic blood pressure. The blood pressure response in all these trials is heterogeneous; that is, while more individuals exhibit a reduction in blood pressure compared to placebo, some may experience a modest blood pressure increase with additional calcium. It recently has been demonstrated that oral calcium supplementation in hypertensive patients on high sodium, low calcium diets may prevent increases in blood pressure by attenuating sodium retention.

The clinical trials of increased dietary calcium intake have produced a number of consistent findings. First, there is a subset of individuals that appears to be more sensitive to the blood pressure-lowering effect of calcium. Reductions in this group may be as great at 20- to 30-mmHg systolic and 10- to 15-mmHg diastolic blood pressure. Second, 30%–45% of hypertensive patients appear to fall into this "calcium-sensitive" subset. Third, the blood pressure response of males to increased calcium seems to be similar with dietary and supplemental calcium, whereas in females, dietary calcium may be more effective. Fourth, increased dietary calcium has been shown to have no adverse effects on serum lipids or total fat intake. Fifth, no negative reactions or compliance problems have been reported in these studies.

Although the effectiveness of increased dietary calcium in reducing blood pressure remains to be determined conclusively, the evidence to date supports the regular consumption of dietary calcium within the range of the recommended dietary allowance of 800–1,200 mg/day. Adequate dietary calcium consumption will prevent calcium deficiency and may afford some protection against the development of hypertension.

Potassium

An inverse relationship between potassium intake and blood pressure or a direct relationship between the urinary sodium-to-potassium ratio and blood pressure has been suggested by the results of several epidemiologic studies. However, the high degree of interactions among dietary factors indicates that the independent role of any specific nutrient, such as potassium, cannot be conclusively determined. The contribution of potassium to blood pressure has been estimated to be approximately an 0.10- to 0.12-mmHg decrease in systolic blood pressure and a 0.3- to 0.07-mmHg decrease in diastolic blood pressure for each 1 mmol increase in potassium intake.

Potassium administration has been reported to reduce blood pressure in human hypertension in several studies. The first double-blind, randomized, cross-over study of the effect of potassium supplementation on blood pressure was performed in 1982. Twenty-three patients with mild to moderate essential hypertension were entered into an eight-week cross-over study comparing the effect of 60 mmol of timed-released potassium as the chloride salt to placebo. At four weeks of potassium therapy, blood pressure decreased by about 4%. In a trial in Italy the effects of potassium on blood pressure were more striking; administration of 40 mmol/day of potassium resulted in a reduction in blood pressure of 14/10.5 mmHg.

In another randomized, double-blind, cross-over trial, mean blood pressure fell by an average of 5.5 mmHg in a group of hypertensive patients who had become hypokalemic while receiving diuretic therapy. In contrast, others have given either 120 mmol/day of potassium or placebo to a large group of hypertensive patients. When corrections were made for differences in blood pressure at entry between the control and intervention groups, no significant effects of potassium were observed.

In a recent study of the effects of potassium depletion on blood pressure in normotensive subjects, both systolic and diastolic blood pressures were significantly increased after nine days on a low versus normal potassium diet. The effect of potassium on blood pressure may be dependent on high sodium intake. In patients who were already on sodium restricted diets, no further blood pressure reduction was observed when potassium supplements were given.

The mechanism of the antihypertensive effect of potassium appears to be related to natriuresis. When normotensive and hypertensive men were placed on a normal sodium diet and dietary potassium was increased from 20 mmol/day to 200 mmol/day, sodium excretion was increased approximately 25% during the first several days of potassium administration. This suggests that increases in dietary potassium are an effective way to cause natriuresis and reduce blood pressure.

An additional factor regarding potassium intake in hypertensive subjects is the mounting evidence that potassium affords protection against the development of stroke. While this effect may be independent of blood pressure control, in persons who by virtue of their increased blood pressure are at risk of suffering a stroke, assuring adequate dietary potassium may offer this additional therapeutic benefit.

An important consideration in increasing potassium intake for the treatment of hypertension is that some individuals are at risk for developing hyperkalemia, including persons with decreased renal function; the elderly; and patients receiving certain potassium-sparing diuretics, converting enzyme inhibitors, nonsteroidal anti-inflammatory drugs, and possibly beta-blockers. Judicious use of potassium in the treatment of hypertension, particularly by dietary adjustment rather than potassium salts, is advised.

Magnesium

Inadequate dietary intake of magnesium may be associated with an increased risk for hypertension. This possibility originally was raised by the observation of increased rates of cardiovascular disease in areas with soft drinking water or magnesium-poor soil. Preliminary studies suggest that there is an inverse relationship between dietary intake of magnesium and blood pressure and that decreased dietary intake of magnesium is associated with an increased risk for hypertension. However, it remains to be determined whether supplemental dietary magnesium will decrease blood pressure in essential hypertension. Only a few well-designed trials have been conducted, and the results have been inconsistent.

Some investigators have found that serum or tissue levels of magnesium are inversely related to blood pressure and that serum levels of magnesium are significantly decreased in patients with hypertension. A striking inverse relationship has been reported between blood pressure and intracellular free magnesium levels in erythrocytes. This observation is consistent with the possibility that magnesium deficiency may contribute to hypertension.

In a recent study of oral magnesium supplementation in subjects with mild to moderate hypertension, Motoyama and co-workers reported that prestudy erythrocyte ouabain-sensitive ^{22}Na efflux rate constant and prestudy intraerythrocyte sodium concentration are valuable indicators of the degree of the hypotensive effect of magnesium. The lower the former or the higher the latter, the greater the decrease in mean blood pressure, suggesting that oral magnesium may lower blood pressure in part by its activating effect on the cell membrane sodium pump that in turn causes decreased intracellular sodium concentration. In certain patients, therefore, magnesium supplementation may be an effective nondrug approach to the treatment of essential hypertension.

Chloride

There is no direct evidence that specifically links chloride intake with hypertension. However, the relationship between chloride intake and sodium intake may be of critical importance. Because most dietary sodium is consumed in the form of sodium chloride, the epidemiologic data relating sodium intake to hypertension might also be reflecting a relationship between chloride intake and hypertension.

Administration of sodium with chloride has been found to exacerbate hypertension in some persons with essential hypertension, whereas nonchloride sodium salts such as sodium citrate, sodium bicarbonate, or sodium phosphate appear to induce little or no change in blood pressure. Recently the effects of sodium chloride and sodium citrate on blood pressure were compared in a double-blind, placebo-controlled, cross-over trial in five men with essential hypertension. The administration of 240 mmol sodium chloride per day for one week induced significant increases in blood pressure, whereas the administration of an equimolar amount of sodium as sodium citrate resulted in no change in blood pressure. Sodium chloride, but not sodium citrate, induced expansion of plasma volume and increases in urinary excretion of calcium.

Thus, for salt to increase blood pressure, both its sodium and chloride components may be necessary. Ingestion of a high sodium, low chloride diet, or a high chloride, low sodium diet, induces little or no increase in blood pressure. Therefore, modification of dietary chloride per se does not appear to be a useful nonpharmacological approach to either the treatment or prevention of hypertension, whereas the role of chloride in combination with sodium must be considered.

Phosphorus

In normotensive humans, serum levels of inorganic phosphorus have been found to be inversely related to blood pressure. In patients with hypertension, serum levels of inorganic phosphorus are significantly decreased compared to those in normotensive persons. These findings suggest that phosphorus deficiency secondary to decreased dietary intake of phosphorus may contribute to hypertension. However, there is only minimal evidence demonstrating that low phosphorus intake is associated with hypertension, and no well-controlled studies examining the effects of supplemental phosphorus on blood pressure in essential hypertension.

Fat

Dietary fat intake, and particularly the dietary polyunsaturated/saturated fat ratio, may contribute to increased blood pressure. Epidemiologic studies suggest that blood pressure is lower in subjects ingesting higher levels of unsaturated fats. An epidemiologic study involving groups of farmers found the percentage of caloric intake from saturated fat was 8.7 in Italy, 17.4 in Maryland, and 24.2 in Finland, with the highest blood pressures being in the latter group.

Intervention studies show little if any effect in normotensive subjects. No effect on blood pressure in normotensive subjects placed on reduced saturated fat (from 21 to 10 g/day) and cholesterol (from 398 to 69 mg/day) diets for three months. Some preliminary evidence suggests that supplementation with unsaturated fats may exert a modest blood pressure-lowering effect in hypertensive patients. However, these data remain inconclusive; the findings have not been consistent and methodological problems have been identified in some studies.

The primary essential fatty acid that has been investigated as to an antihypertensive effect is linoleic acid. It is difficult to ascribe specific functions to polyunsaturated fatty acids because they are more plentiful in plant than in animal foods, and diets consisting of predominantly the former may also be significantly different in their content of other dietary components. Nevertheless, a cross-over study designed to examine the role of essential fatty acids in the reduction of blood pressure indicated that when the ratio of polyunsaturated to saturated fatty acids was changed from 0.3 to 1.0 by the addition of linoleic acid to the controlled diet, blood pressure decreased in both normotensive and mildly hypertensive subjects during periods when the ratio was 1.

Dietary fish and fish oil have received much attention recently in terms of their protective cardiovascular properties as a result of observations that populations consuming large amounts of fish have lower rates of coronary artery disease. Several studies have examined the effect of fish oil on blood pressure, but the results have often been limited by design or methodological flaws. However, a recently published, carefully controlled intervention trial has significant blood pressure-lowering effect of the n-3 fatty acids. Unfortunately, the level of n-3 fat required to achieve the reduction in blood pressure exceeded normal consumption levels and would not be practical for most patients.

Fiber

Assessment of the effect of dietary fiber on hypertension is complicated by the fact that fiber is not a single compound, but a group of indigestible carbohydrates and lignin, and by the presence of the other dietary factors generally inherent in a high fiber diet that may not occur regularly or in abundance in other, more typical diets. Further, individuals consuming high fiber diets are often vegetarians and/or highly health conscious, with the subsequent result of a number of variables in diet and life style that can influence the effect of a specific dietary component on blood pressure.

As with other dietary food groups, there appears to be little if any effect on blood pressure of increasing dietary fiber content in normotensive persons, whereas some modest effects have been noted in hypertensive and hypertensive diabetic patients. However, the number of studies examining the effect of fiber alone in terms of blood pressure is minimal and does not provide sufficient information on which to base dietary recommendations.

Protein

Epidemiologic surveys show few differences in protein intake between normotensive and hypertensive subjects in the United States. In an intervention trial in vegetarians, supplementation with 58 g/day of plant protein for six weeks did not change blood pressure. In a crossover study in normotensive omnivorous subjects fed vegetarian, ovolactovegetarian, and omnivorous diets, blood pressures were highest on the latter. However, as with fiber, there is insufficient evidence that this individual dietary component can be altered to control blood pressure.

Carbohydrate

Because carbohydrate intake stimulates insulin secretion, and insulin inhibits urinary sodium excretion and stimulates the sympathetic nervous system, dietary carbohydrate intake would appear to be a viable factor in the management of high blood pressure. This does not, however, appear to be the case. While an association has been reported in some epidemiologic studies between fasting serum insulin levels, insulin resistance, and essential hypertension, comparison of carbohydrate intake between normotensive and hypertensive individuals in the United States revealed little difference.

Clinical observations provide little definitive information concerning the influence of carbohydrate on blood pressure. In a controlled study in male subjects fed various levels of fructose, 0% to 15% of calories, there was no significant difference in pressures, although pressures were slightly lower when no fructose was consumed. Replacing saturated fat with either carbohydrate or unsaturated fat had no effect on blood pressure in patients with mild hypertension. While carbohydrate would seem to have a role in blood pressure control, there is little if any valid clinical data to support this.

A combination of these nutrients may prove to be a more beneficial approach in reducing blood pressure than manipulations of one nutrient alone. For example, feeding a ovolactovegetarian diet, which was high in fiber and low in protein and fat, modestly but significantly reduced blood pressure in normotensive subjects and in patients with mild essential hypertension. In mildly hypertensive diabetic patients, blood pressure was modestly but significantly reduced with a diet high in fiber and low in fat and sodium. Thus, as was postulated with the Kempner rice diet several decades ago, diets that manipulate several potentially important variables may offer benefit not seen with alteration of one nutrient alone.

Conclusion

The application of nondrug measures to lower blood pressure has entered a new era. In conjunction with an expanding body of information, an appropriate resurgence of interest has emerged. In the current environment of rapid advances toward identifying the molecular mechanisms that are critical to the normal control of arterial pressure, we will soon come to understand, as with pharmaceutical agents, how individual and interactive dietary constituents, as well as other life style factors, directly contribute to the control of blood pressure.

While we await these advances at the molecular level, we can anticipate a significant increase in the clinical data base to support the position that nonpharmacological approaches hold the same promise as drugs to lower blood pressure and could accomplish this at lower risk

114 • HYPERTENSION

and cost to the individual and to society. Additionally, of the two approaches, only nondrug modalities offers the most important potential application, that of primary prevention of high blood pressure.

Acknowledgments: The authors are grateful to the other members of the Organizing Committee of the National Kidney Foundation Physician Education Program on the Nonpharmacological Treatment of Hypertension: Sharon Anderson, M.D., Theodore W. Kurtz, M.D., Stuart L. Linas, M.D., and Friedrich C. Luft, M.D., whose contributions to that program provided the basis of much of the information presented here. We would also like to thank Cynthia D. Morris, Ph.D., M.P.H., for the generous contribution of her expertise to the preparation of this manuscript, which was supported in part by the National Dairy Promotion and Research Board.

Selected References

General

Beilin LJ: Nonpharmacological control of blood pressure. Clin Exp Pharmacol Physiol 15:215–223, 1988.

Blackburn H, Prineas R: Diet and hypertension: anthropolgy, epidemiology, and public health implications. Prog Biochem Pharmacol 19:31–79, 1983.

Joint National Committee on Detection, Evaluation, and Treatment of High Blood Pressure: The 1988 report on detection, evaluation, and treatment of high blood pressure. Arch Intern Med 184:1023–1038, 1988.

Kannel WB: Implications of Framingham Study data for treatment of hypertension: impact of other risk factors. In: Laragh JH, Buhler FR, Seldin DW (eds), Frontiers of Hypertension Research. New York, Springer-Verlag, 1981, pp 17.

Kaplan NM, Meese RB: The calcium deficiency hypothesis of hypertension: a critique. Ann Intern Med 105:947–955, 1986.

McCarron DA, Morris CD, Henry HJ, et al: Blood pressure and nutrient intake in the United States. Science 224:1392–1398, 1984.

Specific

Ades PA, Gunther PGS, Meacham CP, et al: Hypertension, exercise, and beta-adrenergic blockade. Ann Intern Med 109:629–634, 1988.

Altura BT, Altura BM: Cardiovascular actions of magnesium: importance in etiology and treatment of high blood pressure. Magnesium Bull 9:6–21, 1987.

Arkwright PD, Beilin LJ, Rouse I, et al: Effects of alcohol use and other aspects of lifestyle on blood pressure levels and prevalence of hypertension in a working population. Circulation 66: 60–66, 1982.

Chiang BN, Perlman LU, Epstein FH: Overweight and hypertension: a review. Circulation 39:403, 1969.

Criqui MH: Alcohol consumption, blood pressure, lipids, and cardiovascular mortality. Alcoholism. Clin Exp Res 10:564–569, 1986.

Dodson PM, Pacy PJ, Bal P, et al: A controlled trial of a high fiber, low fat, and low sodium diet for mild hypertension in type 2 (non-insulin-dependent) diabetic patients. Diabetologia 27:522–526, 1984.

Nondrug Therapy of Hypertension • 115

Grobee DE, Hofman A: Does sodium restriction lower blood pressure? Br Med J 293:227–229, 1986.

Heyden S, Schneider KA, Fodor TG: Smoking habits and antihypertensive treatment. Nephrol 47(Suppl 1):99–103, 1987.

Iacono JM, Doughterty RM, Puska P. Reduction of blood pressure associated with dietary polyunsaturated fat. Hypertension 4(Suppl III):34–42, 1982.

The Intersalt Cooperative Research Group: Intersalt: an international study of electrolyte excretion and blood pressure. Results for 24-hour urinary sodium and potassium. Br Med J 297:307–308, 1988.

Kaplan NM, Meese RB: The calcium deficiency hypothesis of hypertension: a critique. Ann Intern Med 105:947–955, 1986.

Knapp HR, FitzGerald GA: The antihypertensive effects of fish oil. A controlled study of polyunsaturated fatty acid supplements in essential hypertension. N Engl J Med 320:1037–1043, 1989.

Krishna GG, Miller E, Kapoor S: Increased blood pressure during potassium depletion in normotensive men. N Engl J Med 320:1177–1182, 1989.

Kurtz TW, Al-Bander HA, Morris RC Jr: "Salt-sensitive" essential hypertension in men: is the sodium ion alone important? N Engl J Med 317:1043–1048, 1987.

Little BC, Hayworth J, Benson P, et al: Treatment of hypertension in pregnancy by relaxation and biofeedback. Lancet i:865–867, 1984.

Ljunghall S, Hedstrand H. Serum phosphate inversely related to blood pressure. Br Med J 1:553–554, 1977.

Mac Gregor GA, Markandu ND, Best FE, et al: Double-blind randomized crossover trial of moderate sodium restriction in essential hypertension. Lancet i:351–354, 1982.

Margetts BM, Beilin LF, Armstrong BK, et al: Blood pressure and dietary polyunsaturated and saturated fats: a controlled trial. Clin Sci 69:165–175, 1985.

Margetts BM, Beilin LF, Vandongen R, et al: A randomized controlled trial of the effect of dietary fiber on blood pressure. Clin Sci 72:343–350, 1987.

Margetts BM, Beilin LJ, Vandongen R, et al: Vegetarian diet in mild hypertension: a randomized controlled trial. Br Med J 293:1468–1471, 1986.

Maxwell MH, Kushiro T, Dornfeld LP, et al: Blood pressure changes in obese hypertensive subjects during rapid weight loss: comparison of restricted versus unchanged salt intake. Arch Intern Med 144:1581–1584, 1984.

McCarron DA: Calcium metabolism and hypertension. Kidney Int 35:717–736, 1989.

McCarron DA, Morris CD: Blood pressure response to oral calcium in persons with mild to moderate hypertension: a randomized, double-blind, placebo-controlled, crossover trial. Ann Intern Med 103:825–831, 1985.

McCarron DA, Morris CD: The calcium deficiency hypothesis of hypertension. Ann Intern Med 107:919–922, 1987.

Messerli FH: Cardiovascular effects of obesity and hypertension. Lancet i:1165–1168, 1982.

Motoyama T, Sano H, Fukuzaki H: Oral magnesium supplementation in patients with essential hypertension. Hypertension 13:227–232, 1989.

Nelson L, Esler MC, Jennings GL, et al: Effect of changing levels of physical activity on blood pressure and haemodynamics in essential hypertension. Lancet ii:473–476, 1986.

Nicholson JP, Resnick LM, Laragh JH: The antihypertensive effect of verapamil at extremes of dietary sodium intake. Ann Intern Med 107:329–334, 1987.

Overlack K, Stumpe KO, Moch B, et al: Hemodynamic, renal, and hormonal responses to changes to dietary potassium in normotensive and hypertensive man: long-term antihypertensive effect of potassium supplementation in essential hypertension. Klin Wochenschr 63:352–360, 1985.

Paffenbarger RS, Wing AL, Hyde RT, et al: Physical activity and incidence of hypertension in college alumni. Am J Epidemiol 117:245–257, 1983.

Patel C, Marmot MG, Terry DJ: Controlled trial of biofeedback- aided behavioural methods in reducing mild hypertension. Br Med J 282:2005–2008, 1981.

Peled-Ney R, Sliverberg DS, Rosenfeld JB: A controlled study of group therapy in essential hypertension. Israel J Med Sci 20:12, 1984.

Puddey IB, Beilin LJ, Vandongen R: Regular alcohol use raises blood pressure in treated hypertensive subjects: a randomized controlled trial. Lancet i:647–651, 1987.

Puska P, Nissinen A, Pietinen P, et al: Dietary fat and human blood pressure: results from three controlled intervention studies. Prog Lipid Res 25:495–497, 1986.

Resnick LM, Gupta RK, Laragh JH: Intracellular free magnesium in erythrocytes of essential hypertension: relation to blood pressure and serum divalent cations. Proc Natl Acad Sci 81:6511–6515, 1984.

Rouse IL, Armstrong BK, Beilin LJ, et al: Blood pressure-lowering effect of a vegetarian diet: controlled trial in normotensive subjects. Lancet i:5–10, 1983.

Sacks FM, Rouse IL, Stampfer MJ, et al: Effect of dietary fats and carbohydrate on blood pressure of mildly hypertensive patients. Hypertension 10:452–460, 1987.

Saito K, Sano H, Furuta Y, et al: Effect of oral calcium on blood pressure response in salt-loaded borderline hypertensive patients. Hypertension 13:219–226, 1989.

Schlamowitz P, Hahberg T, Warnoe O, et al: Treatment of mild to moderate hypertension with dietary fiber. Lancet ii:622–623, 1987.

Shore AC, Markandu ND, MacGregor G: A randomized, crossover study to compare the blood pressure response to sodium loading with and without chloride in patients with essential hypertension. J Hypertension 6:613–617, 1988.

Siani A, Strazzullo P, Russo L, et al: Controlled trial of long-term oral potassium supplements in patients with mild hypertension. Br Med J 294:1453–1456, 1987.

Sowers JR, Nyby M, Stern N, et al: Blood pressure and hormone changes associated with weight reduction in the obese. Hypertension 4:686–691, 1982.

Vu Tran Z, Weltman A: Differential effects of exercise on serum lipid and lipoprotein levels seen with changes in body weight. A meta-analysis. JAMA 254:919–924, 1985.

Weinberger MH, Miller JZ, Luft FC, et al: Definitions and characteristics of sodium sensitivity and blood pressure resistance. Hypertension 8(Suppl II):II-127–II-134, 1986.

Willett WC, Green A, Stampfer MJ, et al: Relative and absolute excess risks of coronary heart disease among women who smoke cigarettes. N Engl J Med 317:1303–1309, 1987.

Chapter 6

Diuretics

Barry J. Materson

Introduction

Modern orally and intravenously administered diuretics have had a major impact on the practice of clinical medicine since their introduction beginning in 1957. The treatment of edematous disorders such as congestive heart failure and ascites, hypertension, and a variety of diseases not strictly related to diuretic properties of these drugs has changed dramatically since their introduction.

Although the use of substances with weak diuretic properties dates back to antiquity, it was not until 1937, when the mild diuretic effect of sulfanilamide was recognized, that the development of modern diuretics began. The sulfamoyl group was identified and its carbonic anhydrase-inhibiting properties elucidated. Nearly all of the diuretics in use today possess a sulfamoyl group. Acetazolamide was of limited use as a diuretic, but chlorothiazide became available in 1957 and hydrochlorothiazide, which is still the "gold standard," became available in 1958. The loop-blocking and potassium-sparing diuretics soon followed. Mercurial diuretics made a major therapeutic impact in their day and research into their mechanism of action taught us much about renal physiology and led to the synthesis of ethacrynic acid. They will not be further discussed here.

This chapter is a discussion of thiazides, loop-blockers, and potassium-sparing diuretics as they pertain to the treatment of hypertension.

Strictly speaking, "diuretic" refers to a substance that increases urine flow. Water is technically a diuretic. The clinically important di-

From Punzi HA, Flamenbaum W (eds): *Hypertension*. Mount Kisco, NY, Futura Publishing Co., Inc., © 1989.

uretics are natriuretic; they facilitate the urinary loss of sodium. They are also chloruretic and the chloride loss in the urine may exceed that of sodium.

Thiazide Diuretics

There are two thiazides, six hydrothiazides, and four thiazide-like diuretics currently available in the United States (Table 1). All share a similar mechanism of action in that they bind to receptors in the "cortical diluting segment" of the nephron and block the active transport of sodium across this segment of distal tubular epithelium. Some of them have a proximal tubular effect as well. This probably contributes little to their beneficial effect, but does cause the loss of other cations such as zinc and magnesium. These drugs must be filtered or secreted into the lumen of the proximal tubule in order to be effective. Because most of them are tightly bound to serum proteins, they need to be secreted from the blood to the lumen by means of the proximal tubule organic acid transport mechanism. This may be blocked by competitive drugs such as probenecid. Obviously, there must be some glomerular filtrate

Table 1
Thiazide and Thiazide-like Diuretics

Generic Name	Trade Name
Thiazides	
Benzthiazide	Naclex; Exna
Chlorothiazide	Diuril
Hydrothiazides	
Bendroflumethiazide	Naturetin
Hydrochlorothiazide	Hydrodiuril; Esidrix
Hydroflumethiazide	Saluron; Diucardin
Methyclothiazide	Enduron
Polythiazide	Renese
Trichlormethiazide	Naqua
Thiazide-like	
Indapamide	Lozol
Quinethazone	Hydromox
Metolazone	Zaroxolyn; Diulo; Mykrox
Chlorthalidone	Hygroton; Thalitone

in the tubular lumen in order for the diuretic to effect a diuresis. Generally no more than 20% of the filtered load of sodium reaches the main site of action of the thiazide diuretics. If the patient is dehydrated or the glomerular filtration rate is low, even less sodium is likely to reach the distal tubule. The lower the glomerular filtration rate, the less effective the diuretics will be. Nevertheless, they do not lose their therapeutic efficacy at as high a level of glomerular filtration. There is evidence that even hydrochlorothiazide may remain effective at filtration rates as low as 20 mL/min. The other drugs, particularly metolazone and indapamide may have improved efficacy in the face of decreased GFR by virtue of other properties, but this almost always requires an increase in dosage.

The specific mechanism by which thiazide diuretics reduce elevated blood pressure remains unknown. The diuretic and natriuretic effects certainly play a role early on, and it is important to maintain the net negative sodium balance achieved in order to establish long-term control of blood pressure. That control may be overwhelmed quickly by a dietary or intravenous sodium load. It is clear, however, that diuretics also have a long-term vasodilator effect that appears to be mediated by intracellular mechanisms. For example, vascular smooth muscle cells become less sensitive and less responsive to vasoconstrictor stimuli such as norepinephrine after diuretic administration.

Use in Hypertension

It is now clear that the dose-response curve for arterial pressure reduction by thiazide diuretics is distinct from the dose-response curve for natriuresis and kaliuresis. Early on, diuretic level doses were used to treat hypertension even in the absence of edema. These high doses (e.g., 200 mg of hydrochlorothiazide or 1,000 mg of chlorthalidone) were associated with a moderately high rate of metabolic complications such as hypokalemia and hyperglycemia. In more recent years, it has been recognized that it is not necessary to reach the dose-response plateau for these drugs in order to achieve a therapeutic benefit. The early portion of the dose-response curve is rather steep and the onset of effective arterial pressure reduction is at doses much lower than previously appreciated. It is now known that 25 mg of hydrochlorothiazide will control many mildly hypertensive patients as will 12.5–25 mg of chlorthalidone. Therefore, it makes no sense to start mildly hypertensive patients on larger doses. Using these low doses may achieve the desired beneficial effect while avoiding or minimizing adverse effects. In a Veterans Administration Cooperative Study of hypertension in the elderly, serum potassium was reduced 0.27 mmol/L by 25 mg of hydrochlorothiazide, but 0.50 mmol/L by 50 mg, and 0.70 mmol/L by 100 mg.

The clinician must also keep in mind that the vasodilator effect of the thiazides lags well behind the diuretic effect and that it may take as long as six months for the maximal reduction to be achieved. If goal blood pressure is being approached, it may be appropriate strategy to wait an additional month or two to provide adequate time for a fair therapeutic trial.

Another important point that is often overlooked is that the "low-dose" data were relevant to mildly hypertensive patients and were not obtained for moderately to severely hypertensives. These patients are more likely to have the low set point of their dose-response curve for arterial pressure reduction at a higher level than the mild hypertensives. They are also more likely to require more than one drug.

The indication for the use of a thiazide diuretic as initial therapy in patients with hypertension is undergoing active evolution for several reasons. First, it is now known that there are rational and effective alternatives to diuretics as monotherapy for hypertension. Second, there is a growing body of evidence that suggests that the diuretics may be counteracting some of their beneficial effect by inducing cardiac dysrhythmias and by altering the plasma lipoprotein profile in the direction of greater potential for atherogenesis. Without debating these suggestions, it is evident that there is a move toward alternative nondiuretic selections for initial treatment of hypertensive patients. Black patients and the elderly are particularly responsive to the thiazides and that efficacy usually can be obtained with minimal adverse effects if the dose is kept low.

Even when a thiazide is not selected as the initial treatment, all other antihypertensive drugs may have their beneficial effect greatly enhanced by the addition of a diuretic. Therefore, a shift of the thiazides into a second-step category may be in the making. Nevertheless, when direct drug costs alone are considered, they are extremely inexpensive compared to the nondiuretic alternatives.

Adverse Drug Reactions

Some of the adverse reactions that may be associated with the use of the thiazides have been alluded to. A more detailed discussion from the standpoint that most of the problems can be avoided or at least minimized with proper attention to detail follows.

Hyponatremia

Diuretic-associated hyponatremia has reached some prominence in contemporary medicine due to the permanent neurological damage that can result from hyponatremia and the controversy in the medical literature as to how best to treat it. The very best way to manage diuretic-induced hyponatremia is to avoid it in the first place based on an understanding of the process. Women, particularly middle aged and older, are the prime victims. People who habitually consume large quantities of water or other liquids (e.g., beer) are also at risk. Patients who are taking a thiazide diuretic and experience a problem that either removes sodium, such as protracted vomiting or diarrhea (especially when the fluid losses are replaced with free water), or those who receive large quantities of free water intravenously in the perioperative period are at great risk. Fortunately, clinically important hyponatremia is rare, but that fact also renders many physicians unaware of its lethal potential.

Patients who are started for the first time on treatment with a thiazide diuretic should be cautioned that if they experience headache, nausea, and/or vomiting they should call their physician. The physician should quickly have a serum sodium determination made on the patient and stop the diuretic if there is any evidence of hyponatremia. Even if such patients actually have the "flu" or gastroenteritis most of the time, the consequences of failing to intervene in a timely fashion may be demise of the patient or hyponatremia that eventuates in disabling central pontine myelinolysis.

Details of the treatment of severe hyponatremia are beyond the scope of this chapter. It appears likely that central pontine myelinolysis is a function of damage caused by the hyponatremia itself rather than the absolute rate of correction. There is so much controversy about how quickly (or slowly) to correct. Consultation with a nephrologist or other physician knowledgeable about the treatment of hyponatremia may best serve the treatment goals of avoiding associated morbidity and mortality.

Hypokalemia

For many years, hypokalemia was more or less accepted as an inevitable consequence of thiazide therapy. Some experts advised that this was harmless and that serum potassium levels need not be of concern if they were 2.5 mmol/L or higher. This arbitrary cutoff point was later revised to 3.0, then 3.3 mmol/L, based more on opinion than fact. Other experts contended that any reduction of serum potassium, even below 4.0 mmol/L was likely to be harmful. Strong editorials were written decrying the overuse of potassium supplements to treat a nonproblem at great cost and some documentable harm to a few patients.

The suggestion (and some evidence) that thiazide-induced hypokalemia may be associated with an increase in ventricular dysrhythmias and incidence of sudden death generated considerable attention, but no absolute answers. There is a growing mass of conflicting data as to whether diuretics do or do not induce ventricular ectopy. The suggestion that the phenomenon was limited to those patients with clinically identifiable organic heart disease has been challenged in both directions by claims that "normal" people can get ectopy and by counterclaims that "abnormal" people do not, even when stressed to low levels of serum potassium. Whether or not magnesium has a role in the generation (or prevention) of ectopic activity is also an unanswered question. While a resolution to this conundrum may not be forthcoming in these pages, there is some advice that may be useful.

People who have evidence of organic heart disease, especially if they have evidence of ventricular ectopy, ought to have their hypertension treated with drugs other than thiazide diuretics. Beta-blockers, angiotensin-converting enzyme inhibitors, and calcium channel blockers are reasonable alternatives if not contraindicated for other reasons (e.g., bronchospasm). If a thiazide is needed, the serum potassium should be kept well within the normal range by using potassium chloride supplements or a potassium-sparing diuretic. Consider also the blunting effect on hypokalemia achieved by combination of a thiazide with an angiotensin-converting enzyme inhibitor.

People with uncomplicated hypertension, particularly if they are black or elderly, can be treated with a low dose of thiazide without automatically providing potassium supplementation. They should be advised to consume a no salt added diet (68 to 103 mmol of sodium), eat a reasonable amount of fresh fruit and vegetables, and abstain from the intake of ethanol and large amounts of caffeine. Potassium need not be supplemented unless it falls below normal (usually 3.5 mmol/dL) . Be aware that even this level may be arbitrary and should be considered in the overall clinical context of the patient and their medical problems.

Hypochloremic Metabolic Alkalosis

This common metabolic state is the result of the combination of sustained plasma volume and potassium depletion. It is generally of little clinical consequence unless it is associated with marked potassium depletion or is additive with other causes for alkalosis. Replacement of chloride as well as potassium (and perhaps volume) is important if correction is necessary.

Hyperlipoproteinemia

This has become an important topic as a result of the ability to measure serum lipoproteins and lipoprotein fractions accurately, the documentation that thiazide diuretics do increase total cholesterol and LDL-cholesterol and reduce HDL-cholesterol, the evidence that reduced HDL- and increased LDL-cholesterol is associated with increased cardiac mortality, the evidence that drug-induced reversal of these abnormalities reduces risk of cardiac death, and the availability of alternative antihypertensive drugs that do not alter the lipoprotein profile unfavorably. It has not been proven that the thiazide-induced changes actually are responsible for increased cardiovascular risk, but a great deal has been written about this subject.

Thiazide diuretics probably increase serum cholesterol levels even when prescribed at a low dose, but not nearly as much as higher doses. Drugs such as indapamide and micronized metolazone probably owe their relatively small effect on cholesterol to the very low dose that is generally prescribed. A low fat diet can minimize the serum cholesterol increase. There is no evidence that people with normal levels of serum cholesterol are harmed by the trivial changes associated with thiazide diuretic use for treatment of their hypertension. Combination with other drugs such as an alpha-1-antagonist or angiotensin-converting enzyme inhibitor may blunt the increase in serum cholesterol due to the diuretic.

Phototoxicity

This adverse effect is deemed uncommon by primary care physicians and common by dermatologists who practice in the Sun Belt. The rash is generally maculopapular and can be quite severe. It is most commonly associated with the use of hydrochlorothiazide, but that is the most common diuretic used. We have had success by changing to treatment with metolazone on the hypothesis that this drug did not have an ultraviolet absorption spectrum in the sunlight range. Work done in collaboration with Dr. J. Richard Taylor disproved this hypothesis and left us without explanation for our success.

Sexual Dysfunction

It is extremely difficult to gather accurate data on sexual dysfunction related to antihypertensive drug therapy. It is almost certain that hypertensives have a higher prevalence of sexual dysfunction than do age-matched normotensives. The prevalence of sexual dysfunction varies between different normal populations, and there is an extraordinary placebo effect. All of this makes it nearly impossible to be certain what the true risk of sexual dysfunction is due to treatment with a thiazide diuretic. It is likely, however, that the risk is not trivial and that it is higher than for most other antihypertensive agents (with the exception of the central alpha-2-agonists). There simply have been too many men rendered totally impotent by a placebo only to regain full function on return to active therapy to allow for much faith in the current data. Definitive scientifically derived and verified data do not yet exist.

Calcium Metabolism

When thiazide diuretics are administered to hypertensive patients in controlled clinical trials, there is a very small, but highly statistically significant increase in serum calcium levels. The statistical significance was ascribed to the large numbers of subjects in these trials plus the fact that virtually all patients had a slight increase, rather than the increase being the result of a wide variation of responses that just happened to have a mean value slightly above baseline. This was thought to be an example of statistical significance in the absence of clinical relevance. This may not be accurate. Hypertensive patients as a group have a lower mean serum calcium level than normotensives; the reverse obtains for intracellular calcium concentrations. When patients are treated with a calcium channel blocker, a beta-blocker, or a thiazide diuretic, the serum calcium level is increased and the intracellular calcium decreased toward the level of the normal patients. This suggests that the final common pathway for many antihypertensive drugs may be through either the intracellular calcium-mediated second messenger system or changes in calcium ion flux across cell membranes. This may eventually provide some answers as to the "vasodilator" mechanism of the thiazides.

A small number of patients will increase their serum calcium level into the abnormal range during treatment with a thiazide. They should be investigated for hyperparathyroidism or other syndromes of parathyroid hormone excess.

Thiazide diuretics decrease the amount of calcium excreted in the urine and therefore are useful for the treatment of nephrolithiasis due to calcium stones. It has been observed recently that the calcium not excreted in the urine is deposited in the bones, thereby providing some protection against bone fractures in the elderly and people with osteoporosis.

Allergic Reactions

There are a number of rare immune-mediated reactions associated with thiazide diuretics. These include interstitial nephritis, Stevens-Johnson syndrome, and bone marrow suppression. In general, a patient who is known to be sensitive to any sulfa drug should not be subjected to treatment with any of the thiazides or loop-blocking diuretics. Ethacrynic is an exception because it does not have a sulfamoyl group. Spironolactone may be useful in some patients as well because it is also a nonsulfonamide and may have some blood pressure lowering effect in addition to its potassium-sparing properties.

Hyperuricemia

Any thiazide diuretic can be expected to increase serum uric acid levels about 1 to 2 mg/dL in a dose-related fashion. The vast majority of treated patients still have a uric acid level within the normal range or have asymptomatic hyperuricemia. This elevation should not be treated. Acute gout associated with the use of thiazide diuretics does occur, but is uncommon and rarely the cause for discontinuation of the drug. In a major trial of antihypertensive agents, the only discontinuation from the protocol due to acute gout was a patient who had been randomized to treatment with placebo!

Hyperglycemia

Glucose metabolism is perturbed by administration of thiazide diuretics, but it is unusual for this to be of clinical importance. A few patients who are borderline diabetics may increase their serum glucose concentration level requiring therapy. Rarely will a patient responsive to an oral hypoglycemic agent require insulin instead during treatment with a thiazide. It appears that glucose homeostasis returns to baseline soon after treatment with a thiazide is discontinued, although there is a suggestion that long-term treatment may have more lasting effects.

Summary

Thiazide diuretics, once the cornerstone of modern antihypertensive therapy, are being viewed more cautiously today because of the potential impact of their adverse effects and the availability of alternative drugs for monotherapy. Nevertheless, they are inexpensive, effective, and have an excellent track record over more than three decades of use. Probably 30%–40% of hypertensive patients will require a thiazide alone or in combination with another drug. Adverse effects can be minimized by administering as low a dose as possible.

Loop-Blocking Diuretics

The three loop-blocking diuretics available in the United States are listed in Table 2. All of them work by binding to cell membrane receptor sites on the epithelium of cells in the ascending limb of the loop of Henle. The result is interference with the Na/K/2Cl cotransportor across the lumenal membrane. Because this site is proximal to the cortical diluting segment, which is the site of action of the thiazides, there is considerably more glomerular filtrate available and the impact of blocking its reabsorption is consequently greater. Like the thiazides, these drugs work from the luminal surface and need to be either filtered or transported into the tubular lumen. Competition for the organic acid secretion pathway by probenecid can convert the rapid onset of action characteristics of furosemide to a duration of action curve similar to that of hydro-

Table 2
Loop-blocking Diuretics

Generic Name	*Trade Name*
Bumetanide	Bumex
Ethacrynic acid	Edecrin
Furosemide	Lasix

Diuretics • 127

chlorothiazide. Excessive diuresis with these drugs activates counter-regulatory mechanisms referred to as the "braking phenomenon" to offset the magnitude of induced diuresis and natriuresis.

Use in Hypertension

In general, this class of diuretics is too short acting and too potent for routine use in the patient with uncomplicated hypertension. They should be reserved for that subset of hypertensives who have renal failure, severe edema due to other causes, or who are receiving potent fluid-retaining drugs such as minoxidil. Their short duration of action requires that they be administered at least twice daily. As mentioned above, ethacrynic acid does have a special use in patients who require a diuretic but are allergic to sulfa.

In very unusual circumstances, one of the loop-blocking drugs can be combined extremely cautiously with a thiazide or thiazide-like diuretic (metolazone is often used) for treatment of hypertension in patients with unusually resistant edema. Almost all of these patients have severe renal failure.

Adverse Effects

The adverse effects associated with the loop-blocking diuretics are, in general, similar to those of the thiazides. The shorter the duration of action of the loop blockers makes hypokalemia less of a problem unless the patient also has edema. Overdiuresis with associated orthostatic hypotension is a risk. The doses used for the treatment of hypertension do not convey the risks of higher or intravenous doses such as cardiac dysrhythmias or ototoxicity. Oral ethacrynic acid is associated with more gastric upset than the other drugs. Ethacrynic acid, unlike the sulfonamide-derived loop blockers, has some intrinsic uricosuric effect. This is not generally enough to reduce the serum uric acid level, but it may prevent it from rising as it does with the other drugs.

Summary

The loop-blocking diuretics, although much more potent than the thiazides in regard to sodium excretion, are not as useful for the routine treatment of uncomplicated hypertension. Their role is limited to hypertension complicated by edema, renal failure, or other special problems. Ethacrynic acid can be used in sulfa-sensitive patients.

Potassium-Sparing Diuretics

The potassium-sparing diuretics and their combinations that are available in the United States are listed in Table 3. These drugs exert their pharmacological effect in the far distal portion of the nephron where most of the luminal fluid has already been reabsorbed. Therefore, they cause little net negative balance of sodium and only a trivial reduction, if any, of arterial pressure.

Spironolactone is probably an exception in that it works over a broader range of distal nephron sites and at points more proximal than triamterene and amiloride. It works by competitively inhibiting the binding of aldosterone to its cytosolic receptors. Clinically important reductions in arterial pressure can be obtained by the use of spironolactone alone, although it is mostly used for its potassium-sparing properties. It is particularly effective in patients with hypertension due to primary aldosterone-secreting tumors or adrenal cortical hyperplasia, but can be used in essential hypertension as well. Many patients will respond to as little as 25 mg daily. Some success has been observed using spironolactone in sulfa-sensitive patients. It is important to note that this drug has a long onset and long offset of action of three to five days. There appears to be little rationale to giving it more often than once daily.

Triamterene and amiloride both abolish the electrochemical gradient in the distal nephron and cause sodium ions to be excreted preferentially to potassium and hydrogen. The result is a trivial natriuretic effect, but

Table 3
Potassium-sparing Diuretics

Generic Name	Trade Name
Amiloride	Midamor
Amiloride/hydrochlorothiazide	Moduretic
Spironolactone	Aldactone
Spironolactone/hydrochlorothiazide	Aldactazide
Triamterene	Dyrenium
Triamterene/hydrochlorothiazide	Dyazide; Maxzide

a significant reduction in the amount of potassium excreted. The retention of hydrogen ion may lead to a mild systemic acidosis. This, of course, is useful in countering the metabolic alkalosis associated with the thiazide or the loop-blocking diuretics. Indeed, the major utility of these drugs is in combination with hydrochlorothiazide.

An additional benefit of all of the potassium-sparing diuretics is the sparing magnesium excretion. To what extent this is of value in protecting against ventricular dysrhythmias is highly controversial.

Dyazide brand combination of hydrochlorothiazide 25 mg and triamterene 50 mg was one of the most widely sold antihypertensive agents in the world. More recently, it was discovered that the product is only about 50% bioavailable so that patients were actually getting far less drug than appreciated by the prescribing physician. Nevertheless, one titrates such drugs to a goal blood pressure and there is no doubt that Dyazide was effective for many patients. It also provided a lesson that the minimally effective dose of hydrochlorothiazide might be lower than 25 mg (although one cannot ignore the small effect of the triamterene). Maxzide brand of hydrochlorothiazide 50 mg combined with triamterene 75 mg (there is also a half-strength tablet) was formulated to be more bioavailable than the components of Dyazide. The obvious risk is that patients may receive initial treatment with more drug than they actually need for blood pressure reduction.

Adverse Effects

The principle adverse effect for this group of drugs is hyperkalemia. This is most likely to occur in patients who have decreased renal function, are receiving concomitant potassium supplementation, or who are also receiving angiotensin-converting enzyme inhibitors.

Spironolactone may cause gynecomastia that may be painful. This is particularly distressing to men, but is rather uncommon at the low doses used for the treatment of hypertension in comparison to the amount needed for diuresis of ascitic fluid.

Triamterene is very insoluble in water and has been found as a crystalline component of some renal calculi. It is unclear as to whether triamterene actually causes renal stones to form. Triamterene may also cause acute renal failure when used in combination with indomethacin.

Amiloride is highly water soluble and is renally excreted. Other than the risk of hyperkalemia, its most common adverse effects are related to the gastroenteric tract: nausea, anorexia, vomiting, and diarrhea.

Summary

The potassium-sparing diuretics are also magnesium-sparing and are used primarily as adjuncts to thiazide and loop diuretics. Spironolactone may be used alone as an antihypertensive. The most important adverse effect is hyperkalemia.

Selected Readings

Ashraf N, Locksley R, Arieff AI: Thiazide-induced hyponatremia associated with death or neurologic damage in outpatients. Am J Med 70:1163–1168, 1981.
Brater DC, Pressley RH, Anderson SA: Mechanisms of the synergistic combination of metolazone and bumetanide. J Pharmacol Exp Ther 233:70–74, 1985.
Caralis PV, Materson BJ, Perez-Stable E: Potassium and diuretic-induced ventricular arrhythmias in ambulatory hypertensive patients. Mineral Electrolyte Metabol 10:148–154, 1984.
Cunningham E, Oliveros FH, Nascimento L: Metolazone therapy of active calcium nephrolithiasis. Clin Pharmacol Ther 32:642–645, 1982.
Freis ED: How diuretics lower blood pressure. Am Heart J 106:185–187, 1983.
Gross PA, Ketteler M, Hausmann C, et al: The charted and the uncharted waters of hyponatremia. Kidney Int 32(Suppl 21):S-67–S-75, 1987.
Harrington JT, Isner JM, Kassirer JP: Our national obsession with potassium. Am J Med 73:155–159, 1982.
Materson BJ: Insights into intrarenal sites and mechanisms of action of diuretic agents. Am Heart J 106:188–208, 1983.
Materson BJ: Diuretic-associated hypokalemia. (Invited editorial). Arch Intern Med 145:1966–1967, 1985.
Materson BJ: Sexual dysfunction during antihypertensive treatment. Progress in Pharmacol 6:117–124, 1985.
Materson BJ: Adverse effects of antihypertensive treatment. Cardiol Clinics 4:105–115, 1986.
Materson BJ: Diaretic dose-response relationships. Modern Medicine 56 (Suppl A):47–52, 1988.
Materson BJ, Oster JR, Michael UF, et al: Dose response to chlorthalidone in patients with mild hypertension. Efficacy of a lower dose. Clin Pharmacol Ther 24:192–198, 1978.
Messerli FH, Ventura HO, Elizardi DJ, et al: Hypertension and sudden death: increased ventricular ectopic activity in left ventricular hypertrophy. Am J Med 77:18–22, 1984.
Murphy MB, Kohner E, Lewis PJ, et al: Glucose intolerance in hypertensive patients treated with diuretics; a fourteen-year follow-up. Lancet 2:1293–1295, 1982.
Perez-Stable E, Caralis PV: Thiazide-induced disturbances in carbohydrate, lipid, and potassium metabolism. Am Heart J 106:245–251, 1983.
Tannen RL (Principal Discussant): Diuretic-induced hypokalemia. Kidney Int 28:988–1000, 1985.

Chapter 7

Calcium Antagonists in the Management of Hypertension

Murray Epstein and James R. Oster

Introduction

Calcium antagonists have assumed a very important role in the treatment of patients with ischemic heart disease and in a variety of cardiovascular and noncardiovascular disorders. Similarly, in recent years, calcium antagonists have been used extensively in the United States and elsewhere as antihypertensive agents, and their availability has been an important advance in the management of hypertension. The major hemodynamic abnormality present in most patients with essential hypertension is an increase in peripheral resistance. Considerable evidence suggests that the elevation of peripheral resistance is mediated in part by abnormal transmembrane flux of calcium. Figure 1 summarizes in schematic fashion the known and postulated mechanisms for activation, contraction, and relaxation of vascular smooth muscle. To the extent that abnormal calcium flux constitutes a determinant of elevated peripheral resistance, the major mechanism whereby calcium antagonists lower blood pressure—blockade of calcium-mediated electromechanical coupling in contractile tissue produces arteriolar

---

From Punzi HA, Flamenbaum W (eds): *Hypertension*. Mount Kisco, NY, Futura Publishing Co., Inc., © 1989.
Adapted with permission from Epstein M, Oster JR: Role of calcium channel blockers. In Epstein M, Oster JR: Hypertension, Practical Management, 2nd Edition. Miami, Battersea Medical Publications, 1988, pp 114–126.

132 • HYPERTENSION

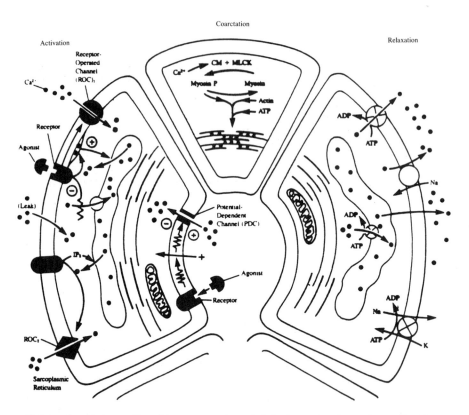

Figure 1. Schematic of known and postulated mechanisms for activation, contraction, and relaxation of vascular smooth muscle. The complex interaction of calcium, myosin, actin, calmodulin (CM), myosin light chain kinase (MLCK), ATP receptor-operated channels (ROC), potential-dependent channels (PDC), etc. are depicted. The PDCs are believed to constitute the primary site of action of calcium blockers. (Modified with permission from a drawing by A. Iselin in Loutzenhiser R, Epstein M: Calcium antagonists and the kidney. Hosp Prac 22:63–76, 1987).

vasodilation—is particularly apropos. As a result of reducing total peripheral resistance (PVR), systemic blood pressure decreases. Calcium antagonists cause widespread arterial and arteriolar vasodilation, but vary in their ability to dilate different vascular beds. In addition to their effects on peripheral blood vessels, the hormonal and renal actions of calcium antagonists have been postulated to contribute to blood pressure lowering.

Differences Among Calcium Antagonists

Calcium antagonists are a heterogeneous group of compounds with diverse chemical structures and pharmacological actions. Presently, four calcium antagonists are available in the United States; more will be marketed soon. The order in which the three prototypic agents were released into the market was verapamil (Calan®), nifedipine (Procardia®), and diltiazem (Cardizem®). The fourth agent, nicardipine (Cardene®) was released recently. All calcium antagonists retard the entry of calcium into the cell—be it cardiac muscle, peripheral vascular smooth muscle, or endocrine. The calcium antagonists are not alpha-blockers, but some prevent the increase in calcium influx resulting from stimulation of alpha-receptors.

Pharmacokinetics

In general, calcium antagonists have short half-lives and extensive hepatic first-pass metabolism. Nevertheless, the three prototypic agents not only differ in their pharmacodynamic effects (discussed below) but also manifest several differences in the way they are handled by the body. Some of these so-called pharmacokinetic variables, which are summarized in Table 1, may importantly influence clinical decisions, including choice of agent, optimum dose, and mode and frequency of administration. For example, the relatively short time to peak blood level for nifedipine accounts in part for its efficacy in patients with severe acute hypertension.

The relatively low bioavailability of verapamil relates mainly to a high hepatic first-pass effect. Careful individual titration of dosage (not only for verapamil but for the other calcium antagonists) is thus required. Verapamil (and to a lesser degree nifedipine and diltiazem) also undergoes unexpected accumulation despite the general rule that a steady-state blood level of a medication usually occurs within three to five half-lives. With chronic treatment, the half-life of the drug may double, perhaps as a result of stereoselective metabolism or from verapamil inducing an effect on it own metabolism. The increased half-life, in part, accounts for the ability, after about two weeks of dosing, to prescribe the conventional(immediate release) preparation of verapamil b.i.d. , instead of t.i.d.

Of the three prototypic agents, nifedipine is the most potent vasodilator and has the least effect on SA and AV nodal function. It is more

Table 1
Some Important Pharmacokinetic Properties of the Three Prototypical Calcium Antagonists

	Nifedipine†	Verapamil†	Diltiazem†
1. Time to peak blood level (min)	30–60	90–120	120–180
2. Systemic bioavailability (%)	60	20	40–50
3. Protein binding (%)	90	95	80
4. Volume of distribution (L/kg)	3	7	4
5. Half-life (hr)	3–5	4–5*	4–5
6. Elimination (major organ)	Liver	Liver	Liver
7. Unexpected accumulation	No	Yes	Yes

* May be substantially prolonged in patients with liver disease; † Conventional formulations.

likely to provoke reflex stimulation of the heart, resulting initially in increases in heart rate, myocardial contractility, and cardiac output. Verapamil has more potent direct negative chronotropic and inotropic actions, so the end result is usually a lack of change in heart rate, myocardial contractility, or cardiac output in normal and hypertensive subjects. In subjects with depressed left ventricular (systolic) function, however, verapamil is more likely to produce undesirable further deterioration. Diltiazem seems to have a somewhat intermediate effect. It produces less peripheral vasodilation and less of a reflex sympathetic response than nifedipine. Diltiazem has mild negative chronotropic activity, which is usually more apparent during exercise than at rest, and relatively little negative inotropic action. The latter is clinically negligible in patients with normal left ventricular function. Although verapamil and diltiazem influence the activity of both the SA and AV nodes, in general, verapamil has a greater effect on AV nodal function and diltiazem has a greater effect on SA function.

Like nifedipine, nicardipine is a short-acting dihydropyridine that is effective for the treatment of angina and hypertension. Its hemodynamic actions are very similar to those of nifedipine. The metabolism of nicardipine is primarily hepatic, and plasma levels may be increased in the patient with hepatic disease. At clinically used dosages, nicardipine does not depress cardiac conduction, and the medication appears to have little or no negative ionotropic effect. Although the latter property is a possible advantage over nifedipine, it probably is of marginal clinical importance. Nicardipine has also been formulated for intravenous use in patients with severe acute hypertension, but this preparation is not yet available in the United States.

Nifedipine, but not diltiazem, reduces pulmonary artery pressure and pulmonary vascular resistance. Calcium antagonists reduce blood pressure without effecting the normal circadian blood pressure variations. They attenuate both isotonic and isometric exercise-induced elevations in blood pressure, but the rate of increase of blood pressure and heart rate induced by exercise is not modified. Preliminary findings, which need confirmation, suggest that, despite its usefulness in patients with radiological cardiomegaly even in the presence of a low ejection fraction, nifedipine somewhat reduces exercise performance and the conditioning response.

Differences between Calcium Antagonists and other Vasodilators

Drugs that directly reduce peripheral vascular resistance, such as hydralazine, have been used for antihypertensive therapy for many years. Nevertheless, the effectiveness of these agents is often limited by the reactive stimulation of renal and hormonal responses that counteract their antihypertensive actions (Fig. 2). These responses tend to produce tolerance to hydralazine's vasodilating action as well as causing volume expansion-induced pseudotolerance to its antihypertensive effects.

The precise mechanism(s) whereby calcium antagonists interfere with angiotensin II or alpha adrenergic-mediated vasoconstriction remains uncertain. Nevertheless, in the presence of calcium antagonists (as indicted in Figure 2 by the interruptions of the arrows), the expected adaptive changes in peripheral vascular resistance, heart rate, cardiac output, and extracellular fluid volume that eventually lead to a reduction in the blood pressure-lowering response to vasodilators are mitigated. An intriguing speculation is the possibility that calcium antagonists might countervail the sodium-retaining renal effects of decreased perfusion and, possibly, of decreased levels of natriuretic hormones.

In contrast to other vasodilators, the calcium antagonists apparently blunt the reflex increase in sympathetic activity by virtue of their indirect alpha-adrenergic inhibitory action. They may also interfere with the action of angiotensin II on vascular smooth muscle. Despite the early in-

Modulation by Calcium Antagonists of Compensatory Responses to Vasodilation

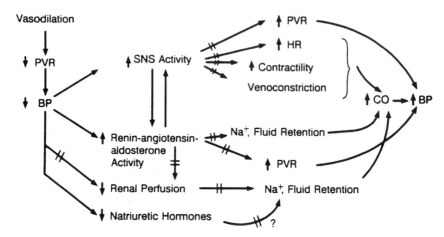

Figure 2. A schematic diagram of the known and postulated compensatory mechanisms whereby vasodilation induced by nonspecific vasodilators such as hydralazine is offset by the reactive stimulation of renal and hormonal responses. These include an increase in the activity of the sympathetic nervous system and RAA areas and a decrease in renal perfusion. Although the precise mechanisms remain uncertain, calcium antagonists attenuate these adaptive changes. (Reproduced with permission from Epstein M, Loutzenhiser R: In Calcium Antagonists and The Kidney. Philadelphia, Hanley and Belfus, 1989).

crease in plasma renin activity (PRA) during calcium antagonist therapy, aldosterone levels fail to rise proportionally (and occasionally decrease), perhaps because of the role of calcium in hormonal release. Recent evidence indicates that acute administration of calcium antagonists, unlike most other nondiuretic antihypertensive medications, produces a diuresis and natriuresis. Additionally, when calcium antagonists are given long term, they are not sodium retaining.

The calcium antagonists differ from previous vasodilators because of their favorable accompanying effects on the heart and kidney. As antihypertensive agents, the calcium antagonists thus appear considerably more versatile than previous vasodilators.

In vitro, all of the calcium antagonists have negative inotropic and chronotropic actions. In patients and in intact animals, these direct effects are balanced variably by reflex sympathetic responses. Table 2 summarizes the typical cardiac and hemodynamic effects of the three prototypic agents.

Table 2
Cardiac and Hemodynamic Effects of Calcium Antagonists

Effect	Nifedipine (Dihydropyridines)	Diltiazem	Verapamil
Arteriolar dilatation	+ + + +	+ +	+ +
Peripheral vasodilation	+ + + +	+ +	+ +
Coronary vasodilation	+ + + +	+ +	+ +
Cardiac preload	↓	—	↓
Cardiac afterload	↓ ↓	↓	↓
Cardiac contractility	0	↓	↓ ↓
Heart rate	↑	↓ or →	↓ or →
AV conduction	0	↓ ↓	↓ ↓ ↓
SA conduction	0	↓ ↓	↓

Use of Calcium Antagonists as Antihypertensive Agents

The three prototypic calcium antagonists have been shown to be similarly effective and safe antihypertensive drugs. For this reason, along with diuretics, beta-blockers, and angiotensin-converting enzyme (ACE) inhibitors, they were recommended in 1988 by the Joint National Committee on High Blood Pressure as initial pharmacological therapy for the treatment of hypertension. Interestingly, calcium antagonists generally have a minimal effect on the blood pressure of normotensive patients. In hypertensive patients, however, there is some evidence that their effect on blood pressure increases with the degree of hypertension. These observations taken together lend support to the notion that these agents act by specifically reversing pathophysiological perturbations.

There are a few contraindications to the use of calcium antagonists (as opposed to beta-blockers) as antihypertensive agents: severely depressed left ventricular systolic function (frank CHF or a history of CHF), sick sinus syndrome, and AV conduction disturbances. In general, a lower dose (given less frequently) of a calcium antagonist is required to achieve blood pressure control than to manage angina. The antihypertensive response demonstrates a dose-response curve, but small doses of the agents have been used with success.

All four calcium antagonists currently available in the United States are efficacious as initial antihypertensive monotherapy. Nifedipine in a dose of 30 to 60 mg/day may lower the systolic and diastolic blood pressures by an average of 28 mmHg and 16 mmHg, respectively. Similarly, the conventional formulation of verapamil administered in a dose of 240 to 720 mg/day may lower the systolic pressure by approximately 22 mmHg and diastolic pressure by 17 mmHg. Diltiazem in a dose of 180 to 360 mg/day may reduce blood pressure by 15/15 mmHg. Similar results have been reported with the administration of nicardipine in doses ranging from 30 to 120 mg/day. Generally, monotherapeutic administration of calcium antagonists reduces blood pressure to goal levels in 40% to 50% of patients, and some lowering of blood pressure occurs in 80% to 90% of patients.

The studies that have compared the antihypertensive effect of calcium antagonists to that of other agents reveal that the various calcium antagonists are equally efficacious in unselected patients with mild to moderate hypertension. Additionally, calcium antagonists appear to be at least as good as beta-blockers in lowering blood pressure in patients with both hypertension and angina. Comparison of conventional nifedipine with hydralazine has shown that the medications are equivalent both in efficacy and side effects. Diltiazem at dosages of 60 to 120 mg t.i.d. has been demonstrated to produce an antihypertensive response similar to that of hydrochlorthiazide.

Pharmacology

The onset of action of the available calcium antagonists differs. Orally administered nifedipine has a more rapid onset of action and attainment of maximal blood pressure reduction than verapamil. Initial response times differ by about 15 minutes. The conventional preparation of verapamil also achieves a maximal lowering of the blood pressure about one hour later than nifedipine. However, the maximum drop in blood pressure and the duration of the hypotensive response after a single dose are similar with either agent. The difference in the rapidity of onset of the antihypertensive actions of these two medications only occasionally dictates the preferential use of one agent. Thus, in a patient with life-threatening hypertension, when a rapid fall in blood pressure is desirable, nifedipine would be preferred. However, when the onset of action is not a consideration and tachycardia is to be avoided, verapamil or diltiazem might be preferable.

The duration of action of the conventional form of all three prototypic drugs is between six and eight hours after a single dose. Therefore, they usually are administered either t.i.d or q.i.d. The sustained-release formulations are administered q.d. or b.i.d.

Verapamil is metabolized in the liver to norverapamil. The half-life of verapamil is prolonged in patients with liver disease, and smaller doses should be used when initiating therapy in such patients. The effective duration of the pharmacological effect of verapamil during chronic therapy is significantly longer than would be predicted based on the plasma half-life, permitting b.i.d. dosing in many patients. Such considerations are becoming moot, however, in view of the marketing in 1986 of a slow-release form of verapamil (Calan-SR®). Very recently, diltiazem has become available in a sustained release formulation (Cardizem SR®). With this preparation, the apparent elimination half-life is 5 to 7 hours. The recommended initial dose is 60 to 120 mg b.i.d., with the usual optimum maintenance dose of 240 to 360 mg/day. The maximal antihypertensive effect of a given dose level is believed to occur in approximately two weeks. A long-acting preparation of nifedipine is expected to be marketed in the United States soon.

In general, the blood-pressure lowering effects of calcium antagonists are sustained. To our knowledge, no resistance has been reported for verapamil or diltiazem during studies lasting for several months. For example, in one trial of verapamil, no tolerance was observed over a 12-month period. Similarly, diltiazem administered over a year to hypertensive subjects was demonstrated not to induce tolerance. Although there have been rare reports of tolerance with calcium antagonists, an increase in dosage re-established blood pressure control, and drug noncompliance could not be excluded. Tolerance to the antihypertensive effects of calcium antagonists, therefore, is not a problem.

Several studies have shown that all calcium antagonists have similar antihypertensive properties. Adverse or salutary effects thus dictate the choice of a specific agent. For example, nifedipine or nicardipine may be preferred in a patient with mild ventricular systolic dysfunction, conduction system disease, or slow heart rate. In contrast, verapamil or diltiazem may be more suitable in a patient with tachycardia.

Demographic Considerations (Age, Race, PRA)

It has been estimated that with calcium antagonist monotherapy, approximately 50% of the general population with essential hypertension can achieve blood pressure control. Calcium antagonists appear to work equally well for men and women. The degree of efficacy of calcium antagonists relates, at least in part, to differing demographic features of the hypertensive patients: age, pretreatment blood pressure, PRA, and perhaps race. First, some preliminary evidence suggested that calcium antagonists are more effective in older patients. In this regard, the response to calcium antagonists would differ from that observed with beta-adrenoceptor blockers (decreased efficacy in patients over 60 years). Subsequently, however, the data indicate that calcium antagonists might be equally efficacious in all age groups. Second, the blood pressure-lowering effect of calcium antagonists may be inversely proportional to the baseline PRA, that is, in general, the lower the PRA, the greater the response to calcium antagonists. In addition, preliminary reports indicate that in patients with low PRA, a high dietary sodium intake does not impair the antihypertensive effect of calcium antagonists and may even enhance it. Perhaps this phenomenon is related to the observation that the combined use of calcium antagonists and diuretics may not provide an additive antihypertensive response. Furthermore, whereas converting enzyme inhibitors (depending on the dose) and beta-blockers tend to work less well as antihypertensive agents in black patients, this is not the case with calcium antagonists. Finally, preliminary evidence also suggests that calcium antagonists preferentially lower blood pressure in salt-sensitive patients and in those with lower levels of serum ionized calcium.

Antihypertensive Therapy in Patients with Accompanying Diseases (Table 3)

Until recently the major therapeutic use of antagonists has been for treatment of coronary artery vasospasm, angina pectoris, and supraventricular arrhythmias. Not surprisingly, it was predominantly in patients with these co-existing problems that much of the initial experience with the calcium antagonists as antihypertensive agents was accumulated. Certainly the concomitant occurrence of hypertension with ischemic heart disease or atrial fibrillation is not uncommon. The calcium antagonists can be used to treat both problems and often provide a welcome alternative for patients who are not good candidates for beta-blockers.

Although the findings require further confirmation, calcium antagonists, like beta-blockers, appear to have a cardioprotective effect in experimental ischemia and infarction. A few intriguing studies also indicate that they may decrease experimental atherogenesis.

Table 3
Complicating Problems that Commend the Selection of Calcium Blockers as Antihypertensive Drugs

1. Ischemic heart disease
2. History of recent non-Q-wave myocardial infarction (diltiazem only?)
3. Left ventricular hypertrophy?
4. Peripheral vascular insufficiency
5. Asthma, chronic pulmonary disease
6. Chronic renal failure?
7. Diabetes (Insulin-dependent or nondependent)

A limited number of studies have been conducted to answer the question of whether calcium antagonists provide secondary protection in patients with myocardial infarction. In this regard, trials with verapamil and nifedipine indicate, at least in the short-term, that the use of these two agents does not reduce postinfarction mortality or reinfarction rates. In contrast, studies carried out by the Multicenter Diltiazem Postinfarction Trial Research Group have shown that in postmyocardial infarction patients without pulmonary congestion, diltiazem reduces the number of cardiac events (deaths from cardiac causes or nonfatal myocardial reinfarction). When pulmonary congestion is present, however, no benefit is conferred. Furthermore, in patients with previous non-Q-wave infarction, diltiazem decreases the rate of early reinfarction, refractory angina, and angina with ECG changes.

Investigations in animals have demonstrated the use of calcium antagonists is associated with regression of left ventricular hypertrophy, and recent studies of hypertensive humans revealed that at least some calcium antagonists induce significant reduction of left ventricular mass, despite appreciable adrenergic stimulation.

All of the above mentioned salutary features, if substantiated, commend the use of calcium antagonists in many patients. In addition, an important observation is that calcium antagonists do not induce the undesirable changes of the serum concentration of lipoproteins, uric acid, or potassium. This, of course, contrasts with the adverse effects characteristically noted with several of the other antihypertensive agents (vide infra).

Calcium antagonists may be particularly desirable antihypertensive agents in other situations. Calcium antagonists are unlikely to worsen symptomatic peripheral vascular disease and may be beneficial in patients with bronchospastic pulmonary disease. Additionally, whereas some data indicate that calcium antagonists inhibit pancreatic insulin release, they appear to cause clinically important metabolic problems in insulin-dependent diabetic patients only rarely. Finally, since calcium antagonists tend to improve ventricular compliance, they may be used with caution advantageously in certain patients with left ventricular diastolic dysfunction (vide infra). Table 4 lists some of the diseases that frequently accompany hypertension and how their presence might effect the selection of an antihypertensive drug. Clearly, the calcium antagonists appear to be useful in many such patients.

An intriguing salutary effect, not fully established, is the influence of calcium antagonists on renal function. Several lines of evidence indicate that calcium antagonists are capable of inducing a dramatic reversal (or protection from) of acute renal ischemia under a number of experimental conditions. Calcium antagonists preferentially attenuate afferent arteriolar vasoconstriction in response to diverse agonists, including norepinephrine, angiotensin II, and thromboxane. This salutary effect of calcium antagonists on intrarenal hemodynamics suggests that they are particularly well suited for the management of hypertension; moreover they may have a future role in managing certain types of acute renal insufficiency. To the extent that renal ischemia underlies many disease states, including hypertension, the potential beneficial effects of such agents in this setting is of great interest.

One final aspect of this class of antihypertensive medications is the atypical action on renal sodium handling. Unlike many nondiuretic antihypertensive drugs, the direct acute renal effect of calcium-entry blockers is to enhance sodium excretion. Whether the natriuretic effects of calcium antagonists are sustained during long-term administration has not been delineated. Nevertheless, it is clear that when taken long term, calcium antagonists are not sodium retentive. It must be emphasized, however, that the net effect of a medication on sodium homeostasis is determined by the sum of the separate effects on blood pressure, cardiac performance, systemic vascular resistance, and renal tubular transport.

Combination Therapy

Calcium antagonists have been used successfully in combination with other antihypertensive drugs as second-line agents in the treatment of hypertension, or as third-step agents in patients with refractory hy-

Table 4
Potential Considerations in Choosing Initial Antihypertensive Therapy

Accompanying Illness	Disadvantages	Advantages
Coronary disease	Hydralazine, alpha-1 blocker, diuretic	Beta-blocker, calcium antagonist
Arrhythmias	Diuretic, hydralazine	Beta-blocker, calcium antagonist
Congestive heart failure	Beta-blocker/calcium antagonist	Diuretic, ACE inhibitor, alpha-1 blocker, calcium antagonist*
Peripheral vascular disease	Beta-blocker, diuretic	Diuretic, ACE inhibitor, calcium antagonist, alpha-1 blocker
Bronchospastic disease	Beta-blocker	Calcium antagonist, ACE inhibitor, alpha-1 blocker, central sympatholytic
Diabetes	Beta-blocker, diuretic	ACE inhibitor, calcium antagonist alpha-1 blocker
Demographics		
Elderly patients	Beta-blocker	Diretic, calcium antagonist, central sympatholytic
Black patients	Beta-blocker, ACE inhibitor (depending on dose)	Diretic, calcium antagonist

* For some patients with diastolic left ventricular dysfunction. (Adapted with permission from Epstein M, Oster JR: Hypertension. Practical Management, 2nd edition, Miami, Battersea Medical Publications, 1988, pp 114–116.)

pertension. There is accumulating evidence the combination of a calcium antagonist and a thiazide diuretic provides less than an additive blood pressure-lowering effect. Nevertheless, patients who are receiving a beta-blocker and a thiazide diuretic may have an additional hypotensive action from a calcium antagonist. In patients with severe hypertension or those with mild left ventricular (diastolic) dysfunction, the combi-

144 • HYPERTENSION

nation of a calcium antagonist and the ACE inhibitor captopril appears to be very efficacious and safe. Several investigators, however, have cautioned against the combined use of an alpha-blocker and calcium antagonist because of an unacceptable risk of hypotension.

Combined Therapy with Beta-Blockers

The topic of the rationale and safety of combined therapy with calcium antagonists and beta-blockers (for the treatment of angina) has been reviewed by Bala Subramanian. Historically, the concomitant use of these two classes of agents (especially using verapamil) was contraindicated. The reservations were based on theoretical factors and data regarding the effect of intravenous, rather than oral, use of these agents. The contraindication was thus due to the putative risk of inducing acute left ventricular failure, advanced heart block (or asystole), severe bradycardia, or hypotension. Current wisdom, however, dictates that beta-blockers and calcium antagonists can be used together when clearly indicated. By following certain guidelines with appropriate monitoring of the patients, this approach may be both efficacious and safe.

The compensatory reflex increase in sympathetic tone induced by a drop in blood pressure is one reason to combine nifedipine with a beta-blocker. This increase in sympathetic tone may produce a symptomatic increase in heart rate and an increment in PRA. These two effects might blunt the antihypertensive effect, but both are preventable with concomitant use of a beta-blocker. Additionally, calcium antagonists may counteract some of the adverse effects induced by beta-blockers (particularly the initial vasoconstriction induced by many). The recent report that beta-blockade might decrease the clearance of verapamil requires confirmation and delineation of its clinical relevance.

Side Effects of Calcium Antagonists

The major adverse reactions to the calcium antagonists are exaggerated pharmacological responses. In striking contrast, the incidence of orthostatic hypotension, CNS side effects, sexual dysfunction, bronchospasm, worsening or masking, or hypoglycemia, is negligible during treatment with calcium antagonists.

As with other potent antihypertensive agents, an excessive decrement in blood pressure is possible when calcium antagonists are used.

Calcium Antagonists • 145

Frank hypotension is rare when calcium antagonists are used as monotherapy, but it may occur during initial titration or at the time of subsequent upward dosage adjustment and may be more likely in patients receiving beta-blockers concomitantly. It appears in part to be on the basis of this hypotension (and the resultant decrease in coronary artery perfusion) that some patients with underlying coronary artery disease paradoxically develop increased frequency, duration, or severity of angina when starting or increasing the dose of nifedipine (or rarely of other calcium antagonists).

An important potential side effect of calcium antagonists, which is most commonly seen with nifedipine, is periorbital and, more commonly, peripheral edema. The edema often relates to arteriolar vasodilation rather than to decreased urinary sodium excretion, but calcium antagonists sometimes cause edema secondary to sodium retention per se.

The major side effects of calcium antagonists can often be predicted from their pharmacological actions. Since nifedipine is the most potent vasodilator, side effects attributable to vasodilation, such as headache, flushing, and edema, are more common with the use of this agent than with verapamil or diltiazem. Although vasodilator side effects are also induced by diltiazem and verapamil, their frequency appears to be less than with nifedipine. Of note, it appears that when nifedipine is ingested with food, its absorption is slowed, resulting in a less abrupt fall in blood pressure (but to a similar nadir level) and fewer "vasodilator type" side effects. As expected, some of the side effects of calcium antagonists, particularly hypotension and peripheral edema, may be dose-related.

The side effects of nicardipine are similar to those of nifedipine, and the important ones, which are dose-related and most frequent early in therapy, are vasodilatory in nature. Vasodilator-type side effects may be reduced by taking the medication with food. Similary, a smoothing out of the peak versus trough blood levels of the medication is the presumed mechanism whereby the new slow release (osmotic pump) form of nifedipine produces fewer vasodilator-related side effects.

Verapamil may produce important effects on cardiac conduction. In most cases, prolongation of atrioventricular conduction time causes no symptoms, but more serious conduction disturbances have been reported. These conduction disturbances (usually induced by the intravenous administration of the drug) include asystole and higher forms of atrioventricular block. Diltiazem effects cardiac conduction similarly. Nifedipine in the doses usually employed has little effect on sinoatrial or atrioventricular conduction. The effects of calcium antagonists on myocardial contractility have been discussed above.

Verapamil has the greatest effect on the gastrointestinal tract; constipation and nausea are more commonly caused by verapamil than by diltiazem or nifedipine.

Reversible renal deterioration in patients with chronic renal failure has been described to occur rarely with both nifedipine and diltiazem. Although the investigators postulated that this effect might be attributable to perturbation of compensatory renal autoregulation, this concept is difficult to reconcile with the above mentioned known ability of calcium antagonists to vasodilate preferentially the preglomerular resistance bed.

Discontinuation Syndrome

The abrupt withdrawal of antihypertensive medications, particularly the central sympatholytic agents, may result in rapid and marked increases in blood pressure. In contrast, there was no rebound in hypertension in several clinical antihypertensive drug trials with calcium antagonists, and it has been stated that a discontinuation syndrome does not occur with the use of calcium antagonists for the treatment of hypertension. Nevertheless, when possible, it seems reasonable to withdraw all antihypertensives, including calcium antagonists, slowly in patients with a background of apparent severe hypertension. In this regard, it has been suggested that nifedipine may exacerbate the increased angina associated with abrupt discontinuation of beta-blocker therapy. Of interest, abrupt discontinuation of calcium antagonist therapy in patients with ischemic heart disease has been reported to result rarely in rebound coronary artery spasm and unstable angina.

Metabolic Effects

Perhaps because we know more about diuretics and their unwanted side effects, they recently have come drawn more criticism than all other antihypertensive agents. The preliminary report of the British Medical Research Council (MRC) trial disclosed a 12% incidence of glucose intolerance in young people followed up for five years of diuretic therapy. Similarly, high incidences of hypokalemia, hyperuricemia, and adverse effects on the lipid profile have also been reported. In light of these

Calcium Antagonists • 147

observations, the metabolic effects of calcium antagonists should be considered in some detail.

Glucose Tolerance

Although calcium plays a role in resulting insulin release and calcium antagonists impair insulin release in animals, the results of recent studies indicate that glucose homeostasis is not adversely affected by clinically used doses of calcium antagonists (whereas anecdotal reports suggest that massive overdose may lead to marked hyperglycemia). For example, Shamoon et al. assessed the influence of oral verapamil on glucoregulatory hormones in humans during hyperglycemic clamp studies. They demonstrated that neither plasma insulin nor glucagon levels were altered in response to verapamil administration.

Lipid Profile

Careful studies in a large group of hypertensive patients disclosed that verapamil does not increase triglycerides or cholesterol; nor does it diminish serum high-density lipoprotein levels. Similar preliminary findings have been observed with diltiazem and nifedipine.

Potassium and Uric Acid

In contrast to the situation obtaining with diuretics, long-term studies have demonstrated that the administration of calciums antagonists does not significantly alter serum potassium or uric acid levels. Indeed, because of the dependence of aldosterone metabolism on calcium flux, calcium antagonists may reduce plasma aldosterone levels in some patients with primary aldosteronism, thereby ameliorating both the hypertension and the hypokalemia.

Dosage

The enormous interindividual variation in the rates of absorption, protein binding, and clearance of calcium antagonists, coupled with the variation in plasma concentration-response relationships preclude "hard

Table 5
Dosages of Calcium Antagonists for the Treatment of Hypertension*

	Form Supplied	Initial Dose (mg/day)	Maximal Dose (mg/day)	Frequency
Verapamil	40, 80, 120 mg tablets	240	480 to 720†	b.i.d. or t.i.d.
Slow-release verapamil	240 mg caplet	120 or 240	480 mg	q.d. or b.i.d.
Nifedipine	10, 20 mg capsules	30	120 to 180	t.i.d.
Diltiazem	30, 60, 90, 120 mg tablets	90	240 to 360?	t.i.d.
Slow-release diltiazem	60, 90, 120 mg capsules	120 to 240	360?	b.i.d.
Nicardipine	20, 30 mg capsules	60	120	t.i.d.

* Recommended or used by investigators reporting their studies and clinical experience.
† Most patients are controlled with no more than 120 mg t.i.d.

and fast" dosing schedules. In practice, the desired therapeutic effect will be arrived at by dose titration in the individual patient. The dosages and schedules that are generally recommended for the administration of calcium antagonists as monotherapeutic antihypertensive agents are shown in Table 5. Of course, as additional data become available concerning dose duration of action and dose side effect interactions, 24-hour blood pressure monitoring, and efficacy of long-acting preparations, these recommendations will undoubtedly change. As is the case with other blood pressure-lowering medications, the dosages needed for combination therapy are often lower than those usually employed for monotherapy.

The manufacturer of nicardipine recommends that the dose not be increased at intervals of less than three days and, because of the short duration of action of the drug, that blood pressure be checked at the time of both presumed peak (1 to 2 hours after dosing) and trough (8 hours after dosing) effects.

Finally, it is suggested that the sustained release form of verapamil be taken with food. This is believed to reduce the differences between the peak and trough blood levels of the agent, which may help limit the occurrence of side effects.

Drug Interactions

Drug interactions between calcium antagonists have been described. In particular, the concomitant use of verapamil and diltiazem is to be avoided because of the considerable risk of marked bradycardia. Drug interactions between calcium antagonists and quinidine, digoxin, phenytoin, theophylline, prazosin, propranolol, and rifampin, have been observed. When verapamil is used together with quinidine, patients may experience severe bradycardia and/or hypotension. Nifedipine and verapamil increase the plasma concentration of co-administered digoxin, and verapamil appears to increase the plasma level of prazosin. Verapamil and diltiazem also reduce the clearance of theophylline. Dilantin and rifampin tend to decrease the blood level of verapamil, and propranolol tends to increase it. Verapamil and diltiazem may enhance the effects of digoxin on atrioventricular conduction. Nicardipine may increase the blood levels of digoxin and cyclosporin. Although there are no absolute contraindications to the use of these combinations of medications, patients who receive them should be closely monitored.

Conclusions

Over the past decade multiple lines of research have implicated transmembrane calcium ion fluxes as an important mediator of the increased systemic vascular resistance that characterizes the majority of hypertensive states. Calcium antagonists exhibit a potent vasodilating effect by directly relaxing vascular smooth muscle. In contrast with previous vasodilators, reflex stimulation of heart rate appears to be minimal. Catecholamine release and the renin-angiotensin-aldosterone system are also minimally affected.

Numerous studies indicate that calcium antagonists effectively lower blood pressure in hypertensive subjects. Calcium antagonists are as effective as the other medications currently used to initiate antihypertensive therapy. They seem to work in all populations and perhaps may have a more pronounced antihypertensive effect when administered to older patients with low renin levels and high vascular resistance. Because of their relatively short half-lives, frequent administration of conventional preparations is required. Slow-release formulations, however, circumvent this problem. Such formulations of verapamil and diltiazem are already marketed, and the availability of such preparations for the other calcium antagonists is imminent.

Calcium antagonists have a unique spectrum of pharmacologic effects as well as actions on the cardiovascular system, so these agents have potentially important advantages in several groups of patients. Included in these categories are patients with co-existing coronary disease, variant angina, supraventricular arrhythmias, and probably some patients with left ventricular diastolic dysfunction ("stiff heart syndrome"). In this regard, it is possible that some of the newly developed and forthcoming calcium antagonists may prove to have less cardiac-pressant properties than do the currently available agents. For example, preliminary observations suggest that the investigational agent isradapine induces little decrease in myocardial contractileforce. Further study is required to determine the role of certain calcium antagonists in patients with previous myocardial infarctions and to determine whether the actions of calcium antagonists on the coronary circulation and their putative ability to reverse the progression of left ventricular hypertrophy and perhaps prevent or delay artherogenesis will prove to be of major clinical importance.

Finally, there is mounting concern that the choice the of an antihypertenisve agent should be predicted in part on its effect on the lipid profile and potassium metabolism. The demonstration that calcium antagonists do not exert adverse effects in this respect has thus assumed considerable importance. This paucity of adverse effects increasingly commends calcium antagonists as initial monotherapy in the management of hypertension.

Acknowledgment: We wish to thank Audrey M. Kincaid for her expert preparation of this manuscript.

Selected References

General

Braunwald E (guest editor): A symposium: calcium antagonists—emerging clinical opportunities. Am J Cardiol 59:1B-187B, 1987.

Epstein W, Oster JR: Hypertensionl Practical Management, 2nd edition. Miami, Battersea Medical Publications, 1988.

Epstein M, Oster JR: Role of calcium channel blockers. In: Epstein M, Oster JR (eds), Hypertension. Practical Management, 2nd edition. Miami, Battersea Medical Publications, 1988, pp 114–126.

Frolich ED (guest editor): A symposium: the calcium ion, cardiac myocyte and

vascular smooth muscle in hypertension and its treatment. Am J Cardiol 59:1A–121A, 1987.
Laragh JH (guest editor): A symposium: calcium antagonists in hypertension—focus on verapamil. Am J Cardiol 57:1D–107D, 1986.
Marone C, Luisoli S, Bomio F, et al: Body sodium-blood volume state, aldosterone, and cardiovascular responsiveness after calcium entry blockade with nifedipine. Kidney Int 28:658–665, 1985.
Murphy MB, Dollery C: Calcium antagonists in the treatment of hypertension. Proceedings of a symposium held in Scheveningen, The Netherlands, September 17–18, 1982. Hypertension 5 (part II):II-1–II-129, 1983.
Sorkin EM, Clissold SP: Nicardipine: a review of its pharmacodynamic and pharmacokinetic properties, and therapeutic efficacy, in the treatment of angina pectoris, hypertension, and related cardiovascular disorders. Drugs 33:296–345, 1987.
Willerson JT (guest editor): New directions in the use of calcium channel blockers. Am J Med 78:1–59, 1985.

Use As Antihypertensive Agents

Frishman WH, Charlap S, Ocken S, et al: Calcium channel blockers and systemic hypertension. J Clin Hyperten 2:107–122, 1985.
Frohlich ED (guest editor): Role of calcium channel blockers in the management of hypertension. Am J Med 79:1–43, 1985.
Halperin AK, Cubeddu LX: The role of calcium channel blockers in the treatment of hypertension. Am Heart J III:363–382, 1986.
Massie BM, Hirsch AT, Inouye IK, Tubau JF: Calcium channel blockers as antihypertensive agents. Am J Med 77:135–142, 1984.
Nicholson JP, Resnick LM, Laragh JH: The antihypertensive effect of verapamil at extremes of dietary sodium intake. Ann Intern Mcd 107:329–334, 1987.
Ram CVS: Southwest Internal Medicine Conference: Calcium antagonists in the treatment of hypertension. Am J Med Sci 290:118–133, 1985.
Resnick L: Calcium metabolism, renin activity, and the anti-hypertensive effects of calcium channel blockade. Am J Med 81:6–14, 1986.

Demographic Considerations

Ben-Ishay D, Leibel B, Stessman J: Calcium channel blockers in the management of hypertension in the elderly. Am J Med 81:30–34, 1986.
Campese VM: Effects of calcium antagonists on deranged modulation of the renal function curve in salt-sensitive patients with essential hypertension. Am J Cardiol 62:856–916, 1988.
Chobanian AV: Treatment of the elderly hypertensive patient. Am J Med 77:22–27, 1984.
Erne P, Bolli P, Bertel O, et al: Factors influencing the hypotensive effects of calcium antagonists. Hypertension 5(Suppl II):II97–II102, 1983.

152 • HYPERTENSION

Garthoff B, Kazda S, Knorr A, et al: Factors involved in the antihypertensive action of calcium antagonists. Hypertension 5(Suppl II):II34-II38, 1985.
Halperin AK, Gross KM, Rogers JF, et al: Verapamil and propranolol in essential hypertension. Clin Pharmacol Ther 36:750–758, 1984.

Salutary Effects In Addition to Lowering of Blood Pressure

Epstein M (guest editor): Calcium antagonists and the kidney. Am J Nephrol 7(Suppl 1):1–66, 1987.
Epstein M, Loutzenhiser R: Potential applicability of calcium antagonists as renal protective agents. In: Epstein M, Loutzenhiser R (eds), Calcium Antagonists and the Kidney. Philadelphia, F Hanley & Belfus, 1989, in press.
Frishman WH, Klein NA, Klein P, et al: Comparison of oral propranolol and verapamil for combined systemic hypertension and angina pectoris. A placebo-controlled double-blind randomized crossover trial. Am J Cardiol 50:1164–1172, 1981.
Hachamovitch R, Sonnenblick EH, Strom JA, et al: Left ventricular hypertrophy in hypertension and the effects of antihypertensive drug therapy. Curr Probl Cardiol 13:371–421, 1988.
Harizi RC, Bianco JA, Alpert JS: Diastolic function of the heart in clinical cardiology. Arch Intern Med 148:99–109, 1988.
Loutzenhiser R, Epstein M: Calcium antagonists and the kidney. Hospital Practice 22:63–76, 1987.
Panidis IP, Kotler MN, Ren JF, et al: Development and regression of left ventricular hypertrophy. J Am Coll Cardiol 3:1309–1320, 1984.
The Multicenter Diltiazem Postinfarction Trial Research Group: The effect of diltiazem on mortality and reinfarction after myocardial infarction. N Engl J Med 319:385–392, 1988.

Use in Patients with Severe or Complicated Hypertension

Epstein M, Oster JR: Antihypertensive agents in acute severe hypertension. In: Epstein M, Oster JR, Hypertension. Practical Management 2nd edition. Miami, Battersea Medical Publications, 1988, pp 175–185.
Murphy MB, Bulpitt CJ, Dollery CT: Role of nifedpine in thee treatment of resistant hypertension. Comparison with hydralazine in hospital outpatients. Am J Med 77:16–21, 1984.
Murphy MB, Scriven AJI, Dollery CT: Efficacy of nifedipine as a step 3 antihypertensive drug. Hypertension 5(Suppl II):118–121, 1983.

Combination Therapy

Bala Subramanian B: Combined therapy with calcium-channel and beta-blockers: facts, fiction, and practical aspects. Cardiovas Rev Rep 7:259–274, 1986.
Epstein M, Oster JR: The role of fixed-dose combination medications. In: Epstein

Calcium Antagonists • 153

M, Oster JR (eds), Hypertension. Practical Management, 2nd edition. Miami, Battersea Medical Publications, 1988, pp 127–135.

Opie LH, Jee L, White D: Antihypertensive effects of nifedipine combined with cardioselective beta-adrenergic receptor antagonism by atenolol. Am Heart J 104:606–612, 1984.

Wolfson P, Abernathy D, Dipetta DJ, et al: Diltiazem and captopril alone or in combination for treatment of mild to moderate systemic hypertension. Am J Cardiol 62:1036–1086, 1988.

Yagil Y, Kobrin I, Stessman J, et al: Effectiveness of combined nifedipine and propranolol treatment in hypertension. Hypertension 5(Suppl II)II:113–117, 1983.

Side Effects and Metabolic Effects

Boden WE, Korn KS, Bough EW: Nifedipine-induced hypotension and myocardial ischemia in refractory angina pectoris. JAMA 253:1131–1135, 1985.

Diamond JR, Cheung JY: Nifedipine-induced renal dysfunction: alterations in renal hemodynamics. Am J Med 77:905–909, 1984.

Enyeart JJ, Pricc WA, Hoffman DA: Profound hyperglycemia and metabolic acidosis after verapamil overdose. JACC 2:1228–1231, 1983.

Epstein M, Oster JR: The choice of an initial antihypertensive agent. J Clin Hyperten 3:1–11, 1986.

Krebs R: Adverse reactions with calcium anatgonists. Hypertension 5(Suppl II):II125–II129, 1983.

Pool PE, Herron JM, Rosenblatt S, et al: Metabolic effects of antihypertensive therapy with a calcium antagonist. Am J Cardiol 62:1096–1136, 1988.

Shamoon H, Baylor P, Kambosos D, et al: Influence of oral verapamil on glucoregulatory hormones in man. J Clin Endocrin Metab 60:536–541, 1985.

Zangerle KF, Wolford R: Syncope and conduction disturbances following sublingual nifedipine for hypertension. Ann Emer Med 14:1005–1006, 1985.

Chapter 8

Converting Enzyme Inhibitors in the Treatment of Hypertension

James A. Schoenberger

Introduction

The treatment of hypertension has evolved over the past 40 years primarily based on the availability of effective antihypertensive drugs but more recently on the emerging knowledge concerning the value of lowering blood pressure and the problems associated with the drugs available for this purpose. Originally there was a clear sense of urgency in lowering blood pressure when severely elevated, such as in malignant hypertension or accelerated hypertension. Under these circumstances, any agent that proved effective was acceptable, providing the side effects were tolerable. Many of the early treatments that lowered blood pressure, such as the rice/fruit diet, sympathectomy, and ganglionic blockade, were effective but the patient paid a high price for the reduction of blood pressure in the form of intolerable side effects and quality of life. A marked change occurred with the advent of diuretic therapy approximately 35 years ago and since that time diuretics have been the mainstay of most antihypertensive regimens. Beginning in 1970, the Joint National Committee on the Detection, Evaluation, and Treatment of High Blood Pressure has published a set of guidelines which have been periodically updated outlining the preferred treatment for high blood pressure. Diuretics were always listed as the drug of choice up

From Punzi HA, Flamenbaum W (eds): *Hypertension*. Mount Kisco, NY, Futura Publishing Co., Inc., © 1989.

to and including the most recent guidelines published in 1988. Additional drugs have been approved for initial therapy over the years and in the current guidelines diuretics, beta-blockers, angiotensin-converting enzyme (ACE) inhibitors, and calcium channel blockers have also been approved for initial or Step I treatment.

Throughout the evolution of the treatment of hypertension, following these guidelines of "stepped-care," therapy was initiated with one drug and a second and third drug was added sequentially when necessary to lower the blood pressure to acceptable limits. This approach has proven to be highly effective as witnessed by the approximately 60% decline in death rates from stroke which has occurred in the United States in the past 15 years. A 40% decline in deaths from coronary heart disease has also occurred during the same period but only some of this decline can be attributed to improved detection and treatment of high blood pressure.

At the same time, as newer drugs have become available, a number of major clinical trials have defined the level of blood pressure above which treatment is clearly superior to no treatment. This critical level for a clear indication of treatment has been declining as clinical trials have studied milder degrees of elevated blood pressure. The Veterans Administration Cooperative Trial, published in 1967, was the first study to show unequivocally the benefit for the treatment of severe hypertension with diastolic blood pressure of 115 mmHg or greater. Subsequent studies including the second portion of the Veterans Administration Cooperative Trial, published in 1970, and the Australian National Trial have shown that patients with a diastolic blood pressure above 95 mmHg are clearly benefited by treatment. Diastolic hypertension with a blood pressure of 90–95 mmHg still is a controversial area since the benefit of treatment shown by many studies is, at best, minimal with short term treatment. It is apparent that only long-term treatment can be of benefit to patients with this mild degree of elevated blood pressure, Under these circumstances, the regimen used to lower the blood pressure becomes of increasing importance since it is possible that adverse effects from the drugs used might outweigh the small benefit to be obtained.

Further, a great deal of attention has been focused in recent years on the quality of life of the hypertensive patient since many drugs available for the treatment of high blood pressure can adversely affect this important aspect of the patient's total well-being. It is becoming increasingly apparent that, at least for mild hypertension, how one lowers the blood pressure is of as great importance as lowering it. Not all drugs have the same impact on quality of life.

Some of the metabolic side effects long known to be associated with antihypertensive treatment have also received increasing attention. Diuretic treatment is known to be associated with hypokalemia, hypomagnesemia, hyperglycemia, hyperuricemia, and hypercholesterolemia. Some of these adverse metabolic effects can have a profound impact on the quality of life and perhaps the duration of life of the patient receiving diuretics. It is now known from the Multiple Risk Factor Intervention Trial (MRFIT) that patients with early left ventricular hypertrophy run an increased risk of sudden death when given large doses of diuretic drugs. This has led to a widespread acceptance of a reduction in the dose of diuretics to levels which are less likely to cause this complication.

Both diuretics and beta-blockers are known to be associated with adverse changes in the blood lipids which are pro-atherogenic. Although there is some controversy about the duration of these effects, the bulk of the evidence favors the view that they are longstanding. Although modest in degree, such changes can be clinically important. This finding may in part explain the generally recognized assumption that current antihypertension therapy based on the stepped-care method, which relies heavily on diuretics and beta-blockers, has failed to prevent one of the major complications of mild hypertension-coronary heart disease. With few exceptions, the clinical trials that have looked at coronary heart disease as an endpoint have failed to show any beneficial impact of antihypertensive treatment. This can be considered to be due perhaps to a reduction in the full benefit of lowering blood pressure because of the adverse metabolic effects associated with the drugs used. Future studies of mild hypertension using different drug regimens, such as the Treatment of Mild Hypertension Study (TOMHS), will address this important question to establish the ideal antihypertensive regimen for the treatment of mild hypertension. The ideal antihypertensive would be free of the adverse metabolic effects noted above and would not have an adverse effect on the quality of life of the patient. One such group of drugs which meets these requirements are the ACE inhibitors; their practical use in the treatment of high blood pressure will be described in the following sections of this chapter.

The Pharmacological Basis for the Antihypertensive Action of ACE Inhibitors

The renin-angiotensin aldersterone system plays a basic role in the regulation of blood volume and blood pressure. ACE inhibitors play an important part in this mechanism by their ability to prevent the conversion of angiotensin I to angiotensin II, a powerful vasoconstrictor which suppresses release of renin and stimulates secretion of aldosterone. Thus, angiotensin II causes a rise in blood pressure, both by its direct vasoconstrictor action and its stimulation of salt and water retention. ACE inhibitors interrupt this conversion, leading to a fall in blood pressure. ACE inhibitors also play an important role in the prevention of the enzymatic degradation of bradykinin to inactive peptides. Bradykinin is a vasodilator and stimulates the conversion of arachidonic acid to vasodilating prostaglandins. There is some evidence that not all ACE inhibitors share this ability to preserve the bradykinin levels and stimulate the production of prostaglandins. It is possible that only those ACE inhibitors containing the sulfhydril group may be capable of this action. In addition to these well-known effects of ACE inhibition, some of the hypotensive action of the ACE inhibitors occurs at the tissue level. The vascular endothelium plays an active role in local vascular regulation and there are tissue mechanisms for the conversion of angiotensin I to angiotensin II. This is of clinical importance insofar as ACE inhibitors have been shown to be effective in lowering blood pressure in patients with low circulating plasma renin, such as elderly and black hypertensives. The fall in blood pressure seen with ACE inhibitors does not, therefore, relate to the circulating plasma renin as specifically as it may to the tissue renin angiotensin system. It has recently been shown that ACE inhibitors containing the sulfhydril (SH) group may activate enzyme systems which potentiate the vasodilatary effect of nitrates and perhaps the effectiveness of endothelial-derived vasodilating constituents such as the endothelial-derived relaxing factor (EDRF) or nitric oxide.

The hemodynamic effects of ACE inhibitors are characterized by a reduction in total peripheral resistance with little change in heart rate or cardiac output. Blood pressure reduction achieved by ACE inhibitors is not associated with reflex tachycardia, possibly because there is simultaneous venodilatation and reduction of preload. It is also important to recognize that converting enzyme inhibitors cause a reduction in left ventricular mass in hypertensive patients, generally considered to be a desirable result of antihypertensive treatment. Finally, ACE inhibitors have a favorable effect on renal function since they increase renal blood flow without a corresponding increase in glomerular filtration rate, because of their preferential vasodilatary effect on the efferent arteriole of the glomerulus.

Currently Available ACE Inhibitors: Similarities and Differences

At the present time, three ACE inhibitors have been approved for use in the United States for treatment of high blood pressure. A large number of other compounds are in various stages of development. All of these share the ability to block the conversion of angiotensin I to angiotensin II. Some are derived from natural peptides, whereas the newer compounds are synthetic. The important clinical differences between these compounds appear to be based on the presence or absence of an SH group, potency, oral absorption, and pharmacokinetic properties, such as the duration of action. These characteristics are summarized in Table 1 for three of the presently available ACE inhibitors.

The significance of the SH group appears to confer on certain ACE inhibitors cardioprotective properties. It appears that those ACE inhibitors containing the SH group are effective in stimulating vasodilator prostaglandin synthesis. These ACE inhibitors also serve as SH donors to cause vasodilatation through the guanylate cyclase pathway. Studies suggest that the SH group potentiates the vasodilatory effect of nitrates and prevents nitrate tolerance in patients taking these drugs for angina. New developments include the use of ACE inhibitors with the SH group in the scavenger of oxygen-free radicals which arise during myocardial reperfusion. Although many of these properties are not fully explored, the presence of the SH group appears to be an advantage to those ACE inhibitors in which it is present.

The other major difference between the ACE inhibitors is their duration of action. It is generally considered desirable that any drug be

Table 1
Characteristics of ACE Inhibitors in Current Use

	Captopril	Enalapril	Lisinopril
Sulfhydril group	yes	no	no
Oral absorption (%)	75	60	30
Bioavailability (%)	70	40	25
Onset of action (h)	0.5–1	1–2	2–4
Duration of action (h)	3–4	12–24	24
Pro-drug	no	yes	no

Modified from Kostis JB: Am J Hypertension 2:57–64, 1989.

capable of administration once a day in order to maximize adherence to the regimen, although studies there is very little fall-off in adherence when a drug is given twice a day. In the case of the three commonly used ACE inhibitors, captopril has a duration of action of 3–4 hours, enalapril 12–24 hours, and lisinopril 24 hours. Captopril is generally administered in a twice a day dose, although some studies have shown that in certain mild hypertensives once a day suffices. This may be due to the fact that the tissue renin-angiotensin system is inhibited for a longer period than the plasma renin-angiotensin system by the administration of ACE inhibitors. These tissue mechanisms appear to play an important role in maintaining elevated blood pressure. Enalapril is generally given in a once or twice a day dose although its duration of action is not invariably a full 24 hours. Of all three currently used ACE inhibitors, lisinopril appears to have the longest duration of action and can be given once a day.

Although the ACE inhibitors vary in their potency, this usually has little clinical significance since it is compensated for by adjusting the dose of the medication. Some of the ACE inhibitors are administered in the form of a pro-drug in order to enhance absorption after oral administration. When administered in this form, there may be some delay in the onset of action but there is a prolongation of action compared to the active analog. The advantage of rapid action versus delayed action must be considered in each individual case. Finally, the route of elimination may differ among the various ACE inhibitors. Most undergo biotransformation in the liver and excretion via the kidneys. This may be of clinical importance in patients with liver disease and renal disease, and there may be some advantage to ACE inhibitors that have alternate routes of excretion both in the urine and the feces.

Practical Guidelines for the Use of ACE Inhibitors in the Treatment of Hypertension

When ACE inhibitors were first introduced for the treatment of high blood pressure, it was recommended that they be used for those patients with moderate to severe hypertension who were resistant to conventional therapy. It was recommended then that only those patients who failed to respond to a combination of three drugs (diuretic, beta-blocker, and vasodilator) would be candidates for converting enzyme inhibitor therapy. As a result, the patients who received ACE inhibitors in these early years were generally more advanced in the severity of their hypertension and in accompanying renal damage. The side effects commonly associated with ACE inhibitors in that era were more likely to occur and there was some concern that the drug had a high side-effect profile. In recent years there has been a dramatic change in the indication for, and the use of, the ACE inhibitors in that they are now commonly used in the management of early hypertension even of milder degree and in considerably smaller doses. In this use of ACE inhibitors in smaller doses, few of the side effects formerly observed are seen, and the drugs have emerged as extremely well-tolerated antihypertensive agents with many potential advantages for the initial treatment of hypertension. This perspective of their role has been recognized in the 1988 guidelines of the Joint National Committee which lists ACE inhibitors as one of the four approved drugs for the initiation of antihypertensive treatment.

Many clinical trials have now shown that ACE inhibitors are effective in the monotherapy of high blood pressure. In this connection, they appear to be as effective as most other antihypertensive agents. About 40%–50% of patients with high blood pressure can be effectively controlled with monotherapy with any of the ACE inhibitors currently available. In these studies, the definition of a good response varies, but the conventional definition of a good blood pressure of less than 90 mmHg diastolic has been the most widely accepted criterion. ACE inhibitors have been compared to diuretics and beta-blockers and found to be equal or superior in efficacy as far as reduction of blood pressure is concerned. It is important to note that, although the ACE inhibitors are effective in reducing blood pressure, no studies have yet evaluated what impact this would have on the long-term effect on the endpoints associated with hypertension, such as heart attack and stroke. All of the clinical trials that have addressed this issue have been limited to antihypertensive treatment with diuretics, beta-blockers, and other adrenergic-inhibiting drugs. Since ACE inhibitors do not cause a change in blood lipids, they may be ideal agents.

The ACE inhibitors have also been evaluated in combination with other antihypertensive agents. Many studies have shown that the addition of a diuretic to treatment of hypertension with an ACE inhibitor will increase the percent of patients who are brought under satisfactory control to as high as 90%–95%. It is important to note that the tendency of ACE inhibitors to cause a slight rise in serum potassium concentration offsets the decrease in serum potassium concentration associated with diuretic therapy, making this an ideal combination. A similar buffering effect on uric acid concentration has also been observed. A number of studies have also shown that there is a synergism of action between ACE inhibitors and calcium blockers. The combination of ACE inhibitors with other agents such as the beta-blockers appears to be less effective.

Studies on the effect of ACE inhibitors on the quality of life of hypertensive patients have been carried out with captopril. It has been shown that the sense of well-being and other parameters improve with captopril but are diminished by treatment with propranolol or methyldopa. This has given rise to some speculation that ACE inhibitors may actually cause an enhanced sense of well-being, although other possible explanations for this effect must be considered. A great deal of interest in the quality of life of hypertensive patients now exists since, the short-term benefit of antihypertensive treatment in patients with mild hypertension is minimal. Drug regimens that permit control of elevated blood pressure without a substantial sacrifice in the quality of life are the only acceptable method of dealing with this important problem. There is some indirect evidence that the addition of a diuretic to patients treated with captopril blunts many of the favorable effects on the quality of life which are observed with captopril therapy alone. Further studies are necessary to compare all major antihypertensive drugs in regard to their effect on the quality of life using similar methodology and with double-blind placebo controls.

The ACE inhibitors have several other important qualities that must be taken into consideration in the treatment of high blood pressure. It has been shown that patients with congestive heart failure not only have symptomatic improvement but prolongation of life when treated with ACE inhibitors. It has also been shown that the use of ACE inhibitors following myocardial infarction prevents ventricular remodeling and dilatation. These findings suggest that patients with coronary artery disease and a history of myocardial infarction or congestive heart failure would benefit with the use of ACE inhibitors as the preferred drug in the treatment of high blood pressure.

There is growing evidence that ACE inhibitors have a beneficial effect on diabetes mellitus. In the experimental animal model, dilatation of the efferent arteriole of the glomerulus leads to reduction of glomerular pressure and preservation of glomerular function and to a decrease in urinary albumin excretion. Studies are now on-going in human diabetics to determine if early treatment with ACE inhibitors will preserve renal function and alter the natural history of type I diabetes by preventing glomerulosclerosis and renal failure. Although the evidence is not complete, it would appear that diabetic hypertensives should be treated with ACE inhibitors. It also appears likely that diabetic patients with proteinuria who are not hypertensive may also benefit from the use of ACE inhibitors.

Because elderly hypertensives and black hypertensives generally have low plasma renin levels, it has been assumed that ACE inhibitors would be ineffective in lowering elevated blood pressure in these groups. In the case of black hypertensives, ACE inhibitors are nearly as effective as in white hypertensives but perhaps a slightly larger dose will be required to control the blood pressure. When combined with a diuretic, there is no difference in the response of blacks and whites in regard to the control of hypertension using ACE inhibitors. Many recent studies have confirmed that ACE inhibitors are as effective in elderly hypertensives as in younger individuals and the dose required to achieve the desired effect does not appear to be any greater. In addition, recent evidence has also established the effectiveness of ACE inhibitors in isolated systolic hypertension.

The dose of ACE inhibitor required to control blood pressure varies from individual to individual and with each of the different ACE inhibitors, captopril has a rapid onset of action and effectively controls blood pressure for a period of 6–10 hours. It is generally given in a dose of 25 mg twice a day to 50 mg twice a day, up to a maximum of 150 mg a day total dose. An occasional patient may be well controlled with 50 mg once a day, and most mild hypertensive patients can be controlled on once a day dosage when the drug is combined with a diuretic. Enalapril has a slightly prolonged onset of action because it is administered as a pro-drug, but it appears to control elevated blood pressure for almost 24 hours. It is generally administered in a dose of 2.5 to 10 mg twice a day with a maximum dose of 40 mg. Lisinopril has a shorter onset of action because it is not administered as a pro-drug but a longer total duration of action, which provides effective control of blood pressure for at least 24 hours. It is generally administered in a dose of 5–20 mg daily up to a maximum of 40 mg daily. When it has been determined that the patient will be started on antihypertensive treatment using an ACE inhibitor, an attempt should be made to maintain monotherapy and to titrate the dose to the maximum recommended. About 40%–50% of hypertensive patients can be controlled on monotherapy with one of these regimens. When monotherapy fails, a combination with a diuretic or a calcium blocker appears to be the best regimen at the present time and will afford control of elevated blood pressure in as high as 90%–95% of patients. These dosage recommendations are shown in Table 2.

Because of their effect on serum potassium concentration, ACE inhibitors should be used with caution when potassium-sparing diuretics

Table 2
Dose Range of ACE Inhibitors

	Initial Dose (mg)	Maximum Total Dose (mg)
Captopril	25–50 BID	150
Enalapril	2.5 BID	40
Lisinopril	10 QD	40

With permission from Williams GH: NEJM 319:1517–1525, 1988.

of potassium supplements are given. Also, the use of nonsteroidal anti-inflammatory agents may diminish the antihypertensive effect of some of the ACE inhibitors but the importance of this in the long term is not fully known.

As with all other antihypertensive drugs, ACE inhibitors have undesirable side effects. In their initial use, problems with rash, taste disturbance, angioneurotic edema, and proteinuria were commonly seen with the doses then used. In more recent years, treating less complicated hypertension with smaller doses, the incidence of these side effects is quite low and the drugs are generally considered to be quite safe and well tolerated. The most clinically significant side effect has been persistent, nonproductive cough. This is more likely to occur with the long-acting ACE inhibitors and there is no effective treatment for it other than cessation of medication. A precise estimation of the incidence of cough is impossible but in a recent study of a large number of patients, it occurred in less than 1% of the cases receiving captopril. Generally, switching from one ACE inhibitor to another does not prevent the cough.

ACE inhibitors can be associated with hypotension. This is more likely to occur in patients with recent heart failure or in hypertensives currently on diuretics, and therefore the initial dose of ACE inhibitor in this setting should be quite low. Shorter-acting ACE inhibitors may have an advantage under these circumstances since hypotension will be of shorter duration. Two relatively rare complications of ACE inhibitor therapy are angioneurotic edema and renal failure in patients with bilateral artery stenosis.

Summary

ACE inhibitors are a class of antihypertensive drugs that have received wide acceptance in recent years because they are effective in

Converting Enzyme Inhibitors • 165

patients of all ages, and in both races, either in monotherapy or in combination treatment with diuretics. They appear to be as effective in lowering blood pressure as other classes of antihypertensive agents but without the adverse side effects seen with the diuretics and beta-blockers. Their use is associated with a preservation or enhancement of the quality of life. It remains to be seen whether their use in the control of elevated blood pressure will prolong life and prevent the complications of hypertension.

Selected References

Brenner BM: The kidney: Therapeutic implications of ACE inhibition. Am J Hypertension 1(4)Part 2:p331s–422s, 1988.
Case DB: ACE Inhibitors: Are they all alike? J Clin Hypertension 3(3):243–256, 1987.
Croog SH, Levine S, Sudilovsky A, et al: Sexual symptoms in hypertensive patients: A clinical trial of antihypertensive medications. Arch Int Med 148:788–794, 1988.
Croog SH, Levine S, Testa MA, et al: The effects of antihypertensive therapy on the quality of life. N Engl J Med 314(26):1657–1664, 1986.
Curb JD, Borhani NO, Blaszkowski TT, et al: Long-term surveillance for adverse effects of antihypertensive drugs. JAMA 253(22):3263–3268, 1985.
The Captopril-Digoxin Multicenter Research Group: Comparative effects of captopril and digoxin in patients with mild to moderate heart failure. JAMA 259(4):539–544, 1988.
DiBianco R: Survival in patients with heart failure: Focus on captopril. Clin Ther 10(2):204–215, 1988.
Dzau VJ: Evolving concepts of the renin-angiotensin system: Focus on renal and vascular mechanisms. Am J Hypertension 1:3345–3375, 1988.
Dzau VJ: Significance of the vascular renin-agiotension pathway. Hypertension 8(7):553–559, 1986.
Hollenberg NK (ed): Experience, progress and clinical perspectives on angiotensin converting enzyme inhibition. Am J Med 84(4A):1–46, 1988.
Hollenberg NK, Rapaport E (eds): Regional hemodynamics following captopril therapy. Am J Med 76(5B) 1–118, 1984.
The Management Committee: The Australian Therapeutic Trial in Mild Hypertension. Lancet 1:1261–1267, 1980.
Multiple Risk Factor Intervention Trial Research Group: Risk factor changes and mortality results. JAMA 248:1165–1477, 1982.
Parving H-H, Andersen AR, Smidt UM, et al: Early aggressive antihypertensive treatment reduces rate of decline in kidney function in diabetic nephropathy. Lancet 1:1175, 1983.
Parving HH, Hommel E, Smidt UM, et al: Protection of kidney function and decrease in albuminuria by captopril in insulin-dependent diabetics with nephropathy. Br Med J 297:1086–1091, 1988.
Reyes AJ, Leary WP, Acosta-Barrios, TN et al: Further experience with once-

daily captopril monotherapy in essential hypertension. Curr Ther Res 43(4):698–706, 1988.

Sharpe N, Murphy J, Smith H, et al: Treatment of patients with symptomless left ventricular dysfunction after myocardial infarction. Lancet 1:255–259, 1988.

Sleight P, Zanchetti A (eds): The renin-agiotensin system and the heart. Am J Med 84(3A):1–162, 1988.

1988 Report of the Joint National Committee on Detection, Evaluation, and Treatment of High Blood Pressure. Arch Int Med 148:1023–1038, 1988.

Tuck ML, Katz LA, Kirkendall WM, et al: Low dose captopril in mild to moderate geriatric hypertension. J Am Geriatr Soc 34:693–696, 1986.

Veterans Administration Cooperative Study Group on Antihypertensive Agents: Effects of treatment on morbidity in hypertension. II. Results of patients with diastolic blood pressures averaging 115 through 129 mmHg. JAMA 202:1028–1034, 1967.

Veterans Administration Cooperative Study Group on Antihypertensive Agents: Effects of treatment on morbidity in hypertension. II. Results in patients with diastolic blood pressure averaging 90 through 114 mmHg. JAMA 213:1114–1152, 1970.

Veterans Administration Cooperative Study Group on Antihypertensive Agents: Racial differences in response to low dose captopril are abolished by the addition of hydrochlorothizide. Br J Clin Pharmacol 14(S2):97s–101s, 1985.

Viberti GC, Wiseman MJ: The kidney in diabetes: significance of the early abnormalities. Clin Endocrinol Med 15:753, 1986.

Williams GH: Converting-enzyme inhibitors in the treatment of hypertension. N Engl J Med 319(23):1517–1525, 1988.

Williams GH: Quality of life and its impact on hypertensive patients. Am J Med 82:98–105, 1987.

Working Group on Hypertension in Diabetes: Statement on hypertension in diabetes mellitus—Final Report. Arch Int Med 147:8320–842, 1987.

Working Group on Renovascular Hypertension, Detection, Evaluation, and Treatment of Renovascular Hypertension—Final Report. Arch Int Med 147:820–829, 1987.

Zusman RM: Effects of converting enzyme inhibitors on the renin-angiotensin, aldosterone, bradykinin, and arachidonic acid prostaglandin systems: Correlation of the chemical structure and biologic activity. Am J Kidney Dis X(1)(S1):13–23, 1987.

Chapter 9

Beta-Adrenergic Blockade in Systemic Hypertension

William H. Frishman

Introduction

It is now well recognized that beta-blockers are effective in reducing the blood pressure of many patients with systemic hypertension. Although there is no consensus as to the mechanism whereby the beta-blocker drugs lower blood pressure, it is probable that some, or all, of the mechanisms referred to in Table 1 are involved.

The various beta-blockers differ in terms of the presence or absence of intrinsic sympathomimetic activity (ISA), membrane-stabilizing activity (MSA), beta-1-selectivity, alpha-blocking properties, and relative potencies and duration of action. Nevertheless, all beta-blockers to date appear to have blood pressure-lowering effects. This chapter reviews the pharmacological differences among the various beta-blockers, their circulatory and noncirculatory effects, and finally, their use in different population groups.

Pharmacodynamic and Pharmacokinetic Properties

As a class of drugs, the beta-blockers have been so successful that many of them have been synthesized, and over 20 are available on the world market. The application of these agents has been accelerated by

From Punzi HA, Flamenbaum W (eds): *Hypertension*. Mount Kisco, NY, Futura Publishing Co., Inc., © 1989.

Table 1
Proposed Mechanisms to Explain the Antihypertensive Actions of Beta-Blockers

1. Reduction in cardiac output
2. Central nervous system effect
3. Inhibition of renin
4. Reduction in venous return and plasma volume
5. Reduction in peripheral vascular resistance
6. Resetting of baroreceptor levels
7. Effects on prejunctional beta-receptors; reduction in norepinephrine release
8. Prevent the pressor response to catecholamines with exercise and stress

(With permission from Frishman WH: Clinical Pharmacology of the Beta-Adrenoceptor Blocking Drugs, 2nd ed. Norwalk, Appleton-Century-Crofts, 1984, p 28.)

the development of drugs possessing a degree of selectivity for two beta-adrenoceptor subgroups: beta-1-receptors in the heart and beta-2-receptors in the peripheral circulation and bronchi. More controversial has been the introduction of beta-blocking drugs with alpha-adrenergic blocking action, varying amounts of ISA, and nonspecific membrane stabilizing effects. There also are pharmacokinetic differences among beta-blocking drugs that may be of clinical importance.

Pharmacodynamic Properties

Potency

Beta-blocking drugs are competitive inhibitors of catecholamine binding at beta-adrenoceptor sites. They reduce the effect of any concentration of catecholamine agent on a sensitive tissue. The dose-response curve of the agonist is shifted to the right; a given tissue response requires a higher concentration of agonist in the presence of beta-blocking drugs. Beta-blocker potency can be assessed by the inhibition of tachycardia produced by isoproterenol or exercise; potency varies from compound to compound (Table 2).

These differences in potency are of no therapeutic relevance. However, they do explain the different drug dosages needed to achieve ef-

Table 2
Pharmacodynamic Properties of Beta-Adrenoceptor Blocking Drugs

Drug	β-Blockade Potency Ratio (Propranolol = 1.0)	Relative β₁-Selectivity	Intrinsic Sympatho-mimetic Activity	Membrane-Stabilizing Activity
Acebutolol	0.3	+	+	+
Atenolol	1.0	+ +	0	0
Bevantolol	0.3	+ +	0	0
Bisoprolol	10.3	+ +	0	0
Bucindolol††		0	+	0
Carteolol	10.0	0	+	0
Carvedilol*	10.0	0	0	+ +
Celiprolol**	9.4	+	+ ?	0
Dilevalol†	1.0	0	+ ?	0
Esmolol	0.02	+ +	0	0
Labetalol††	0.3	0	0	0
Metoprolol	1.0	+ +	0	+
Nadolol	1.0	0	0	0
Oxprenolol	0.5–1.0	0	+	+
Penbutolol	1.0	0	+ +	0
Pindolol	6.0	0	+ +	+
Propranolol	1.0	0	0	+ +
Sotalol§	0.3	0	0	0
Tertatolol		0	0	0
Timolol	6.0	0	0	+ +

Isomer: d-propranolol

* = carvedilol has additional α₁-adrenergic-blocking activity without peripheral β₂-agonism; ** = celiprolol may have additional peripheral α₂-adrenergic blocking activity at high doses; † = dilevalol is an isomer of labetalol adrenergic with peripheral β₂-agonism but no α₁-blocking activity; †† = bucindolol and labetalol have additional α₁-adrenergic blocking activity and direct vasodilatory actions (β₂-agonism); § = sotalol has additional types of antiarrhythmic activity. (With permission from Frishman WH: Clinical Pharmacology of the Beta-Adrenoceptor Blocking Drugs, 2nd ed. Norwalk, Appleton-Century-Crofts, 1984, p 15, and Frishman WH: the beta-adrenergic blockers. Med Clin N Amer 72:41, 1988.)

fective beta-adrenergic blockade when initiating therapy in patients or when switching from one agent to another.

MSA

In concentrations well above therapeutic levels, certain beta-blockers have a quinidinelike or "local anesthetic" effect on the cardiac action potential. There is no evidence that MSA is responsible for any direct negative inotropic effects of beta-blocking drugs since both drugs with and without this property equally depress left ventricular function. MSA can manifest itself clinically during massive beta-blocker intoxications.

Selectivity

The beta-adrenoceptor blockers may be classified as selective or nonselective, according to their relative abilities to antagonize the actions of sympathomimetic amines in some tissues at lower doses than those required in other tissues. When used in low doses, beta-1-selective blocking agents, such as atenolol and metoprolol, inhibit cardiac beta-1-receptors but have less influence on bronchial and vascular beta-adrenoceptors (beta-2).

Because selective beta-1-blockers have less of an inhibitory effect on the beta-2-receptors, they have two theoretical advantages. The first is that beta-1-selective agents may be safer than nonselective ones in patients with obstructive pulmonary disease because beta-2-receptors remain available to mediate adrenergic bronchodilation. In some clinical trials on patients with asthma, relatively low doses of beta-1-selective agents caused a lower incidence of side effects than did similar doses of propranolol. However, even selective beta-blockers may aggravate bronchospasm in certain patients, so that these drugs generally should not be used in patients with bronchospastic disease.

The second theoretical advantage is that unlike nonselective beta-blockers, beta-1-selective blockers in low doses may not block the beta-2-receptors that mediate dilation of arterioles. This property might be advantageous in the treatment of hypertension with relatively low doses of beta-1-adrenergic drugs, but this possibility has not been demonstrated. During infusion of epinephrine, nonselective beta-blockers can cause a pressor response by blocking beta-2-receptor-mediated vasodilation, since alpha-adrenergic vasoconstrictor receptors are still operative. Selective beta-1-antagonists may not induce this pressor effect in the presence of epinephrine and may lessen the impairment of peripheral blood flow.

It is possible that leaving the beta-receptors unblocked and responsive to epinephrine may be functionally important in some patients with asthma, hypoglycemia, hypertension, or peripheral vascular disease treated with beta-adrenergic blocking drugs.

ISA (Partial Agonist Activity)

Certain beta-blockers (acebutolol, alprenolol, carteolol, oxprenolol, penbutolol, pindolol) possess partial agonist activity (PAA). These drugs cause a slight-to-moderate activation of the beta-receptor, even as they prevent the access of natural and synthetic catecholamines to the receptor sites. The result is a weak stimulation of the receptor.

Quantitative assessment of the PAA of a beta-blocker is made by observing the action of the drug in animals whose resting sympathetic tone has been abolished by adrenalectomy and retreatment with reserpine or syringoserpine. If the beta-blocker increases the heart rate or force of myocardial contraction, the drug has PAA. The effects are known to be mediated through beta-adrenergic stimulation because they can be antagonized by propranolol. Whether or not PAA in a beta-blocker offers an overall advantage in cardiac therapy remains a matter of controversy. Some investigators suggest that drugs with this property may reduce peripheral vascular resistance, and may depress atrioventricular conduction less than other beta-blockers. Other investigators claims that PAA in a beta-blocker protects against myocardial depression, bronchial asthma, and peripheral vascular complications in patients receiving therapy. However, these claims have not yet been substantiated by definitive clinical trials.

Alpha-Adrenergic Activity

Labetalol is a beta-blocker with antagonistic properties at both alpha- and beta-adrenoceptors. Labetalol is 4–16 times more potent at beta- than at alpha-adrenoceptors. In a series of tests, the drug has been shown to be 6–10 times less potent than phentolamine at alpha-adrenoceptors and 1.5–4 times less potent than propranolol at beta-adrenoceptors. A stereoisomer of labetalol, dilevalol, with peripheral beta-2-agonist properties, is now being evaluated in hypertension and angina.

Whether or not concomitant alpha-adrenergic activity is generally advantageous in a beta-blocker has not yet been determined. In the case of labetalol, alpha-adrenergic blocking action does result in a reduction of peripheral vascular resistance, and unlike most other beta-blockers, labetalol may maintain cardiac output in patients.

Pharmacokinetic Properties

Although the beta-adrenergic blocking drugs have similar pharmacotherapeutics, their pharmacokinetic properties differ significantly (Tables 3, 4) in ways that may influence their clinical usefulness in some patients. Among individual drugs, there are differences in completion of gastrointestinal absorption, amount of first-pass hepatic metabolism, lipid solubility, protein binding, extent of distribution in the body, penetration into the brain, concentration in the heart, rate of hepatic biotransformation, pharmacological activity of metabolite, and renal clearance of the drug and its metabolites.

On the basis of their pharmacokinetic properties, the beta-blockers can be classified into two broad categories: those eliminated by hepatic metabolism and those eliminated unchanged by the kidney. Drugs in the first group, propranolol and metoprolol, for example, are lipid-soluble, are almost completely absorbed by the small intestine, and are largely metabolized by the liver. They tend to have highly variable bioavailability and relatively short plasma half-lives. In contrast, drugs in the second category are more water-soluble, are incompletely absorbed throughout the gut, and are excreted unchanged by the kidney. They show less variable bioavailability and have longer half-lives.

Many of the beta-blockers, including those with short plasma half-lives, can be administered as infrequently as twice daily. The longer the half-life, of course, the more useful the drug is likely to be for patients who experience difficulty in compliance.

In medical practice, the pharmacokinetic properties of the different beta-adrenergic blockers are important. The clinician who is administering a drug must be knowledgeable about the extent of first-pass metabolism, its active metabolites, and its lipid solubility. Oral agents with extensive first-pass effect necessitate a larger dosage than the intravenous dosage. Knowing if the drug is transformed into active metabolites (acebutolol) as opposed to inactive metabolites is important in gauging the total pharmacological effect.

Finally, for some beta-blockers, lipid solubility has been associated

Table 3
Pharmacokinetic Properties of Various Beta-Adrenoceptor-Blocking Drugs

Drug	Extent of Absorption (% of Dose)	Extent of Bioavailability (% of Dose)	Dose-Dependent Bioavailability (major First-Pass Hepatic Metabolism)	Interpatient Variations in Plasma Levels	β-Blocking Plasma Concentrations	Protein Binding (%)	Lipid Solubility†
Acebutolol	≈70	≈40	No	7-fold	0.2–2.0 µg/mL	25	Moderate
Atenolol	≈50	≈40	No	4-fold	0.2–5.0 µg/mL	<5	Weak
Bevantolol	≈90	≈55	No	4-fold	0.13–3.0 µg/mL	95	Moderate
Carteolol	≈90	≈90	No	2-fold	40–160 ng/mL	20–30	Weak
Celiprolol	≈30	≈30	No	3-fold		≈30	Weak
Esmolol‡	NA	NA	NA	5-fold	0.15–1.0 µg/mL	55	Weak
Labetalol	>90	≈33	Yes	10-fold	0.7–3.0 µg/mL	≈50	Weak
Metoprolol	>90	≈50	No	7-fold	50–100 ng/mL	12	Moderate
Nadolol	≈30	≈30	No	7-fold	50–100 ng/mL	≈30	Weak
Oxprenolol	≈90	≈40	No	5-fold	80–100 ng/mL	80	Moderate
Penbutolol	>90	≈90	No	4-fold		98	High
Pindolol	>90	≈90	No	4-fold	5–15 ng/mL	57	Moderate
Propranolol	>90	≈30	Yes	20-fold	50–100 ng/mL	93	High
Long-acting propranolol	>90	≈20	Yes	10- to 20-fold	20–100 ng/mL	93	High
Sotalol	≈70	≈60	No	4-fold	0.5–4.0 µg/mL	0	Weak
Timolol	>90	≈75	No	7-fold	5–10 ng/mL	≈10	Weak

† Determined by the distribution ratio between octanol and water; ‡ ultrashort-acting β-blocker only available in intravenous form; NA = not applicable. (With permission from Frishman WH: Clinical Pharmacology of the β-Adrenoceptor Blocking Drugs. Edition 2. Norwalk, CT, Appleton-Century-Crofts, 1984, and Frishman WH: the beta-adrenergic blockers. Med Clin N Amer 72:46, 1988.)

Table 4
Elimination Characteristics of Beta-Adrenoceptor-Blocking Drugs

Drug	Elimination Half-life (H)	Total Body Clearance (mL H/Min)	Urinary Recovery of Unchanged Drug (% of Dose)	Total Urinary Recovery (% of Dose)	Predominant Route of Elimination†	Active Metabolites	Drug Accumulation in Renal Disease
Acebutolol	3–4‡	6–15	≈40	>90	RE (≈40% unchanged and HM)	Yes	Yes
Atenolol	6–9	130	≈40	>95	RE	No	Yes
Bevantolol	2–4	960	1	74	HM	No	No
Carteolol	5–6	497	40–68	90	RE	Yes	Yes
Celiprolol	5	500	≈90	≈30	RE (≈50% unchanged and HM)	Yes	No
Esmolol§	9 min	27,000	<2	70–90	BE‖	No	No
Labetalol	3–4	2,700	<1	>90	HM	No	No
Metoprolol	3–4	1,100	≈3	>95	HM	No	No
Nadolol	14–24	200	70	70	RE	No	Yes
Oxyprenolol	2–3	380	2–5	70–95	HM	No	No
Penbutolol	27	350	50–70	>90	RE	No	No
Pindolol	3–4	400	≈40	>90	RE (≈40% unchanged and HM)	No	No
Propranolol	3–4	1,000	<1	>90	HM	Yes	No
Long-acting propranolol	10	1,000	<1	>90	HM	Yes	No
Sotalol	9–10	150	≈60	>90	RE	No	Yes
Timolol	4–5	660	≈20	65	RE U (≈20% unchanged and HM)	No	No

† RE = renal excretion; HM = hepatic metabolism; ‡ Acebutolol has an active metabolite with elimination half-life of 8 to 13 hours; § Ultrashort-acting β-blocker only available in intravenous form; ‖ Metabolized by blood esterases. (With permission from Frishman WH: Clinical Pharmacology of the β-Adrenoceptor Blocking Drugs. Edition 2. Norwalk, Appleton-Century-Crofts, 1981, p 2, and Frishman WH: the beta-adrenergic blockers. Med Clin N Amer 72:47, 1988.)

with the entry of these drugs into the brain, resulting in side effects that are probably unrelated to beta-blockade, such as lethargy, mental depression, and even hallucinations. Whether or not drugs that are less lipid-soluble cause fewer of these adverse reactions remains to be determined.

Cardiovascular Effects

Blood Pressure

It is now well recognized that beta-adrenergic blockers are effective in reducing the blood pressure of many patients with systemic hypertension. At the present time there is no consensus of opinion as to the mechanism(s) whereby these drugs lower blood pressure. It is probable that some or all of the mechanisms proposed in the following sections play a part.

Negative Chronotropic and Inotropic Effects

Slowing of the heart rate and some decrease in myocardial contractility with beta-blockers lead to a decrease in cardiac output that in both the short and long term may lead to a reduction in blood pressure. It might be expected that these factors would be of particular importance in the treatment of hypertension related to high cardiac output and increased sympathetic tone.

Central Nervous System Effect

There is now good clinical and experimental evidence to suggest that most beta-blockers cross the blood-brain barrier and enter the central nervous system. The occurrence of dreams, insomnia, hallucinations, and depression during therapy with many beta-blockers supports this conjecture.

Infusion of 1- and d,l-propranolol into the cerebral ventricles of conscious rabbits was reported to cause a marked antihypertensive effect, whereas d-propranolol alone caused the blood pressure to rise. By injecting drugs into the vertebral arteries of anesthetized dogs, other investigators found a central antihypertensive action for alprenolol but not for propranolol. Although there is little doubt that beta-blockers with high lipophilicity (e.g., metoprolol, propranolol) enter the central nervous system in high concentrations, a direct antihypertensive effect mediated by this property is not well defined. Also, beta-blockers that are less lipid-soluble and less likely to concentrate in the brain appear to be as effective in lowering blood pressure as propranolol.

Differences in Effects on Plasma Renin

The relationship between the hypotensive action of beta-blocking drugs and their ability to reduce plasma renin activity remains one of the more controversial areas in hypertension research. There is no doubt that some beta-blocking drugs can antagonize sympathetically mediated renin release. Adrenergic activity is not the only mechanism whereby renin release is mediated, however. Other major determinants are sodium balance, posture, and renal perfusion pressure.

Laragh and co-workers have suggested that a decrease in renin output by the kidney is the major factor contributing to the antihypertensive effects of beta-blockers. Propranolol lowers plasma renin activity in normal and hypertensive subjects and blocks the orthostatic rise in plasma renin activity while standing. The dextroisomer of propranolol has no effect on renin release, unlike the inhibitory action of racemic propranolol in the same patient. The suppressant effect of racemic propranolol is therefore dependent on the beta-blocking action of the levoisomer.

The effect of different beta-blockers on resting and orthostatic renin release is variable. Among the nonselective beta-blockers, propranolol causes the greatest reduction of both resting and orthostatic renin release, timolol causes significant reduction, oxprenolol has less effect (especially on orthostatic renin release), and pindolol has the least effect. Weber and co-workers found that in the rabbit, pindolol causes a rise in plasma renin activity; Stokes and co-workers found that when patients were switched from propranolol to pindolol, they continued to have good control of their blood pressure despite a rise in plasma renin activity. It has been suggested that oxprenolol and pindolol have a lesser effect on renin than propranolol because of their partial agonist properties.

Beta-1-selective blockers show similar variation in their effects on renin; metoprolol lowers resting and furosemide-induced renin release, while the reports are conflicting for atenolol (Amery and coworkers showed no effect, whereas Aberg demonstrated a significant decrease in resting renin). The effectiveness of some beta-1-selective adrenergic blockers in reducing renin suggests that in humans renin release is mediated by a beta-1-receptor-mediated mechanism.

The important question remains whether there is a clinical correlation between the beta-blocker effect on plasma renin activity and the lowering of blood pressure. Laragh and associates found that "high renin" patients respond well to propranolol, "low renin" patients do not respond or may even show a rise in blood pressure, and "normal renin" patients have less predictable responses. Other investigators have been unable to confirm this relationship with either propranolol or other beta-blockers. In the "high renin" hypertensive patient, it has been suggested that renin may not be the only factor responsible for the high blood pressure. At present, the exact role of renin reduction in blood pressure control is not well defined.

Venous Tone

Reduced plasma volume and venous return may play a role in the control of blood pressure by beta-blockers. A few studies have demonstrated these actions of beta-blockers when heart failure was not present in acute and long-term clinical trials. Since one would expect an impaired cardiac output with beta-blockade to cause a reflex increase in plasma volume, these observations, although not yet fully substantiated, are of interest.

Vascular Resistance and Peripheral Blood Flow

Isoproterenol mediates its effect on cardiac contractility through the beta-1-receptor and its peripheral vasodilating effects through the beta-2-receptor. Propranolol blocks both receptors but leaves the peripheral alpa-adrenergic one uninhibited. Peripheral vascular resistance increases through catecholamine stimulation and is clearly apparent with propranolol. The increase in peripheral resistance also potentiates propranolol's rate-slowing effects and negates some of the antihypertensive benefits. The increase in peripheral resistance also affects blood flow to the extremities, coronary arteries, renal circulation, splanchnic vessels, and brain. Beta-1-selective drugs (metoprolol) have little or no effect on peripheral vessels (at normal doses), and they do not increase peripheral resistance. Drugs with PAA (pindolol) or alpha-adrenergic blocking properties (labetalol) reduce the peripheral vascular resistance.

178 • HYPERTENSION

"Quinidine Effect" (MSA)

Some early clinical investigations indicated that the antihypertensive effect of propranolol paralleled the antihypertensive effect of quinidine, suggesting that the MSA in the beta-blocker might be important. Subsequent studies refuted these early findings. All beta-blockers appear to reduce blood pressure, regardless of the presence or absence of "membrane" effects. d-propranolol, with predominant membrane effects, does not affect blood pressure.

Resetting of Baroreceptors

It has been suggested that the baroreceptors in long-standing hypertension react less strongly to a reduction in blood pressure than in normal subjects and that baroreceptor sensitivity can be increased by beta-blockade. The clinical significance of this proposed mechanism remains unknown.

Effects on Prejunctional Beta-Receptors

Apart from their effects on postjunctional tissue beta-receptors, it is believed that blockade of prejunctional beta-receptors may be involved in the hemodynamic actions of beta-blocking drugs. The stimulation of prejunctional alpha-2-receptors leads to a reduction in the quantity of norepinephrine released by the postganglionic sympathetic fibers. Conversely, stimulation of prejunctional beta-receptors is followed by an increase in the quantity of noradrenaline released by postganglionic sympathetic fibers. Blockade of the prejunctional beta-receptors should, therefore, diminish the amount of norepinephrine released, leading to a weaker stimulation of postjunctional alpha-receptors, an effect that would produce less vasoconstriction. Opinions differ, however, on the contributions of presynaptic beta-blockade to a reduction in the peripheral vascular resistance and the antihypertensive effects of beta-blocking drugs.

In summary, beta-blockers have been found to be useful in treating systemic hypertension, although their precise mechanism of action remains unclear. Whether beta-blockers with beta-1-selectivity, partial agonist activity, or alpa-adrenergic blocking activity will ultimately prove more advantageous than nonselective beta-blocking drugs for treating hypertension must still be determined.

Conclusion

It is now well recognized that beta-blockers are effective in reducing the blood pressure of many patients with systemic hypertension. The various beta-blockers differ in terms of the presence or absence of ISA, MSA, beta-1-selectivity, alpha-blocking properties, and relative potency and duration of action. All beta-blockers appear to have blood pressure lowering effects.

The choice of which beta-blocker to use in an individual patient is determined by the pharmacodynamic and pharmacokinetic differences between the drugs in conjunction with the patient's other medical condition(s).

Selected References

Aberg H: Beta receptors and renin release. N Engl J Med 290:1025, 1974.
Achong MR, Piafsky KM, Ogilvie RI: The effects of timolol (MK950) and propranolol on peripheral vessels in man. Clin Pharmacol & Ther 17:228, 1975 (abstr).
Amery A, Billiet L, Fagard R: Beta receptors and renin release. N Engl J Med 290:284, 1974.
Cocco G, Burkart F, Chu D, et al: Intrinsic sympathomimetic activity of β-adrenoceptor blocking agents. Europ J Clin Pharmacol 13:1–4, 1978.
Cruickshank JM: The clinical importance of cardioselectivity and lipophilicity in beta blockers. Am Heart J 100:160–78, 1980.
Frishman W: Acebutolol. Cardiovasc Rev & Rep 6:979–82, 1985.
Frishman WH: Atenolol and timolol: two new systemic β-adrenoceptor antagonists. N Engl J Med 306:1456–62, 1982.
Frishman WH: Beta-adrenoceptor antagonists: new drugs and new indications. N Engl J Med 305:500–06, 1981.
Frishman WH: Clinical Pharmacology of the Beta-Adrenoceptor Blocking Drugs, 2nd ed. Norwalk, Appleton-Century-Crofts, 1984.
Frishman WH: Clinical pharmacology of the new beta-adrenergic blocking drugs. Part 1. Pharmacodynamic and pharmacokinetic properties. Am Heart J 97:663–70, 1979.
Frishman WH: Pindolol: A new β-adrenoceptor antagonist with partial agonist activity. N Engl J Med 308:940–44, 1983.
Frishman WH: Nadolol: A new β-adrenoceptor antagonists. N Engl J Med 305:678–82, 1981.
Frishman WH: Beta-adrenergic blockers. Med Clinics N Amer 72:37–81, 1988.

Frishman W, Halprin S: Clinical pharmacoloyg of the new beta-adrenergic blocking drugs. Part 7. New horizons in beta- adrenoceptor blockade therapy: labetalol. Am Heart J 98:660–65, 1979.
Frishman W, Jacob H, Eisenberg E, et al: Clinical pharmacology of the new β-blocking drugs. Self-poisoning with beta-adrenoceptor blocking drugs: recognition and management. Am Heart J 98:798–811, 1979.
Frishman WH, Kostis J, Strom J, et al: Clinical pharmacology of the new beta-adrenergic blocking drugs. Part 6. A comparison of pindolol and propranolol in treatment of patients with angina pectoris. The role of intrinsic sympathomimetic activity. Am Heart J 98:526–35, 1979.
Frishman WH, Razin A, Swencionis C, et al: Beta-adrenergic blockade in anxiety states: a new approach to therapy? Cardiovasc Rev & Rep 2:447–59, 1981.
Frishman W, Silverman R: Clinical pharmacology of the new beta-adrenergic blocking drugs. Part 3. Comparative clinical experience and new therapeutic applications. Am Heart J 98:119–31, 1979.
Frohlich ED: Hyperdynamic circulation and hypertension. Postgrad Med 52:64, 1972.
Hansson L, Zweifler AJ, Julius S, et al: Hemodynamic effects of acute and prolonged β-adrenergic blockade in essential hypertension. Acta Med Scand 196:27–34, 1974.
Imhof PR: Characterization of beta blockers as antihypertensive agents in the light of human pharmacology studies. In: Schweizer W (ed), Beta-Blockers—Present Status and Future Prospects. Bern, Huber, 1974, pp 40–50.
Johnsson G, Regardh CG: Clinical pharmacokinetics of β adrenoceptor blocking drugs. Clin Pharmacokin 1:233–63, 1976.
Koch-Weser J: Metoprolol. N Engl J Med 301:698–703, 1979.
Kuramoto K, Kurihara H, Murata K, et al: Haemodynamic effects and variations in plasma activity after oral administration of oxprenolol. J Intern Med Res 2:448, 1973.
Langer SZ: Presynaptic receptors and their role in the regulation of transmitter release. Br J Pharmacol 60:481–497, 1977.
Laragh JH: Vasoconstriction-volume analysis for understanding and treating hypertension: the use of renin and aldosterone profiles. Am J Med 55:261–74, 1973.
Leonetti G, Mayer G, Morganti A, et al: Hypotensive and renin suppressing activities of propranolol in hypertensive patients. Clin Sci Mol Med 48:491–99, 1975.
Lydtin H, Schuchard J, Wober W, et al: The effect of timolol on renin, angiotensin II, plasma catecholamines, and blood pressure in the human. In: Magnani B (ed), Beta-Adrenergic Blocking Agents in the Management of Hypertension and Angina Pectoris. New York, Raven Press, 1974, p 81.
Meyer JS, Okamoto S, Shimazu K, et al: Cerebral metabolic changes during treatment of subacute cerebral infarction by alpha and beta adrenergic blockade with phenoxybenzamine and propranolol. Stroke 5:180–95, 1974.
Michelakis AM, McAllister RG: The effect of chronic adrenergic receptor blockade on plasma renin activity in man. J Clin Endocrinol Metab 34:386–94, 1972.
Myers MG, Lewis PJ, Reid JL, et al: Brain concentration of propranolol in relation to hypotensive effects in the rabbit with observations on brain propranolol levels in man. J Pharmacol & Exp Therap 192:327–35, 1975.

Nies AS, McNeil JS, Schrier R: Mechanisms of increased sodium reabsorption during propranolol administration. Circulation 44:596–604, 1976.

Offerhaus L, VanZweiten PA: Comparative studies on central factors contributing to the hypotensive action of propranolol, alprenolol and their enantiomers. Cardiovasc Res 8:488–495, 1974.

Pickering TG, Gribbin B, Petersen E, et al: Effects of autonomic blockade on the baroreflex in man at rest and during exercise. Circ Res 30:177–185, 1972.

Price HL, Cooperman LH, Warden JC: Control of the splanchnic circulation in man. Circ Res 21:333–40, 1967.

Rahn KH, Hawlina A, Kersting F, et al: Studies on the antihypertensive action of the optical isomers of propranolol in man. Naunyn Schmiedebergs Arch Pharmacol 286:319, 1974.

Reid JL, Lewis PJ, Myers MG, et al: Cardiovascular effects of intracerebroventricular d-, l-, and dl-propranolol in the conscious rabbit. J Pharmacol & Exp Therap 188:394–99, 1974.

Stokes GS, Weber MS, Thornell IR: β-Blockers and plasma renin activity in hypertension. Br Med J 1:60–62, 1974.

Taylor SH, Silke B, Lee PS: Intravenous beta-blockade in coronary heart disease. Is cardioselectivity or intrinsic sympathomimetic activity hemodynamically useful? N Engl J Med 306:631–35, 1982.

Tobert JA, Slater JDH, Fogelman F, et al: The effect in man of (+) propranolol and racemic propranolol on renin secretion stimulated by orthostatic stress. Clin Sci 44:291, 1973.

Waal HJ: Hypotensive action of propranolol. Clin Pharmacol Ther 7:588–598, 1966.

Waal-Manning HJ: Hypertension. Which beta-blocker? Drugs 12:412–41, 1976.

Waal-Manning HJ: Metabolic effects of β-adrenoceptor blockade. In: Simpson FO (ed), Proceedings Queenstown Symposium. Drugs II:121, 1976.

Weber MA, Stokes GS, Gain JM: Comparison of the effects of renin release of beta-adrenergic antagonists with differing properties. J Clin Invest 54:1413–19, 1974.

Winer N, Chokshi DS, Yoon MS, et al: Adrenergic receptor mediation of renin secretion. J Clin Endocrinol Metab 29:1168–75, 1969.

Wolfson S, Gorlin R: Cardiovascular pharmacology of propranolol in man. Circulation 40:501–11, 1969.

Yamaguchi N, deChamplain J, Nadeau RL: Regulation of norepinephrine release from cardiac sympathetic fibers in the dog by presynaptic α- and β-receptors. Circ Res 41:108–117, 1977.

Chapter 10

Vasodilators

E. Paul MacCarthy

Introduction

Vasodilator drugs relax vascular smooth muscle either directly at the level of the vascular smooth muscle cell or indirectly (e.g., via blockade of the adrenergic nervous system). Drugs that induce vascular relaxation have proved useful in the treatment of a variety of disorders including hypertension, angina pectoris, and cardiac failure. Vasodilators, which decrease vascular resistance, appear to be the most logical agents for the treatment of hypertension, since the principle hemodynamic abnormality in this condition is an increased total peripheral resistance. In the strictest sense, one may define a vasodilator as a drug that acts directly on vascular smooth muscle to induce relaxation. However, the definition may be expanded to include any drug that lowers blood pressure by reducing peripheral resistance. The term "specific" vasodilator is often applied to this latter type of drug. Such agents include drugs that inhibit vascular smooth muscle contraction by blocking the conversion of an inactive precursor to an active agonist (e.g., angiotensin-converting enzyme inhibitors), drugs that interfere with the binding of an agonist to its receptor (e.g., alpha-1-adrenoceptor antagonists), or drugs that block voltage-dependent calcium channels. A method for classifying vasodilators that incorporates the concept of this expanded definition is outlined in Table 1. This chapter focuses on the directly acting vasodilators.

From Punzi HA, Flamenbaum W (eds): *Hypertension.* Mount Kisco, NY, Futura Publishing Co., Inc., © 1989.

Table 1
Classification of Vasodilators

1. Direct-acting vasodilators
   (e.g., hydralazine, minoxidil, diazoxide, nitroprusside, nitroglycerin, pinacidil, etc.)
2. Sympatholytics
   (e.g., clonidine, prazosin, terazosin, etc.)
3. Calcium antagonists
   (e.g., nifedipine, diltiazem, verapamil, nicardipine, etc.)
4. Angiotensin-converting enzyme inhibitors
   (e.g., captopril, enalapril, lisinopril, etc.)
5. Other
   (e.g., ketanserin)

Control of Vascular Smooth Muscle Tone

In order to understand the mechanism of action of vasodilator drugs it is important to review the factors that control vascular smooth muscle tone. Many extracellular factors, hormones, and drugs are capable of modulating vascular tone by regulating the contraction-relaxation cycle of the vascular smooth muscle cell.

At a tissue level, sympathetic nerve impulses release norepinephrine from nerve endings, and this neurotransmitter stimulates postsynaptic alpha-adrenoreceptors located on vascular smooth muscle cells, resulting in vasoconstriction. The resting tone in the peripheral vasculature may be modified by many other factors. Circulating humoral agents such as angiotensin II, catecholamines, and vasopressin may regulate vascular tone via a variety of direct and indirect mechanisms. Locally released vasoactive substances such as prostacyclin, serotonin, endothelium-derived relaxing factor (EDRF), and the potent vasoconstrictor endothelin are important local regulators of vascular tone.

At the level of the vascular smooth muscle cell, calcium ions are of central importance in the contractile process. It is now widely accepted that contraction of vascular smooth muscle is initiated by an increase of cytosolic calcium and subsequent calcium-calmodulin complex-dependent phosphorylation of myosin light chains. This phosphorylation enables myosin to interact with actin to form actomyosin ATPase which provides the energy for contraction. The intracellular concentration of free calcium is regulated primarily by calcium channels and by ATP-

Vasodilators • 185

dependent calcium pumps present in the plasmalemma and sarcoplasmic reticulum.

Intracellular free calcium is increased by an activation of plasmalemmal channels including the voltage- and receptor-dependent calcium channels. Many hormones and drugs capable of activating the receptor-dependent calcium channel also activate phospholipase C and increase the intracellular levels of inositol-1,4,5-trisphosphate (IP_3) and of 1,2-diacylglycerol DAG), resulting in release of calcium from intracellular calcium stores and activation of protein kinase C, respectively. Both events may participate in mediating receptor-induced contraction.

Vasodilator drugs may interfere with many of the foregoing processes to relax vascular smooth muscle and lower blood pressure. The local regulation of vascular smooth muscle cell tone by hormones, drugs, and other factors is shown in Figure 1.

Mode and Site of Action of Vasodilators

Vasodilators (other than ACE inhibitors) that act directly at the level of the vasculature may be classified as either endothelium-dependent or endothelium-independent agents (Table 2). Endothelium-dependent agents stimulate the endothelium to produce endothelium-derived relaxing factor (recently identified as nitric oxide), which increases cyclic GMP (cGMP) levels in vascular smooth muscle and produces vascular relaxation. Endothelium-independent vasodilators may be divided into calcium antagonists, alpha-1-adrenergic antagonists, cyclic AMP (cAMP)-elevating agents, and cGMP-elevating agents. A variety of evidence suggests that certain direct-acting vasodilators inhibit calcium-dependent phosphorylation of myosin light chains and contraction of vascular smooth muscle via activation of cAMP- and cGMP-dependent protein phosphorylation.

Some of the oldest and clinically still very important vasodilators are drugs that contain nitrogen oxides, including the organic nitrates and nitroprusside. Substantial evidence has accumulated that shows that these agents achieve their effects by increasing cGMP via activation of a soluble guanylate cyclase. Atrial natriuretic factor (also a potent vasodilator) has been shown to activate particulate guanylate cyclase in vascular smooth muscle and also to increase cGMP. A variety of endothelial-dependent vasodilating substances (including acetylcholine, histamine, and bradykinin) stimulate the endothelium to produce EDRF, which increases cGMP and relaxes vascular smooth muscle. The vaso-

186 • HYPERTENSION

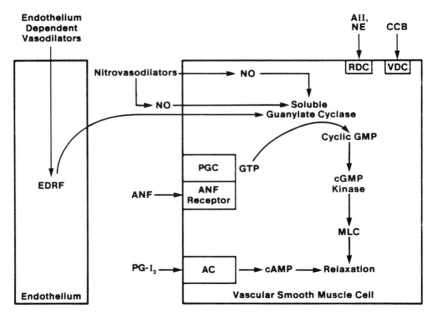

Figure 1. Schematic illustration of factors that regulate vascular smooth muscle cell tone. A variety of endothelium-dependent vasodilators lead to the synthesis and release of EDRF. Nitric oxide (NO) derived from the nitrovasodilators and EDRF activate guanylate cylcase and result in increases cyclic GMP synthesis. These events result in the dephosphorylation of myosin light chain (MCL) and vascular relaxation. Atrial natriuretic factor (ANF) activates particulate guanylate cylcase (PGC), which results in cyclic GMP synthesis and vascular relaxation. Prostacyclin (PG-I$_2$) activates cyclase (AC), which leads to increased synthesis of cyclic AMP and vascular relaxation. Angiotensin II (AII) and norepinephrine (NE) stimulate the receptor-dependent channel (RDC) and vasoconstrict, whereas calcium channel blockers (CCB) antagonize the voltage-dependent calcium channel (VDC) and vasodilate.

dilating drug hydralazine has been shown to cause maximal vascular relaxation in the presence of intact endothelium, which is suggestive evidence for a role of EDRF in the action of this drug.

The intracellular effects of cGMP in vascular smooth muscle are not very well defined, although the high concentration of cGMP- dependent protein kinase and its activation by nitrogen oxide-containing and endothelium-dependent vasodilators suggest that regulation of cGMP-dependent protein phosphorylation is of central importance for this class of vasodilators. Substrates and potential targets for the cGMP-depen-

Table 2
Locally Acting Vasodilators

1. Endothelium-dependent agents
   (e.g., acetylcholine, histamine, hydralazine, bradykinin)
2. Endothelium-independent agents
   Calcium antagonists (e.g., nifedipine, verapamil, diltiazem, nicardipine)
   Alpha-1-adrenoceptor antagonists (e.g., prazosin, terazosin, doxazosin)
   cAMP-elevating agents (e.g., prostacyclin, forskolin)
   cGMP-elevating agents (e.g., nitroprusside, nitrates, ANF, EDRF, minoxidil, diazoxide)

dent protein kinase could be calcium ATPase, regulatory proteins of the contractile apparatus, or components of the phosphatidylinositol cycle.

Another class of direct-acting vasodilators includes prostacyclin, which is produced by the endothelium, and increases cAMP in vascular smooth muscle and subsequently activates cAMP-dependent protein kinase. Cyclic AMP-dependent phosphorylation may inhibit myosin light chain kinase, or cAMP may relax vascular smooth muscle by regulating calcium release and/or calcium pumps.

Recently a new class of directly acting vasodilators, potassium channel openers or potassium channel agonists, have been developed. Compounds in this class include pinacidil, cromakalim, and nicorandil. These agents produce vasodilation by opening plasmalemmal potassium channels in vascular smooth muscle cells, allowing increased potassium efflux with consequent plasmalemmal potassium channels. This results in a reduction in the availability of calcium for the contractile process and reduced sensitivity of blood vessels to depolarizing stimuli. At least four types of potassium channels have been identified in mammalian smooth muscle, but the channel that pinacidil modulates has not yet been identified. Recent evidence suggests that the potassium channels opened by pinacidil in cardiac muscle may be different from that in peripheral blood vessels.

Site of Action of Vasodilators

Different vasodilators may act principally on arteries, principally on veins, or on both arteries and veins. The ability of drugs to act selectively on blood vessels of different types reflects differences in the functional properties of the smooth muscle in the vessel wall.

The smooth muscle in the limb veins has little capacity for spontaneous activity and depends on stimulation by agonists such as norepinephrine for activation. The alpha-adrenoceptor antagonists, such as prazosin and phentolamine, inhibit contractile activity of this type. Such contractile activity is mediated by receptor-operated mechanisms that are also inhibited by such agents as nitroprusside or nitroglycerin. Venous relaxation causes a fall in central venous pressure with a consequent reduction in pulmonary venous pressure, left ventricular dimensions, cardiac output, and arterial pressure. Since these effects depend on venous pooling, they are more pronounced in the upright position and postural hypotension may occur. This pattern of action can cause a large reduction in the work and oxygen needs of the left ventricle and is thus of particular value in the management of angina pectoris. Venodilation may also be of value in the treatment of cardiac failure when elevation of pulmonary venous pressure is a conspicuous feature.

The smooth muscle of the arteriolar resistance vessels possesses intrinsic tone and, in some circumstances, exhibits rhythmic contractile behavior. Dilation of these arterioles reduces peripheral resistance and hence lowers blood pressure. Hydralazine is an example of a direct-acting vasodilator that is highly selective for the arteriolar resistance vessels. Most vasodilator drugs do not act solely on vessels of one type, but act to some extent both on veins and resistance vessels. The pattern of their circulatory effects will thus depend upon their relative effects

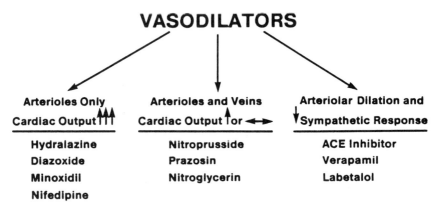

Figure 2. Schematic presentation of the effects of vasodilators on arterioles and veins and their subsequent hemodynamic effects.

on venous capacitance and peripheral resistance. Figure 2 outlines the effects of different vasodilators on arterioles and veins and their subsequent hemodynamic effects.

Compensatory Responses to Vasodilators

Vasodilator drugs invariably produce neurohumoral responses that tend to offset their blood pressure-lowering action (Fig. 3). Sympathetic activation via arterial baroreceptors elicits tachycardia and contributes to a reflex increase in cardiac output. The increase in cardiac output is mediated largely by a reflex increase in sympathetic nervous system activity but also is due to a lesser extent to withdrawal of parasympathetic tone and alterations in intrinsic myocardial properties.

All directly acting vasodilators may induce a rise in plasma renin activity and increased concentrations of angiotensin II, which oppose their dilator effect. Prolonged administration of vasodilators induces retention of sodium and water. The extent of sodium retention varies

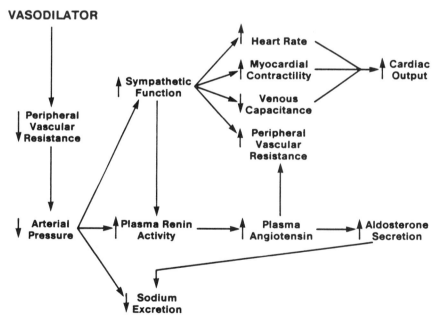

Figure 3. Primary and secondary effects of vasodilator therapy.

widely between drugs and is most marked with minoxidil and diazoxide. Frequently the sodium retention is of such a magnitude that large doses of loop diuretics are required to reverse it. The mechanism of this sodium retention is not entirely clear but may involve hyperaldosteronism, a direct effect of angiotensin II or the drug itself on the renal tubule, or a combination of these factors.

Chronic monotherapy with directly acting vasodilator drugs such as hydralazine and minoxidil is usually ineffective in the treatment of hypertension because of the compensatory increase in cardiac output, hypereninemia and sodium retention. Long-term therapy with such vasodilators usually requires the concurrent administration of beta-blockers or other sympatholytic drugs in addition to diuretics in order to sustain an effective antihypertensive response.

The Effect of Vasodilators on Large Arteries

Recent studies have demonstrated that the hemodynamic abnormalities in hypertension are not confined to the arterioles but also involve the large arteries, resulting in a decrease in arterial compliance. This observation is potentially important since cardiovascular morbidity and mortality in treated hypertensive patients is related to ischemic events involving large arteries in the coronary and cerebral circulations. Therefore the effects of vasodilating drugs on the large arteries of hypertensive patients may be an important influence on subsequent cardiovascular morbidity and mortality.

Antihypertensive drugs may have different (and even opposite) effects on small and larger arteries. For a given degree of arteriolar dilation, the caliber of large arteries may be unchanged (alpha- and beta-adrenoceptor antagonists), decreased (dihydralazine), or increased (angiotensin-converting enzyme inhibitors and calcium channel antagonists). Different effects of these agents on arterial compliance have also been observed. Because arterial compliance is decreased in patients with untreated essential hypertension, a possible improvement in the functional capacity of large arteries may be extremely important, with possible consequences on cardiac performance and vascular damage.

Vasodilators and Structural Alterations in Hypertension

Since left ventricular hypertrophy is a relatively common structural alteration in hypertension and is associated with an increased risk of

Table 3
Factors That May Influence Left Ventricular Hypertrophy

Favoring prevention or regression

Reduced arterial systolic pressure (integrated)
Reduced ventricular volume
Reduced ventricular diastolic pressure
Slowed heart
Reduced myocardial contractility
Decreased cardiac sympathetic drive
Decreased angiotensin levels

Favoring persistence

Selective reduction of diastolic pressure
Uncontrolled blood pressure during exercise or stress
Reflex cardiac sympathetic stimulation
Cardiac dilation
Tachycardia
Renin-angiotensin stimulation

cardiovascular morbidity and mortality, regression of left ventricular hypertrophy is considered a desirable goal of antihypertensive therapy. Control of blood pressure is the most important factor leading to regression of cardiac hypertrophy during antihypertensive therapy. However, nonhemodynamic or humoral factors may also be important since similar degrees of blood pressure reduction with different classes of antihypertensive drugs can result in different degrees of regression of left ventricuLar hypertrophy. The factors that may influence left ventricular hypertrophy are summarized in Table 3.

Regression of left ventricular hypertrophy due to systemic hypertension has been shown to occur in both humans and experimental animals after control of blood pressure by a variety of drugs including α-methyldopa, other sympatholytic agents, angiotensin-converting enzyme inhibitors, and calcium channel antagonists. Several studies have suggested that when blood pressure is controlled by directly acting vasodilators such as hydralazine or minoxidil, regression of left ventricular hypertrophy either does not occur or occurs to a lesser degree. This is not surprising since the compensatory responses to vasodilator monotherapy involve many of the factors that favor the persistence of hypertrophy.

Sympathetic nervous system stimulation may be an important pathogenetic factor in the process of vascular hypertrophy that is observed in hypertension. This vascular hypertrophy may contribute to the increase in peripheral resistance and also result in ischemia of the brain, heart and kidneys. Evidence that sympathetic stimulation might influence vascular hypertrophy comes from several studies showing that denervated arteries do not develop a similar degree of hypertrophy as those with intact sympathetic innervation. Since direct-acting vasodilator monotherapy produces a reflex increase in sympathetic nervous activity, it may fail to cause regression of vascular hypertrophy. However, concerns that vasodilator drugs may fail to cause regression of the cardiovascular structural alterations in hypertension may not be appropriate when these agents are used as combination therapy (e.g., in combination with beta-blockers and diuretics).

Individual Vasodilator Drugs

Hydralazine

Hydralazine (l-hydrazinophthalazine) has been available for the treatment of hypertension for 40 years. After early disappointing results when the drug was used as a single agent, it subsequently found favor in the 1970s and 1980s when used in combination therapy.

Hydralazine exerts its hypotensive action by reducing vascular resistance through direct relaxation of arteriolar smooth muscle. Previous studies suggest that some of the vasodilatory activity in at least some vascular beds may be due to formation of prostaglandins, inhibitors of dopamine, beta-hydroxylase, and interference with purinergic mechanisms. The precise subcellular mechanism of action remains uncertain. It has been suggested that hydralazine interferes with calcium entry into the vascular smooth muscle cell, or it inhibits the release of tightly bound calcium. Recently, convincing evidence has been presented that rabbit aortic rings, deprived of their endothelium, were substantially less sensitive to hydralazine than were unaltered preparations, indicating that the endothelial component of the hydralazine response represents a major contribution of the net relaxant effect on vascular smooth muscle.

The peripheral vasodilation induced by hydralazine is not uniform; vascular resistance in the coronary, cerebral, splanchnic, and renal circulations is decreased more than in skin and muscle. Hydralazine affects postcapillary capacitance vessels much less than precapillary resistance

Vasodilators • 193

vessels and has no appreciable effects on nonvascular smooth muscle. Since the drug does not interfere with the autonomic nervous system, it is devoid of appreciable orthostatic hypotension and lowers blood pressure equally in the supine and upright positions.

The magnitude of the antihypertensive effect of hydralazine depends on the dose, route of administration, duration of therapy, and the patient's acetylator phenotype. Following intravenous administration, the onset of action occurs between 5–20 minutes and lasts 2–9 hours, whereas after oral administration, the onset of action is between 20–30 minutes and lasts 2–6 hours. Rapid acetylators require a higher dose of the drug.

The compensatory responses to vasodilators outlined earlier in this chapter render hydralazine less effective as a single agent for the long-term treatment of hypertension. However, the reflex increase in heart rate and cardiac output can be counteracted by concomitant therapy with a beta-adrenoceptor antagonist, reserpine, or a centrally acting alpha-adrenoceptor agonist such as clonidine, while the sodium and water retention can be corrected by concomitant diuretic therapy. Thus the drug is generally used clinically as a step-3 agent in combination with a beta-blocker and diuretic. Since elderly patients appear to show a reduced baroreflex-mediated increase in heart rate, it has been suggested that hydralazine may be effective and well tolerated when used alone in small doses in these patients.

Much of the earlier literature on hydralazine pharmacokinetics is misleading because acid-labile conjugates of the drug (mainly its principal circulating metabolite, the inactive pyruvic acid hydrazone) are known to interfere with many nonspecific hydralazine assays. These assays significantly overestimate the peak plasma level, half-life, plasma clearance, and volume of distribution of hydralazine as measured using specific assays.

Hydralazine has low oral bioavailability and food interferes with the bioavailability of the drug. There is extensive acetylator phenotype-dependent presystemic metabolism, with hydroxylation, acetylation, and glucuronide conjugation by the gastrointestinal mucosa and the liver. Both hypotension and the incidence of toxicity are greater with the slow acetylator phenotype. After intravenous administration, metabolism of the drug differs, with most of it being converted intravascularly to the pyruvic acid hydrazone. This action is independent of the acetylator phenotype. Following administration by either route, approximately 75% of the metabolites and 1%–2% of the remaining parent drug are eliminated in the urine, with a half-life of 4–5 hours.

The usual initial dose of hydralazine orally is 10–25 mg two to four times daily. Dose increments should be guided by the clinical response and acetylator phenotype, if the latter information is available. It is probably unjustified to exceed 300 mg/d of hydralazine on a long-term basis even in rapid acetylators unless special circumstances exist. Dosage reduction may be needed in patients with renal failure to prevent drug accumulation. The usual intravenous dose of hydralazine is 10–20 mg but the dose and frequency of administration required for satisfactory blood pressure control are highly variable. The long duration of action makes titration of dose against hypotensive effect difficult, and many patients with hypertensive crises do not respond adequately to any dose of hydralazine.

Many of the adverse reactions to hydralazine are related to its direct or reflex-mediated hemodynamic actions including headache, flushing, dizziness, palpitations, and anginal attacks. Drug-induced retention of salt and water can be countered by diuretic therapy. Chronic administration of hydralazine may result in the development of systemic lupus erythematosus. The overall incidence of this adverse event is approximately 7% and it is dose-related (greater than 10% incidence in those receiving 200 mg/d more of the drug). Known risk factors for this adverse reaction are female gender, Caucasian race, slow acetylator phenotype, and possibly the histocompatibility locus DR4. With the current availability of highly tolerable and effective alternative antihypertensive drugs it would seem prudent to avoid using hydralazine in patients with a past or present history of systemic lupus erythematosus or rheumatoid arthritis.

Minoxidil

Minoxidil is a piperidino-pyrimidine derivative and is a very potent orally active vasodilator. The drug is reserved for the treatment of severe or malignant hypertension or for those patients who are resistant to other antihypertensive agents.

Minoxidil acts primarily on arterioles to reduce peripheral vascular resistance, and it exerts little or no effect on venous capacitance vessels. In this respect, it resembles hydralazine, but minoxidil is considerably more potent and longer-acting. The exact subcellular mechanism of action of minoxidil is not clear but the drug appears to increase cGMP concentration and to limit the availability of intracellular calcium in the vascular smooth muscle cell. Minoxidil is an endothelium-independent

Vasodilators • 195

vasodilator. A recent study suggested that the metabolite of minoxidil, minoxidil sulfate, acts as a potassium channel opener.

Minoxidil is at least 90% absorbed from the gastrointestinal tract with a peak plasma concentration at about one hour. The drug is metabolized by the liver and along with its metabolites is then excreted by the kidney. About 15% of the parent compound is excreted in the urine, while 85% is metabolized by the liver and is then excreted by the kidney predominantly as the glucuronide conjugate of minoxidil. Minoxidil is not protein bound, and renal excretion depends on glomerular filtration since the drug does not appear to be either reabsorbed or secreted within the renal tubule. Little or no dosage adjustment is required in renal failure. In patients receiving peritoneal dialysis or hemodialysis, minoxidil is best given after dialysis since it is easily dialyzed. The maximal effect of minoxidil on blood pressure is observed approximately four hours after administration of the drug. The plasma half-life is four hours, but the effect on blood pressure is prolonged for up to three days owing to tissue binding of the drug.

The powerful systemic vasodilation produced by minoxidil triggers activation of the peripheral sympathetic nervous system, which results in renin secretion, increased heart rate and cardiac output, and an increase in norepinephrine output. Marked sodium and water retention also ensues. Beta-adrenoceptor blockade and large doses of loop diuretics usually are used to counteract these responses. In resistant cases of hypertension, clonidine may be added to the treatment regimen to suppress increased plasma norepinephrine levels that result from minoxidil therapy.

The initial dose of minoxidil is 2.5 or 5 mg once daily. This dose can be doubled every 3 or 4 days to achieve the desired effect. The usual daily dose is 2.5–10 mg once or twice a day, and the maximum approved daily dose is 100 mg in adults. After hypertension is controlled with minoxidil, there are frequent reports of stabilization or improvement in function of hypertensive target organs such as the kidney and heart. Indeed, several patients with end-stage renal disease have recovered sufficient kidney function to enable them to discontinue chronic hemodialysis. Minoxidil's effectiveness generally is independent of the underlying mechanism of hypertension including renovascular hypertension.

The most common side effects of minoxidil are fluid retention and edema. Therefore, all patients must be monitored for edema, weight gain, and evidence of congestive heart failure. Increased hair growth (hypertrichosis) especially involving the face and extremities occurs in

80% of patients after 3–6 weeks of therapy. The mechanism of hypertrichosis is not established, but no hormonal changes have been reported. Some women and children control excess hair growth with depilatories or by shaving exposed areas. Tachycardia is to be expected as is edema and should be counteracted with concurrent beta-blockers and diuretics. Many patients develop changes in the T wave on electrocardiography. These ECG changes are usually asymtomatic and disappear with continued treatment. In patients with underlying coronary artery disease, angina or even myocardial infarction can be precipitated if tachycardia is not controlled. Pericardial effusions that rarely progress to tamponade have been reported in patients receiving minoxidil, especially when congestive heart failure or kidney failure complicated the hypertension. Pathological lesions of the heart have been reported in animals treated with minoxidil. However, similar lesions have not been observed in an autopsy study of patients treated with the drug. In contrast to hydralazine, which can cause a lupuslike syndrome, there have been no reports of positive antinuclear antibody tests developing during minoxidil treatment.

Diazoxide

Diazoxide, a benzothiadiazine derivative, which is closely related chemically to the thiazide diuretics, is a potent direct-acting vasodilator with a rapid action. It is available for intravenous treatment of hypertensive crisis. However, in recent years the drug has been largely replaced by other parenteral agents such as sodium nitroprusside, nitroglycerine, and labetalol in the management of this condition.

The cellular mechanism by which diazoxide produces arteriolar dilation is not fully understood. The drug probably influences cellular calcium movement or depletes cellular calcium stores. Diazoxide has also been shown to reduce vascular reactivity to calcium ions. Recent studies have shown that diazoxide increased cGMP levels in the vascular smooth muscle, which may result in vascular relaxation. The vasodilatory action of diazoxide is also independent of the endothelium.

Diazoxide is predominantly an arteriolar dilator with only a small relaxing effect on veins. Like other vasodilators of this type, diazoxide causes a reflex stimulation of the sympathetic nervous system, inducing cardiac stimulation, a rise in the plasma renin and catecholamines, and sodium and water retention. After intravenous administration of diazoxide, arterial pressure falls within 1 minute, reaches its lowest level within 5 minutes, and the antihypertensive effect persists for 4–12 hours. Diazoxide is well absorbed after oral administration, but the drug is rarely administered by this route. The major portion of the drug (70%–90%) is bound to plasma proteins, and the bound portion is inactive. The drug usually is given as an intravenous bolus to reduce the time available for protein binding, but the rationale for this approach is controversial. Approximately half of the dose is metabolized to inactive forms by oxidation and sulfate conjugation; and both metabolites and unchanged drug are renally excreted. The elimination half-life ranges from 10–72 hours.

In the past it was recommended that 150–300 mg of diazoxide should be administered as a rapid (within 30 sec) intravenous bolus in adults. Reduction of the dosage is required in patients with renal failure. Recently, however, concern for the potential of rapid large boluses of diazoxide to induce myocardial or cerebral infarction has led to trials of repeated small (1 mg/kg) injections and of slow continuous infusions. The results of these studies have been favorable.

Adverse reactions to diazoxide include hyperglycemia, mild hyperuricemia, local cellulitis, uterine atony, and excessive hypotension. This latter complication has resulted in cerebral and myocardial infarction. Edema and hirsutism, which are uncommon during intravenous administration, have also been reported as side effects of therapy. Diazoxide can displace warfarin and phenytoin from albumin-binding sites and may produce a transient increase in the pharmacological activity of both drugs. In addition to the caution needed in patients with cerebral or coronary artery disease, diazoxide should be avoided in patients with dissecting aortic aneurysm since the drug-induced reflex cardiac stimulation increases mechanical stress on the aortic wall.

Nitroprusside

Sodium nitroprusside is the most potent blood pressure-lowering drug and has proved to be the most effective and best-tolerated vasodilator for the management of acute hypertension and heart failure as well as for the indication of controlled hypertension during surgery. The hypotensive response occurs within seconds after the infusion is started and dissipates almost as rapidly when the infusion is discontinued. This rapid onset and decline in activity permits close titration of the infusion rate against hypotensive effect.

The actions of nitroprusside are almost exclusively confined to the vascular smooth muscle, where it relaxes both the arteries and veins, reducing systemic arterial and venous pressures along with the systemic and pulmonary vascular resistance. Like other vasodilators with a direct action on vascular smooth muscle, nitroprusside causes hypotension that is accompanied by a reflex activation of the sympathetic nervous system. The exact cellular mechanism of action of nitroprusside is not entirely known, but recent studies suggest that involves release of nitric oxide, which activates soluble guanylate cyclase and stimulates cyclic GMP formation in the vascular smooth muscle cell. The cardiac output response to nitroprusside is variable and depends largely on the pre-existing hemodynamic status of the patient. In hypertensive patients not in cardiac failure, cardiac output usually falls; in patients with low cardiac output states, it consistently increases. However, nitroprusside may cause redistribution of blood flow away from ischemic areas and potentially could increase the extent of myocardial damage in patients with coronary disease. In patients with congestive heart failure, nitroprusside increases renal blood flow and decreases renovascular resistance. However, a marked reduction in arterial pressure in the absence of heart failure may decrease the glomerular filtration rate and sodium excretion.

Sodium nitroprusside is only given by the intravenous route, always as an infusion. The hypotensive effect of the drug begins 1–2 minutes after commencing the infusion and starts to dissipate within a few minutes after the infusion is stopped. Since nitroprusside is photosensitive the solution must be protected from light. The usual initial dose is 0.5 µg/kg/min, and the dose may be increased every 5 minutes according to blood pressure response up to a dose of 10 µg/kg/min. Almost all patients will respond to nitroprusside if a large enough dose is given. Because of its rapid onset of action and potency, nitroprusside infusion must be monitored closely and accurately by an infusion pump or microdrop regulator, along with frequent blood pressure measurements. Intra-arterial monitoring of blood pressure during infusion is desirable, but not essential in all cases.

The metabolism of nitroprusside is complex and not fully understood. Nitroprusside promptly reacts with sulfhydryl groups in blood and tissues to produce free cyanide ions. These cyanide groups are then converted to thiocyanate by the enzyme rhodanase, which is primarily found in the liver. The rate of conversion of cyanide to thiocyanate is limited by the availability of thiosulfate, and in cases of cyanide toxicity, addition of thiosulfate may be therapeutic. Acute cyanide toxicity (causing inhibition of mitochondrial oxygen transport and lactic acidosis) and

Vasodilators • 199

chronic thiocyanate toxicity leading to weakness, nausea, and confusion are the principal hazards of nitroprusside administration. These symptoms tend to occur at plasma thiocyanate levels of 50–100 mg/L, and death may occur if the plasma level exceeds 200 mg/L. Chronic thiocyanate toxicity is more likely in uremic patients since the elimination half-life of thiocyanate is markedly increased in renal failure. Thiocyanate may interfere with iodine trapping in the thyroid gland and produce hypothyroidism. Since hydroxocobalamin is an antidote for cyanide it may be used to treat cyanide or thiocyanate toxicity resulting from nitroprusside therapy.

Additional problems encountered during nitroprusside therapy include hypotension, methemoglobinemia, metabolic acidosis, ventilation perfusion mismatch, increased intracranial pressure, and abnormalities in platelet function.

Nitroglycerin

Nitroglycerin has been used for over 100 years in the treatment of angina, but recently has been applied to the management of congestive heart failure and acute myocardial infarction. Intravenous nitroglycerin has also been found to be useful for the treatment of accelerated hypertension and the control of blood pressure during the perioperative period, especially during coronary artery bypass procedures. Continuous intravenous administration of nitroglycerin provides predictable and quickly reversible control of preload and afterload and offers advantages over other vasodilators because of its unique effects on the coronary circulation and regional myocardial blood flow. The drug differs from nitroprusside in being less hypotensive, more active in relaxing the large arteries, and more active on the venous than the arterial side of the circulation. This latter property makes it a logical choice for the treatment of hypertensive left ventricular failure. The net hemodynamic alterations resulting from infusion of nitroglycerin depend on the dose administered and the basal preload and peripheral vascular resistance.

Nitroglycerin also dilates the large coronary arteries; including possibly the collateral vessels. This renders the drug safer than nitroprusside for the management of hypertension in patients with unstable angina or acute myocardial infarction; nitroprusside may produce a coronary steal syndrome in such patients.

The cellular mechanism of the vasodilating action of nitroglycerin is similar to that of nitroprusside in that it involves the formation of nitric oxide or S-nitrosothiol, which activates guanylate cyclase leading to an increase in cylic GMP levels in the vascular smooth muscle cell.

Nitroglycerin is rapidly metabolized by reductive hydrolysis under the influence of the hepatic enzyme glutathione organic nitrate reductase. The liver has an enormous capacity to catalyze this reaction, and therefore the biotransformation of nitroglycerin is the principal determinant of the drug's duration of action in vivo and its relative efficacy when given by various routes of administration.

The usual initial dose of nitroglycerin is 5 µg/minute by continuous infusion, and this may be increased by 5-10 µg/minute every 3-5 minutes until the desired therapeutic response has been obtained. There is no fixed optimum dose of nitroglycerin and therefore blood pressure and other hemodynamic parameters should be closely monitored during the infusion. Doses in excess of 200 µg/minute may be required for optimum blood pressure control in severe cases of hypertension.

Since nitroglycerin may adsorb to polyvinylchloride-type plastic intravenous bags and infusion sets, the drug should be mixed in glass or polyolefin containers and, ideally, administered via nonpolyvinylchloride-type infusion sets.

Intravenous nitroglycerin, if carefully monitored, is generally well tolerated. Excessive hypotension, which is the most common and potentially serious side effect, can be controlled by decreasing the rate of infusion or by drug withdrawal. Other side effects include headache, nausea, vomiting, tachycardia, restlessness, increased intracranial pressure, methemoglobinemia (rare), and diluent toxicity from ethanol or propylene glycol.

Other organic nitrates in addition to nitroglycerin have also been used in the treatment of hypertension. Isosorbide dinitrate has been administered intravenously in perioperative hypertension and via the oral route for the management of systolic hypertension.

Pinacidil

Pinacidil is a cyanoguanidine derivative that has a potent vasodilating action on precapillary resistance vessels by opening potassium channels. The drug does not alter cAMP or cGMP levels and its vasodilating action is independent of the endothelium. Pinacidil is distinguishable from hydralazine by its different mechanism of action, its potency, and the apparent absence of intrinsic positive inotropic and chronotropic activity. In addition to causing vasodilation, pinacidil has been found to inhibit human platelet thromboxane synthetase. Whether this effect on platelet aggregation is related to potassium channel opening activity is unknown. Clinical trials have shown the drug to be effective in the treatment of mild, moderate, and severe hypertension, and it has been recommended by the FDA advisory committee for acceptance as an antihypertensive agent. The antihypertensive effect of pinacidil is enhanced by combination with a diuretic or beta-adrenoceptor antagonist, or both. Pinacidil has also been reported to lower total serum cholesterol and triglycerides and raise HDL cholesterol concentrations in humans.

Pharmacokinetic studies in man have shown that pinacidil is rapidly and almost completely absorbed following oral administration. Concomitant food ingestion can enhance absorption leading to an increase in peak serum concentration of the drug and a decrease in the terminal elimination half-life. The plasma half-life is normally 3–4 hours. The drug is eliminated by hepatic metabolism to pinacidil-N-oxide followed by renal excretion, and the N-oxidation is partly reversible. Pinacidil-N-oxide has been shown in animals to have one quarter the hypotensive effect of pinacidil. Elimination of pinacidil and pinacidil-N-oxide is reduced in patients with hepatic and renal disease. The drug is 40% bound to plasma protein.

The oral therapeutic dose range of pinacidil is 25 to 150 mg/d with a maximum of 200 mg/d, and the drug is administered twice or three times daily. Side effects of pinacidil are those commonly reported with directly acting vasodilators and include edema (30%), headache (20%), and dizziness and palpitations (10%–12%). Because of the frequent occurrence of edema and palpitations, the drug is optimally administered concomitantly with diuretics and beta-adrenceptor blockers. Hypertrichosis has been reported in 2% of males and 13% of females treated with pinacidil, which is a lower frequency than that observed with minoxidil therapy. ECG changes consisting of T-wave inversion or flattening have also been reported during pinacidil treatment.

Uses of Vasodilators in Hypertension

Mild-to-Moderate Hypertension

Hydralazine is the most commonly used direct-acting vasodilator in mild-to-moderate hypertension. It is used predominantly as a step-3 agent in this instance, usually in combination with a beta-adrenoceptor blocker and diuretic. A recent comparative clinical trial has shown that pinacidil is at least as effective and well tolerated as hydralazine in patients with this category of hypertension.

Severe or Resistant Hypertension

Minoxidil has proven to be an extremely useful agent for controlling blood pressure in severe or resistant cases of hypertension. In hemodialysis patients with severe renin-mediated hypertension, minoxidil has permitted blood pressure to be controlled without having to resort to bilateral nephrectomy. Minoxidil has also been found to be useful in the control of some cases of scleroderma renal crisis, and the addition of captopril to minoxidil has aided in blood pressure control in this and other forms of severe important hypertension.

Hypertensive Emergencies

Hypertensive emergencies usually are characterized by a marked increase in peripheral vascular resistance, and direct-acting vasodilators have proven to be a logical treatment for these conditions. Hypertensive emergencies that develop in the setting of a myocardial infarction or left ventricular failure are most appropriately managed with intravenous nitroglycerin or nitroprusside. Eclampsia or severe pre-eclampsia is best managed with parenteral hydralazine or diazoxide. In certain hypertensive emergencies, however, the use of some direct-acting arteriolar dilators, e.g., hydralazine or diazoxide is contraindicated. The use of hydralazine or diazoxide in aortic dissection may increase the shear force on the aorta because of reflex increments in heart rate and cardiac output, and this may extend the dissection.

Nitroprusside, because of its additional action on venules, is a more appropriate therapy for aortic dissection especially when administered in combination with a beta-blocker. When hypertensive emergencies develop in the setting of a cerebrovascular accident, nitroprusside or nitroglycerin are the most suitable agents because adjustment of the infusion rate provides very fine control of blood pressure. Both of these agents, however, may increase intracranial pressure and should be avoided in cases with raised intracranial pressure.

Vasodilators • 203

Secondary Hypertension

Direct-acting vasodilators, especially minoxidil, has been very successful in the management of hypertension in patients with a variety of renal diseases. These agents have not only been found to be helpful in controlling blood pressure in renovascular hypertension but they have also been used to stimulate renal vein secretion in the evaluation of patients with this condition.

Direct-acting vasodilators with the exception of nitroprusside should be avoided in cases of pheochromocytoma because they reflexly increase sympathetic nervous activity and may induce a pheochromocytoma crisis.

Summary

The direct-acting vasodilators have proven to be an extremely important part of the antihypertensive drug armanentarium and will remain so for many years to come. Although they have not been effective as single agents for chronic therapy because of reflex increments in sympathetic nervous activity and fluid retention, they combine very well with sympatholytics and diuretics. In most cases of severe hypertension and hypertensive emergencies, vasodilators remain the agents of choice for treatment because they counteract the markedly increased peripheral resistance. The extensive list of new vasodilators that currently are being developed by the pharmaceutical industry is further evidence of the usefulness and bright future for this category of therapeutic agents.

Selected References

Anderson KP: Sudden death, hypertension and hypertrophy. J Cardiovasc Pharmacol 6:S498–S503, 1984.
Bevan RD: Effect of sympathetic denervation on smooth muscle cell proliferation in the growing rabbit ear artery. Circ Res 37:14–19, 1975.
Byyny RF, Nies AS, LoVerde ME, et al: A double-blind, randomized, controlled trial comparing pinacidil to hydralazine in essential hypertension. Clin Pharmacol Ther 42:50–57, 1987.
Cohn JN, Burke LP: Nitroprusside. Ann Int Med 91:752–757, 1979.
Cook NS: The pharmacology of potassium channels and their therapeutic potential. Trends Pharmac Sci 9:21–28, 1988.
Cook NS, Quast V, Hof RP, et al: Similarities in the mechanism of action of two

new vasodilator drugs: pinacidil and BRL34915. J Cardiovasc Pharmacol 11:90–99, 1988.
Cottrell JE, Turndorf H: Intravenous nitroglycerin. Am Heart J 96:550–553, 1978.
Dzau VJ: Evolution of the clinical management of hypertension. Emerging role of "specific" vasodilators as initial therapy. Am J Med 82 (Suppl 1A):36–43, 1987.
Frohlich ED: Pathophysiological considerations in left ventricular hypertrophy. J Clin Hypertens 3:54–65, 1987.
Fung HL, Chong S, Kowaluk E: Mechanisms of nitrate action and vascular tolerance. Eur Heart J 10(Suppl A):2–6, 1989.
Goldberg MR: Clinical pharmacology of pinacidil, prototype for drugs that affect potassium channels. J Cardiovasc Pharmacol 12(Suppl 2):S41–S47, 1988.
Hart MN, Heistad DD, Brody MJ: Effect of chronic hypertension and sympathetic denervation on wall/lumen ratio of cerebral vessels. Hypertension 2:419–28, 1980.
Herline IM: Intrvenous nitroglycerin: clinical pharmacology and therapeutic considerations. Am Heart J 108:141–149, 1984.
Ignarro LJ: Biological actions and properties of endothelium-derived nitric oxide formation formed and released from artery and vein. Circ Res 65:1–21, 1989.
Levenson J, Simon A: Heterogeneity of response of peripheral arteries to antihypertensive drugs in essential hypertension. Basic effects and functional consequence. Drugs 35(Suppl 5):34–39, 1988.
Linas SL, Nies AS: Minoxidil. Ann Int Med 94:61–65, 1981.
Lund-Johansen P: Haemodynamics in essential hypertension. Clin Sci 59:343s–354s, 1980.
Koch-Weser J: Diazoxide. N Engl J Med 294:1271–1274, 1976.
Koch-Weser J: Hydralazine. N Engl J Med 295:320–323, 1976.
Kreye VAW: Direct vasodilators with unknown modes of action: the nitro-compounds and hydralazine. J Cardiovasc Pharmacol 6:S646–S655, 1984.
Lipe S, Moulds RFW: In vitro differences between human arteries and veins in their responses to hydralazine. J Pharmacol Exp Ther 217:204–208, 1981.
McLean AJ, Barron K, Du Somuch P, et al: Interaction of hydralazine derivatives with contractile mechanisms in rabbit aortic smooth muscle. J Pharmacol Exp Ther 205:418–425, 1978.
Meisheri KD, Cipkus LA, Taylor CJ: Mechanism of action of minoxidil sulfate-induced vasodilation: a role for increased K+ permeability. J Pharmacol Exp Ther 245:751–760, 1988.
Miller RR, Fennell WH, Young JB, et al: Differential systemic arterial and venous actions and consequent cardiac effects of vasodilator drugs. Prog Cardiovasc Dis 24:353–374, 1982.
Morgan KG: Calcium and vascular smooth muscle tone. Am J Med 82(Suppl 3B):9–15, 1987.
Murphy RA, Mras S: Control of tone in vascular smooth muscle. Arch Intern Med 143:1001–1006, 1983.
Palmer RF, Lasseter KC: Sodium nitroprusside. N Engl J Med 292:294–297, 1975.
Pettinger WA: Minoxidil and the treatment of severe hypertension. N Engl J Med 303:922–926, 1980.
Pettinger WA, Mitchell HC: Minoxidil—an alternative to nephrectomy for refractory hypertension. N Engl J Med 289:167, 1973.

Robinson BF: Drugs acting directly on vascular smooth muscle: circulatory actions and secondary effects. Br J Clin Pharmacol 12:5S–9S, 1981.
Safar ME: Focus on the large arteries in hypertension. J Cardiovasc Pharmacol 7:S1–S4, 1985.
Safar ME, Levenson JA: Vasodilating drugs and the large arteries in essential hypertension. Artery 14:1–27, 1986.
Safar ME: Therapeutic trials and large arteries in hypertension. Am Heart J 115:702–710, 1988.
Songkittiguna P, Majewski H, Rand MJ: Inhibition by hydralazine of conversion of dopamine to noradrenaline in rat atria in vitro and in vivo. Clin Exp Pharmacol Physiol 7:509–514, 1980.
Sorkin EM, Brogden RE, Romankiewicz JA: Intravenous glyceryl trinitrate (nitroglycerin). A review of its pharmacological properties and therapeutic efficacy. Drugs 27:45–80, 1984.
Spokas EG, Folco G, Quilley J, et al: Endothelial mechanism in the vascular action of hydralazine. Hypertension 5(Suppl I):I-107–I-111, 1983.
Strauer BE, Bayer F, Brecht HM, et al: The influence of sympathetic nervous activity on regression of cardiac hypertrophy. J Hypertens 3(Suppl 4):S39–S44, 1985.
Tarazi RC, Fouad FM: Reversal of cardiac hypertrophy by medical treatment. Ann Rev Med 36:407–14, 1985.
Tobia AJ, Giardino EC: Modification of renal vasodilator responses of hydralazine in dogs pretreated with inhibitors of prostaglandin synthesis. Fed Proc 41:1662, 1982.
Walter V, Waldmann R, Nieberding M: Intracellular mechanism of action of vasodilators. Eur Heart J 9(Suppl H):1–6, 1988.
Worcel M, Saiag B, Chevillard C: An unexpected mode of action for hydralazine (HYD). Trends Pharm Sci 136, 1980.

Chapter 11

Centrally Acting Antihypertensive Agents

H. Mitchell Perry, Jr.

Introduction

There are four adrenergic inhibitors with a primarily central effect: methyldopa, clonidine, guanabenz, and guanafacine. In addition, reserpine, is an adrenergic inhibitor with a primarily peripheral effect but with a significant central effect as well. These agents have all been available for considerable periods of time and so have lost the sheen of newness. As such, their use has decreased, although each continues to be used by some patients who, over a period of years, have obtained adequate diastolic pressure control without unacceptable side effects. Only methyldopa, clonidine, and reserpine, however, continue as important antihypertensive agents, and they do this primarily by filling specific niches.

The major specific use of methyldopa is as the adrenergic inhibitor in the three-drug regimen which is usually needed in order to obtain long-term control of moderate and severe systolic-diastolic hypertension (SDH). A thiazide diuretic in this regimen is used, not because of its antihypertensive efficacy, but to potentiate the other two antihypertensive agents, thus diminishing by about half the required dosage, and thereby markedly reducing side effects and making long-term treatment acceptable. Although the original adrenergic inhibitor was reserpine, presumably any similarly acting drug could presumably serve as the second agent; certainly methyldopa and clonidine can be used effectively

From Punzi HA, Flamenbaum W (eds): *Hypertension*. Mount Kisco, NY, Futura Publishing Co., Inc., © 1989.

in this capacity. The third agent in the three-drug regimen is a peripheral vasodilator, such as hydralazine. A drug like hydralazine can only be used after a sympatholytic agent is in place to prevent the reflex tachycardia which otherwise is annoying and which counteracts the antihypertensive effect of the vasodilator. There has been no definitive demonstration that replacing hydralazine in this regimen by either of the newest types of agents, converting enzymes inhibitors and calcium channel blockers, produces the same decrease in mortality or morbidity; on the other hand, there are no data indicating that they are less effective in this regard than the older agents.

Methyldopa was also used as the second drug as a two-drug regimen by the European Working Party on High Blood Pressure in the Elderly (EWPHE). The other drug was a potassium-sparing diuretic. This regimen was reported to lower morbidity and mortality for elderly patients in a multicenter, double-blind placebo-controlled trial of antihypertensive treatment in patients over 60 years old with diastolic pressures from 90 to 119 mmHg. A total of 480 patients were randomized to diuretic, plus methyldopa if needed, or to placebo. A significant reduction in cardiovascular mortality of 27% was reported. This was due to reduced cardiac mortality (38%) and reduced cerebral vascular mortality (32%). The major reduction in deaths from myocardial infarction in this trial was unusual and unexplained. The decrease in morbidity and mortality was most marked in the patients with moderate and severe hypertension, but it was reported to be considerable in patients with mild hypertension as well.

Clonidine can also be used very effectively as the adrenergic inhibitor in the three-drug regimen for moderate and severe SDH. Because of its prompt and considerable effect, clonidine is frequently used when there is need for a sizable and quick response.

In a minimum dose (0.1 mg b.i.d.), clonidine has also been reported to be an effective monotherapy for mild SDH. For mild SDH where the effective treatment on mortality and morbidity has been less clearly demonstrated, apparently all available antihypertensive agents will lower the blood pressure in most patients and none will lower it in all, even though some agents are more potent than others and various mechanisms of action are involved.

Finally, clonidine can be administered transdermally. This route provides a constant supply of drug with once a week dosage. The transdermal patch produces a marked lowering of blood in a convenient manner and without the wide fluctuations associated with intermittent oral dosage.

Because of its very long duration of action, reserpine is uniquely able to provide a significant and constant antihypertensive effect for the patient who cannot remember to take medication regularly or who for any reason does not take medication daily. The fact that the usual daily dose of reserpine is 0.1–0.25 mg, which is significantly in excess of 0.05 mg per day needed for the antihypertensive effect, coupled with a very prolonged effect, means that patients who only take the drug every few days or even only once or twice a week obtain a significant antihypertensive effect—and it is a constant effect rather than the markedly oscillating effect that results from the irregular use of other antihypertensive agents.

Methyldopa

Methyldopa (1-α-methyl-3,4-dihydroxyphenylalanine) was described as antihypertensive in man in 1960. It quickly gained widespread popularity in the treatment of essential hypertension. It was effective and had a much better side effect profile than the drugs it replaced, the ganglioplegic agents.

Mechanisms of Action

Methyldopa's postulated mechanisms of antihypertensive action have undergone considerable revision through the years. It was originally postulated that it reduced blood pressure by inhibiting the decarboxylation of 5-hydroxytryptamine, dopamine, and norepinephrine. This was thought to decrease the concentrations of these compounds in the central nervous system as well as in most peripheral tissues and therefore to decrease in the stores of norepinephrine and hence vasomotor tone. However, the depletion of catecholamines does not correlate with the antihypertensive effect of the drug.

Because methyldopa is itself metabolized to α-methylnorepinephrine, which can be stored in sympathetic nerve endings, it was next hypothesized that the substituted neurotransmitter displaced norepinephrine and acted as an inadequate "false transmitter." The antihypertensive effect of methyldopa is not, however, well correlated with the production or tissue content of α-methylnorepinephrine. Moreover, the α-methylnorepinephrine formed is readily released by sympathetic nerve activity and effectively constricts peripheral blood vessels in most circumstances.

Currently, it is generally accepted that methyldopa lowers blood pressure via an effect of α-methylnorepinephrine on the central nervous system. The theory holds that this compound stimulates central alpha-adrenergic receptors and thereby inhibits sympathetic outflow. This is an expansion of the false-transmitter hypothesis and accounts for many otherwise unexplained observations about methyldopa.

Several peripheral mechanisms probably also contribute to the antihypertensive effect of methyldopa. There is reduction in renal vascular resistance which may be related to the fact that α-norepinephrine is a much weaker vasoconstrictor in this vascular bed than is norepinephrine. In addition, methyldopa lowers the blood pressure effectively in immunosympathectomized rats, suggesting a more direct peripheral action. Finally, a methyldopa-induced decrease is renin secretion may contribute to the antihypertensive effect, but this action certainly is not the dominant one.

The predominant chronic antihypertensive effect of methyldopa is to decrease cardiac output. There is no compromise of the functional competence of sympathetic nerves as manifested by normal responses to nerve stimulation and the maintenance of most cardiovascular reflexes. Thus, a moderate decrease in supine blood pressure is seldom accompanied by orthostatic hypotension, and post-exercise hypotension is also unusual.

Clinical Pharmacology

There is considerable variability in the absorption of unchanged methyldopa, but it averages about 25%. The decrease in blood pressure is maximal 4 to 6 hours after an oral dose and persists for as long as 24 hours. Since renal excretion accounts for about two-thirds of the ingested dose, some accumulation may occur in patients with impaired renal function, but this is usually not sufficient to require adjusting the dosage.

Methyldopa and its metabolites may interfere with some of the standard chemical tests for catecholamines and so can cause false-positive tests for pheochromocytoma.

Methyldopa is available for oral administration in 125, 250, and 500 mg tablets. The current average daily oral dose of methyldopa approximates 1,000 mg. It is usually given in divided doses, two or three times per day, although in some patients, with moderate or mild hyperten-

Centrally Acting Antihypertensive Agents • 211

sion, one daily dose may be adequate. In the past, doses as large as 5,000 mg have been given, and a 3,000 mg dose was common. These larger doses were used when the only other sympatholytic antihypertensive agents were ganglioplegic agents and rauwolfia alkaloids, and when severe hypertension was more frequent. With these larger doses, the side effects were increased, but there was little additional antihypertensive effect with doses over 2,000 mg. Retention of salt and water with resultant weight gain and edema may occur in association with methyldopa, as with most other antihypertensive drugs. When they do occur, previously controlled blood pressure may become uncontrolled. Correcting salt and water balance usually restores control.

Methyldopa is also available for intravenous use as the ester, but there is little need for it. Disappearance of the drug from the plasma after intravenous administration is biphasic, with the half-time of disappearance being about 2 hours for the second phase.

Side Effects

The most disturbing side effect is sedation, lethargy, or some variant thereof. Like many side effects, this tends to decrease with time, particularly if the blood pressure is adequately controlled, but it frequently does not disappear. It can be incapacitating to those who require mental acuity. Rarely it can progress to significant mental depression.

Nasal stuffiness, dry mouth, and decreased salivation can also be very disturbing. Sexual dysfunction, primarily impotence, can be a major problem for some men. Gastrointestinal symptoms have been reported, but they are uncommon and seldom severe. Rare effects referable to the central nervous system include vertigo, extrapyramidal signs and nightmares. Methyldopa-induced lactation is a very unusual side effect which can appear in either sex and is associated with high concentrations of prolactin in plasma.

Toxicity

Methyldopa has several very unusual toxic effects. First, rare but severe drug fever shortly after starting therapy can mimic sepsis, with shaking chills and high, spiking temperatures. Second, later less dramatic fever can be associated with hepatic dysfunction, reflected by elevated plasma levels of hepatic enzymes and occasionally by the appearance of jaundice. Although usually reversible, the hepatic injury caused by the drug can progress to hepatic necrosis. Some workers have reported relatively frequent elevations of hepatic enzymes which have been sufficiently disturbing to discourage use of the drug, although there are usually no other symptoms or serious sequella and eventual resolution is the rule. Other investigators, however, have denied seeing this. Third, methyldopa can also prevent the rise in body temperature usually induced by bacterial and leukocytic pyrogens; moreover, in large doses, it can cause hypothermia.

A few patients taking 1,000 mg of methyldopa daily for 6 months and about a third of those taking 3,000 mg develop a positive direct Coombs' test. Other than causing difficulties in the crossmatching of blood, this by itself does not cause clinical problems; however, hemolytic anemia can occur in those with a positive Coombs' test. It is very rare, with an estimated incidence of 1 in 30,000 exposed patients. In the few cases of methyldopa-induced hemolytic anemia, the antibody responsible for the positive Coombs' test is an IgG directed at the red-cell membrane; such patients are almost always white and have a low acetyl transferase level. Methyldopa should be discontinued if hemolysis is detected. In most methyldopa-treated patients, however, the anemia is nonhemolytic and unrelated to the drug; while, even in those with a positive direct Coombs' test, it is usually of the non-IgG type. The positive Coombs' test and the hemolytic anemia induced by methyldopa are considered to be reversible, but reversal may be slow and require weeks or months after discontinuation of the drug. In the rare instances when hemolysis is severe, corticosteroids may be useful.

Clonidine

Clonidine hydrochloride is a potent centrally acting antihypertensive agent with many diverse actions.

Mechanisms of Action

The chronic antihypertensive action of oral clonidine results from direct stimulation by unchanged drug of alpha-adrenergic receptors in the vasomotor center of the brain, with resultant inhibition of peripheral sympathetic activity.

Small amounts of intravenous drug produce a biphasic response with a brief rise and a subsequent persistant fall in blood pressure. The initial acute pressor response results from direct stimulation of peripheral alpha-adrenergic receptors; this is followed by peripheral alpha-adrenergic blockade. After oral administration, the pressor response is rarely seen, and the depressor effect is primarily central rather than peripheral. The decrease in blood pressure is apparently due to decreased cardiac output, but there is usually some decrease in peripheral resistence as well. Reflex control of capacitance vessels is not abolished; thus postural hypotension is considerably less marked than with some other adrenergic inhibitors. Oral clonidine decreases renal vascular resistance so that renal blood flow is characteristically maintained despite the lowered blood pressure; however, sodium excretion is considerably reduced. Renin activity in plasma is decreased, apparently primarily through a central action of clonidine, although a direct effect on the kidney may also be important.

The tricyclic antidepressants, imipramine and desipramine, antagonize the effects of clonidine and therefore should not be prescribed when clonidine is being used. In general clonidine should not be employed in patients with depression. Withdrawal of clonidine has occasionally triggered rapid return of marked hypertension. Since elective surgery requires withdrawal, other antihypertensive drugs should be substituted well in advance.

Clinical Pharmacology

The bioavailability of clonidine in normal volunteers following a single oral dose averaged 75%. Plasma was cleared at a rate of 3 mL/kg per minute, and 60% of the clearance was due to renal elimination of the unchanged drug. The duration of a significant hypotensive effect after a single oral dose approximated 8 hours in normal volunteers and varied from 4 to more than 24 hours in hypertensive patients.

Oral clonidine is marketed in 0.1 and 0.2 mg tablets. The usual oral dose ranges from 0.2 to 1.2 mg/day, with a few patients requiring as much as 2 mg/day. Except for patients with mild SDH, a single daily dose of clonidine is seldom adequate to control blood pressure. Unwanted effects, especially drowsiness, can be significantly lessened by administering the drug twice daily; side effects can be lessened even further if the drug is given in two unequal doses, the larger one at bedtime and the other at noon. The likelihood of added control of blood pressure can be increased by adding a thiazide diuretic and if necessary a peripheral vasodilator as well.

In a randomized double-blind comparison, 0.45 mg clonidine and 750 mg of methyldopa were equally effective in controlling the 6% of patients with moderate and severe hypertension who were uncontrolled on diuretics alone. Doubling this ratio of clonidine to methyldopa made clonidine the more effective of the two.

Clonidine can also be given transdermally providing continuous systemic delivery for 1 week at an approximately constant rate. Therapeutic plasma clonidine levels are achieved 2–3 days after the initial application. Patches with an area of 3.5, 7.0, and 10.5 cm^2 are marketed; they deliver 0.1, 0.2, and 0.3 mg of clonidine per day. They can be combined or cut to provide whatever area, and hence dose, is desirable. To ensure constant release over 7 days, the patch contains an excess of drug. At the end of 7 days, the patch should be removed. If no new patch is placed, the plasma clonidine level will persist unchanged for 8 hours after removal and then decline slowly for several days. Over this interval, blood pressure returns gradually to pretreatment levels.

Side Effects

The most frequent side effects of clonidine are dry mouth and sedation. They are very common and frequently severe, but they usually improve significantly when therapy is continued, particularly if it is effective; however, they seldom disappear completely unless the dose is small. Impotence occurs occasionally and orthostatic hypotension rarely. As with other antihypertensive drugs, retention of sodium and fluid, with resultant loss of blood pressure control, often occurs with long-term use of clonidine alone. The addition of sufficient diuretic ordinarily restores blood pressure control; hence the combination of diuretic plus clonidine is usually necessary for optimal care. With transdermal clonidine, transient localized skin reactions, consisting primarily of pruritus and/or arrythmia, occur in 25% of patients.

Sudden withdrawal of clonidine has been reported to induce a hypertensive crisis that can be life-threatening. This "crisis" has been associated with initial symptoms of nervousness, headache, abdominal pain, tachycardia, and sweating, followed by increased blood pressure 8 to 12 hours after the last dose of clonidine. In a true "crisis," the increased pressure overshoots the pretreatment level, but this is very rare. Concentrations of catecholamines in the plasma and urine are elevated in symptomatic patients. It is much more common to have a return to the original pretreatment pressure with prodromal symptoms. This latter clinical picture is primarily a reflection of the fact that the drug is potent and short-acting so that when it is discontinued the blood pressure reverts to its original level.

Guanabenz

Guanabenz is an orally active central alpha-2-adrenergic agonist. The antihypertensive action is mediated by stimulation of central alpha-adrenergic receptors with a resultant decrease of sympathetic outflow from the brain to the peripheral vasculature.

Mechanisms of Action

In man, 75% of oral guanabenz is absorbed and metabolized with less than 1% of the unchanged drug being recovered from urine. Peak plasma concentrations occur 2–5 hours after an oral dose. The average half-life of guanabenz is 6 hours. The sites of metabolism and the effects of meals on absorption are poorly defined. The onset of antihypertensive activity begins 1 hour after a single oral dose, reaches a peak within 2–4 hours, is appreciably reduced in 6–8 hours, and is gone after 12 hours.

Acutely guanabenz does not change peripheral resistance but chronically there is a decrease. Cardiac output is decreased acutely, but cardiac output and left ventricular ejection fraction are both said to be unchanged during long-term therapy. Postural hypotension is said not to occur, and there is reported to be no effect on glomerular filtration rate, renal blood flow, or body fluid volume. Tolerance is rare. The most frequent and significant adverse effects are drowsiness or sedation and dry mouth.

Clinical Pharmacology

Tablets are available in 4 mg and 8 mg doses. A starting dose of 4 mg twice a day is recommended although some people are controlled on a total daily dose of 4 mg. The usual maximum dose is 64 mg a day. It can be given with a thiazide diuretic.

Guanafacine

Mechanisms of Action

Guanafacine is reported to be a centrally acting alpha-2 adrenergic agonist with the same mechanism of action as guanabenz.

Clinical Pharmacology

Eighty percent of an oral dose was found to be bioavailable. Following an oral dose, the half-life of drug in the plasma was 17 hours, with the antihypertensive effect persisting for 24 hours. The drug is 70% bound to plasma protein. Younger patients tended to eliminate the drug more rapidly. About half of the drug is eliminated unchanged in urine; most of the rest being excreted in urine as metabolites. There is suggestion that the drug is secreted by the tubule as well as being filtered by the glomerulus. Both a single oral dose and long-term oral treatment produce significant decrease in peripheral resistance, but cardiac output is not altered. It is recommended that guanafacine be used in combination with a thiazide diuretic. It is supplied as 2 mg tablets and the recommended dose ranges from 1–3 mg daily; it need be given only once daily.

Reserpine

Mechanisms of Action

The antihypertensive effect of reserpine results from depletion of stored catecholamines and 5-hydroxytryptamine in many organs, including the brain and the adrenal medulla.

Clinical Pharmacology

Although it is currently believed that most of reserpine's antihypertensive effect is peripheral, there probably is a significant central component. Therefore, the drug is briefly considered here since it is not discussed elsewhere. Reserpine is unique in that its effect is slow to develop, but it persists for at least a month. As has been mentioned,

Centrally Acting Antihypertensive Agents • 217

this has major advantages for certain patients. The currently recommended maximum dosage is no more than 0.25 mg per day; however, a Veterans Administration Cooperative Study demonstrated that 80% of the antihypertensive effect was eventually achieved with a dose as small as 0.05 mg per day, the smallest dose tested. It is important to realize that if toxicity is to be avoided, small doses should be used with the results that the antihypertensive effect will not become maximal for at least a month and perhaps 6 weeks or 2 months.

In the United States, little reserpine is used by itself, although it is used in combination particularly with a thiazide diuretic. The decrease in usage may also be related to the fact that the drug is very cheap and therefore has no pharmaceutical company constituency which advertises it. In addition, it is an old drug and therefore has less appeal than newer and presumably better drugs. Finally because of its slow onset of action, it is frequently felt to be ineffective.

Side Effects

The most bothersome side effects have been stuffy nose and lethargy. Other side effects include nightmares, extrapyramidal disturbances, and increased gastrointestinal motility, with cramps, diarrhea, and increased gastric acid secretion. Thus it is generally contraindicated in patients with a history of peptic ulceration. Finally, reserpine has been frequently associated with a weight gain of as much as 25 pounds, presumably due to its generally sedative effect and the lowering of overall activity; this is certainly an undesirable therapeutic result in a mild hypertensive.

Toxicity

Reserpine has achieved a bad reputation because of the serious depressions it induced when it was first used in the mid-1950's at which time it was given in massive doses. In 1954, ganglion blocking agents were the primary antihypertensive agents. The patients for whom they were being used had severe hypertension and needed a prompt antihypertensive effect; the ganglion blocking agent provided such an effect. Reserpine can also provide a prompt antihypertensive response, even when given orally; however, to do this, it must be given in massive doses—and the early doses were indeed massive, ranging from 2.5 mg to 25 mg per day, i.e., from 10 to 100 times the maximum currently recommended dosage. With such dosages, severe depression occurred in a significant number of cases. There is no evidence, however, that depression has been induced with doses of 0.5 mg per day or less. Therefore, the current dosage recommendation is for no more than 0. 25 mg per day. Even with this limit on dose size, it is still recommended that the drug not be given to patients with a history of depression. Moreover, both the patient and his family should be warned that if there is any evidence of depression, the physician should be notified promptly.

In addition to being accused of inducing depression, reserpine was accused of inducing carcinoma of the breast in postmenopausal women. Suffice it to say that the original report has been completely discredited and there is no evidence of such an association.

Summary

Several older antihypertensive agents—methyldopa, clonidine, guanabenz, guanfacine, and reserpine—act by central adrenergic inhibition. These agents continue to be useful in combination with thiazides and vasodilators in providing long-term control of moderate and severe hypertension. Three of these agents have additional considerable usage in particular situations: (1) Methyldopa has had long-standing wide usage as an antihypertensive agent, and this continues. (2) Clonidine, which has a prompt and marked effect, is used in urgent situations. In a minimum dose, it has also been used an monotherapy for mild hypertension. Transdermal clonidine provides a constant blood level with once a week dosage, thus obviating the fluctuations in blood pressure which characterize intermittent oral dosage. (3) Reserpine provides a constant effect, even when taken irregularly. Moreover, since the usual daily dose is two to five times the antihypertensive dose of 0.05 mg per day, several doses per week are effective for patients who take medication irregularly.

The two most important adverse effects of these agents are depression of the central nervous system and sympathetic blockade with widespread autonomic, particularly sexual, dysfunction. Severe psychotic depression attributed to reserpine has only been observed with ten to one hundred times the currently recommended daily dose.

Selected References

Altura BM: Pharmacological effect of alpha-methyldopa, alpha-methylnorepinephrine, and octopamine on rat arteriolar, arterial and terminal vascular smooth muscle. Circ Res 36(Suppl 1):223–246, 1975.

Ayitey-Smith E, Varma DR: Mechanism of the hypotensive action of methyldopa in normal and immunosympathectomized rats. Br J Pharmacol 40:186–193, 1970.

Elkington SG, Schreiber WM, Conn HO: Hepatic injury caused by L-alpha-methyldopa. Circulation 40:589–594, 1969.

Finch L, Haeusler G: Further evidence for a central hypotensive action of a-methyldopa in both the rat and cat. Br J Pharmacol 47:217–228, 1973.

Freed CR, Quintero E, Murphy C: Hypotension and hypothalamic amine metabolism after long-term a-methyldopa infusions. Life Sci 23:313–322, 1978.

Glontz GE, Saslaw S: Methyldopa fever. Arch Intern Med 122:445–447, 1968.

Kopin IJ: False adrenergic transmitters. Ann Rev Pharmacol 8:337–394, 1968.

Kwan KC, Foltz EL, Breault GP, et al: Pharmacokinetics of methyldopa in man. J Pharmacol Exp Ther 198:264–277, 1976.

LoBuglio AF, Jandl JH: Nature of alpha-methyldopa red cell antibody. N Engl J Med 276:658–665, 1967.

Lowder SC, Liddle GW: Effects of guanethidine and methyldopa on a standardized test for renin responsiveness. Ann Intern Med 82:757–760, 1975.

Lund-Johansen P: Hemodynamic changes at rest and during exercise in long-term clonidine therapy of essential hypertension. Ann Intern Med 195:111–115, 1975.

Lund-Johansen P: Hemodynamic changes in long-term a-methyldopa therapy of essential hypertension. Act Med Scand 192:221–226, 1972.

Myhre E, Brodwall EK, Stenbaek O, et al: Plasma turnover of methyldopa in advanced renal failure. Acta Med Scand 191:343–347, 1972.

Oates JH, Gillespie L, Udenfriend S, et al: Decarboxylase inhibition and blood pressure reduction by a-methyl-3, 4-dihydroxy-DL-phenylalanine. Science 131:1890–1891, 1960.

Oates JA, Seligman AW, Clark MA, et al: The relative efficacy of guanethidine, methyldopa and pargyline as antihypertensive agents. N Engl J Med 273:729–734, 1965.

Perry HM Jr, Chaplin H, Carmody S, et al: Immunologic findings in patients receiving methyldopa: A prospective study. J Lab Clin Med 78:905, 1971.

Rehman OU, Keith TA, Gall EA: Methyldopa-induced submassive hepatic necrosis. JAMA 224:1390–1392, 1973.

Chapter 12

Quality of Life and the Hypertensive Patient: Clinical Aspects

Sydney H. Croog

Quality of Life: Tasks of Evaluation and Refinement

In the treatment of the hypertensive patient, consideration of quality of life is emerging as an important factor in the selection of therapy and in patient management. This point was underlined in the 1988 Report of the Joint National Committee on Detection, Evaluation, and Treatment of High Blood Pressure which noted that in order to continue progress in the control of hypertension, clinicians must address the impact of treatment on the quality of life of the patient.

This chapter examines some principal aspects of quality of life as a concept, problems of measurement and assessment, and various emergent controversies in the field of quality of life studies insofar as these have relevance for the clinical care of the hypertension patient. Selected aspects of the clinical use of quality of life as a tool in the treatment and management of the patient with mild to moderate hypertension will also be reviewed.

Emergence of the Recent Trend

Over the past 15 years, the concept of quality of life has received increasing attention as an issue in many areas of medicine and health

---

From Punzi HA, Flamenbaum W (eds): *Hypertension*. Mount Kisco, NY, Futura Publishing Co., Inc., © 1989.

care. In 1989 the Medline Service of the National Library of Medicine listed approximately 400 articles relating to the topic in the medical literature which appeared during the previous year. The effects of therapies on quality of life have been examined with illnesses as diverse as hypertension, heart disease, cancer, diabetes, renal disease, asthma, stroke, and many others.

We are now seeing the emergence of research which uses quality of life as a scientific concept in evaluating health care. This is reflected in part in the increasing number of large, randomized clinical trials in which quality of life is an important component. Along with this development, efforts are being made to incorporate the systematic use of quality of life as a tool in clinical practice as well.

As part of this work on quality of life, new attention is being given to the conceptualization and measurement of the concept, its utility in clinical studies, and its application in clinical practice. The number of scales and indices designed to measure quality of life continues to proliferate. Numerous reviews have been appearing that report on the many instruments and measures that have been employed to assess this complex phenomenon and its subdimensions.

Given the current attention to quality of life in medicine and health care, it is perhaps not surprising that there are broadly ranging views on its value and utility. Its strongest partisans assert that in the future, virtually every evaluation of a new treatment or every evaluation of a major new technology in health care will include an evaluation of the impact of these innovations on quality of life. Detractors maintain that the concept is only a metaphor that has an attractive sound, but that it is essentially amorphous, too global, and of minimal use for purposes of scientific research. Further, according to this perspective, physicians are already aware of the importance of consideration of the "whole patient" in treatment, and concerns with quality of life constitute only an elaboration of the obvious and well known.

Considering the current trajectory of research interest, work in this area will proliferate over the next decades. However, as with any conceptual and methodological tool, it is important to keep a critical eye and to maintain a continued effort at evaluation and possible refinement. Equally important is the need for continued evaluation of the clinical aspects and the applications of quality of life in the treatment of the patient. They should be grounded on sound conceptual and methodological bases if they are to be integrated into the clinical armamentarium.

Quality of Life and the Patient • 223

Quality of Life and the Treatment of Hypertension

Why is the systematic consideration of quality of life of the patient becoming increasingly recognized as important in the treatment of mild to moderate hypertension?

As with other chronic diseases, in the absence of potential for cure, the treatment of the hypertensive patient is directed toward controlling the illness, prolonging life, and maintaining function. However, along with control of blood pressure and other physiological sequelae, the therapy itself can have major effects on quality of life. These effects can extend over a period of many years of the remaining life of the patient.

Today there are numerous antihypertensive drugs that are effective in controlling blood pressure but that differ in their impact on various areas of the quality of life of the patient. The physician now has a range of choices among the many antihypertensive drugs that both lower blood pressure and have minimal impact on quality of life. Hence, quality-of-life assessment can have special utility in clinical care: in screening and evaluation of the hypertensive patient, in monitoring of how well the treatment is accomplishing its goals, and in documenting the condition and health of the patient. During continuous therapy, changes in quality of life can provide signals for change of medication if necessary.

In the treatment of hypertension, the problem of nonadherence to the medical regimen has long been recognized as a major potential barrier to effective care. Noncompliance can be costly in terms of endangering the health and life of the patient, wasting the time of the practitioner, and wasting the health care dollar. Because mild to moderate hypertension is usually asymptomatic, the treatment and its side effects may be perceived by the patient as "worse" than the disease. Consequently, noncompliance may often be due to the patient's unwillingness to tolerate the negative impact of antihypertensive medications on quality of life. So in a major sense, whether or not the patient takes medication and has blood pressure control can be mediated by quality-of-life considerations.

The rise of the "consumer movement" in the United States had led to increasing expectations about medical care. Patients have become increasingly critical about the quality of treatment that they receive from their physicians. In addition, various news media report from time to time about the prospect that antihypertensive medications can be selected which will not impair quality of life but may in some instances even improve it. As information on these issues disseminates among the public through the media, the level of expectations of patients has been rising concerning antihypertensive treatment. In fact, it appears that many patients have come to expect that their physicians will take quality of life into consideration when prescribing antihypertensive medications.

Increasingly there are hypertensive patients who change physicians because of dissatisfaction with their antihypertensive medications and with the attitude of their physicians in seemingly minimizing or disparaging their reports of side effects. In a more global sense, hypertensive patients satisfied with their quality of life on antihypertensive medications may generalize these positive affect to their feelings about their physicians and to the health care he or she provides. Conversely, feeling "poorly" can be identified, rightly or wrongly, by the hypertensive patient as the product of being treated by a "poor" physician.

In clinical practice, there is increased documentation that developing information about the quality of life of patients may be handicapped by problems of physician-patient communication. Hence, the need for systematic, reliable, and valid methods of assessment is becoming even more evident.

The role of differing perceptions in complicating assessment of quality of life can be seen in some data on reported sexual symptoms. These were collected for a large multicenter clinical trial on the effects of antihypertensive medications in which I took part. In the course of that research, we asked the study population of 626 hypertensive men to report through a confidential, self-administered questionnaire about their degree of distress, if any, over certain major sexual symptoms. These symptoms are commonly associated with a diagnosis of impotence (i.e., erectile and ejaculatory problems) as well as suppression of sexual desire. Among those 487 men who completed the study, nearly half (47% or 233 men) reported one or more symptoms at the study baseline prior to beginning the treatment phase of the trial (Fig. 1). Six months later, 260 men (53%) reported one or more symptoms. These were not necessarily the same men reporting at the beginning, of course. In all, 362 men reported sexual symptoms on questionnaires at some point during the clinical trial.

As part of the usual procedures of the clinical trial, the physicians collected data from the 626 patients on adverse effects and reported them in the medical case reports. Physicians noted in the medical case reports that a total of 31 patients reported some degree of sexual symptoms: 17 had completed the study, and 14 were among those who withdrew from the study citing sexual problems. Thus, the number of patients with

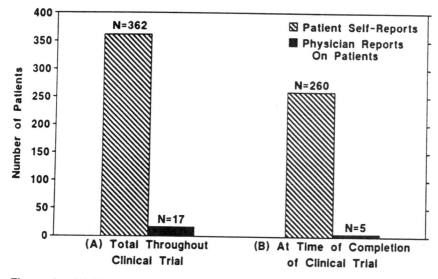

Figure 1. (A) Total male patients who reported distress over sexual symptoms during the course of the clinical trial, as indicated by quality of life questionnaires and by their physicians in medical case reports. (B) Total male patients who reported distress over sexual symptoms at the final interview of the clinical trial after 24 weeks, as indicated by self-reports and by physician reports.

sexual symptoms as reported by their physicians was only one-tenth of the total number of patients reporting symptoms on questionnaires.

Further, at the six months' assessment following inception of treatment, we found 260 patients with distressing sexual symptoms. The number cited in physician case reports at that time point was five. Numerous other reports in the current literature also outline how the clinical picture of the quality of life of the patient can vary markedly, depending on who is doing the assessment and how it is performed.

Summary

Numerous factors have combined in recent years to promote attention to the quality of life of the hypertensive patient. The application of clinical approaches incorporating quality-of-life considerations presents expanded opportunities for monitoring the responses of hypertensive patients to treatment. Thus, it aids in assessing not only the effectiveness of the treatment in blood pressure control but in understanding the full physical, psychological, and social impact of the treatment as well. Considerations of quality of life can provide the clinician with additional tools and cues to aid in the selection of the appropriate therapy for each patient, based on the patient's lifestyle as well as physical and biochemical characteristics.

In a period when compliance and even withdrawal from the antihypertensive drug regimen constitute important problems in the treatment of the hypertensive population, the focus on quality of life can improve adherence to the regimen and aid in achieving blood pressure control. Further, physician concerns with quality of life may itself have a favorable impact on the doctor-patient relationship and on the quality of mutual communication. Beyond this, studies of the placebo effect suggest the challenging notion that the demonstration of support and interest from the physician concerned with the patient's quality-of-life concerns may itself have a salutary impact on the outcomes of therapy.

Progress and Issues in Assessment of Quality of Life

Effective tools and techniques for quality-of-life assessment have been demonstrated in clinical trials of antihypertensive medications. However, the use of quality-of-life measurements in clinical care of hypertensive patients presents another set of dimensions and problems that must be evaluated separately and specifically in relation to medical practice. Of course, many of these problems and issues for clinical practice are relevant to clinical trials and research concerns as well.

Conceptualization

A first and fundamental problem in the assessment of quality of life is the wide variation in how the construct is conceptualized. The definition of quality of life varies from one study to another. These definitions in their relatively simpler forms maintain that quality of life is represented by such dimensions as good health, well-being, the degree to which an individual fulfills his personal needs and aspirations, or the ability to work and have freedom from symptoms. More complex formulations seek to incorporate a series of physical, social, psychological, and environmental variables as well.

Conceptualizations of the approach to quality-of-life evaluation

Quality of Life and the Patient • 227

range from considerations that quality-of-life measures in clinical research must be solely and specifically health-related, to concerns that they should be based on broader, relevant elements of life conditions as well, such as housing, income level, environmental pollution, racial or ethnic prejudice, unemployment, or the level of political control in a society. In the case of hypertension in particular, selection of the appropriate conceptualization of quality of life for measure is complicated by studies suggesting the relevance of social stress, living conditions, intergroup hostility and prejudice, overcrowding, and other factors that may affect blood pressure level and the course of treatment.

Efforts are now underway to properly conceptualize quality of life and to provide a coherent framework for use in research. However, many studies do not attempt to define the concept at all, leaving it to the reader to infer that the measures reported on are assessing quality of life. Obviously, if research in this area is to progress, consensus must be achieved among investigators in regard to conceptualization of the core construct.

Measurement

Other issues relate to the validity and reliability of measures of quality of life and its components. Questions on validity and reliability are pervasive, of course, and are standard concerns in regard to any measurement instrument. In addition, in regard to quality-of-life assessment, there is much discussion about the relative merit of using *specific, focused measures* versus using those that are *generic* and applicable to broad populations. Among the different approaches, one can select measures *specific to the disease* one is studying, such as hypertension, heart disease, diabetes, or arthritis, or measure that are *population-specific*, such as those for elderly females or middle-aged black males. However, such instruments are not usually applicable beyond the groups for which they are specifically focused. Broad categories of measures—generic measures—are designed for use across diverse populations. Examples are the Rand General Well-Being Index, the Sickness Impact Profile, the McMaster Health Index, or the Nottingham Health Profile. Hypertension is in many ways an optimal illness for the use of generic measures. Since the patient with mild to moderate hypertension feels no symptoms that would distinguish him from the general population, generic instruments developed for assessment of aspects of quality of life with broad populations can be employed.

Because much work has been done in refining and testing generic instruments relevant to quality-of-life measurements, they have advantages in use as far as reliability and validity are concerned. In addition, scores for the hypertensive patients in particular can be evaluated in relation to norms for the general populations previously assessed. A disadvantage of generic instruments is that they often contain questions that are irrelevant or inappropriate when applied to the specific illness groups with which the clinician is concerned. Quality-of-life studies often use conglomerate generic and specific indices and questions from various sources, shaping them for the operational needs at hand—a condition that leads, of course, to noncomparability between studies.

Objective Versus Subjective Measures

Discussion of the value of using either objective measures or subjective measures involves consideration of the relative merit of reporting on the patient's subjective perceptions of his condition—his reporting of symptoms of depression or anxiety, his life satisfaction or feelings of vitality—*versus* those which can be measured objectively, that is, whether or not the patient had returned to work after illness, whether he can climb a flight of stairs, or his income level. In general, critics are suspicious of subjective measures, viewing them as "soft," and unreliable.

Yet how the patient *feels* is obviously an important element in assessing quality of life. The data reported earlier in this chapter on sexual symptoms illustrates how much would have been missed if we had not asked patients directly about their symptoms.

It appears that neither objective nor subjective measures alone are sufficient in adequately documenting quality of life. Numerous studies have shown a lack of congruence between objective measures and subjective measures in characterizing quality of life. Hence, one cannot assume that in knowing about one area, one is also informed about the other. In response to a common criticism of quality-of-life assessments that they are based too much on subjective measures, one obvious solution in clinical practice is to use both subjective and objective indicators.

Aggregate Score Versus Profile Score

Another set of issues involves the continuing controversy over the desirability of using an *aggregate score* to characterize quality of life versus the position that one should use a *profile score*, characterizing each of the separate dimensions which are being measured. Given the complex, multidimensional nature of the construct, can a single, aggregate score adequately characterize the nature of quality of life? A single score summarizing a series of measures of differing areas of quality of life may be useful and economical in making comparisons between groups—but what does it mean?

The aggregate score does not provide the clinician with information about problem areas among the dimensions of quality of life of the patient or about specific progress in particular areas. Changes in one area or another, while they may be clinically important, may be masked by the fact that different configurations in scores on individual areas may nevertheless add up to be the same total score at different points in time. The profile score has an advantage in reviewing separate relevant areas, each of which may constitute a separate, clinically relevant domain. However, it may provide the clinician with more than he or she needs to know and is more complex than the single score for purposes of making comparisons.

Clinical Relevance and Quality-of-Life Measures

An important current debate centers on the potential for transfer of quality-of-life scales and indices from clinical trials and other research to clinical care. In randomized trials with groups of patients, the quality-of-life instruments may be effective in distinguishing whether one treatment or intervention has more salutary effects than another. However, the efficacy of measures in clinical research programs does not mean that they can automatically meet criteria for use in the treatment of the individual patient. If one drug in a clinical trial causes a significant reduction in symptoms of depression of 1.5 on a 16-point scale compared with a 0.5 reduction by another drug within large study populations, what does this mean *clinically*?

With regard to monitoring the long-term progress of the individual hypertensive patient, the meaning of changes in scores is unclear on many available measures of areas of quality of life. On a single scale of well-being or life satisfaction, for example, what degree of change in a score is meaningful in terms of the real world of the patient's quality of life? As yet, these problems of clinical relevance of quality-of-life measures are unresolved.

At present, few quality-of-life instruments have received the systematic evaluation that is necessary if they are to serve as scientific tools in the context of clinical care. There is no substantial body of literature based on comparative studies in clinical practice through which the merits of quality-of-life instruments are evaluated and rated. While such clinical practice studies will be pursued in the future, currently the physician who wishes to employ standardized quality-of-life measures in treatment of individual hypertension patients has only a few guidelines.

The Press Toward Parsimony in Measurement: Short Forms and Quality of Life

Recently there has been special interest in preparation of "short forms" to measure quality of life, reflecting a need for refining and reducing instruments to the basic elements most effective in analysis. There are many pressures underlying the demand for measures that are brief, easily administered, and easily scored. For example, federal and pharmaceutical sponsors of clinical trials increasingly wish to include quality of life in their studies. At the same time, they seek the most economical way in terms of patient time, personnel time, and monetary cost, and they look for minimal intrusion on the clinical, biomedical parts of the clinical trial. Physicians who wish to include quality-of-life measures in their treatment of patients also usually wish to minimize time, effort, and expense. Typically, such physicians express the need for a short form that will provide a single, summary score that indicates how well the patient is doing from visit to visit. It must also be easy to complete and acceptable to patients. Numerous short forms have become available over recent years, and there are many indications that this trend of production will accelerate.

A danger in the use of short forms lies in reductionism, in measurement of complex areas in ways that will not fulfill goals of obtaining valid and reliable assessment. In the field of tests and measurements, assessment of complex quality-of-life phenomena requires a sufficient number of scale items for each dimension in order to ensure satisfactory reliability and validity. A short form often aims to measure complex dimensions of quality of life with only one or several questions for each, a procedure that may preclude scientifically sound assessments. The problem currently is inherently a difficult one to solve, for if each relevant dimension of quality of life is to be measured in a valid way, the conceptual and statistical requirements tend to militate against a short form. As Donald Patrick and Richard Deyo noted in an article in 1989,

"The trade-off between short, simple measures and more comprehensive, complex measures in terms of reliability, validity, and responsiveness remains to be assessed for many generic and disease-specific instruments."

Sources of Information on Quality of Life of the Patient: Whose Assessment Should Guide Treatment?

In treating the hypertensive patient, when quality of life is part of the input into the clinical decisions, upon whose assessment of the quality of life of the patient should the physician most rely? Should information be collected from the patient only? While the patient is the key informant, processes of conscious or unconscious denial may block valid reporting on aspects of quality of life. Further, illness-relevant or medication-relevant changes may occur, but the patient may not make the connection and may thus not report them. Should the physicians add their own perspective? Should information be obtained from spouse or relatives of the patient? Though the perceptions of each of these potential sources of information may vary greatly, there often may be some advantages to putting them into the mix on which clinical decisions concerning the patient can be based.

The advantages of multiple reporters or observers must be balanced against the fact that the use of persons other than the patient to provide information can produce biased perspectives, as illustrated earlier (Fig. 1). In clinical care, some physicians may feel a temptation to evaluate the quality of life of the patient through using their own personal criteria and values, although these may differ from those of patients from other cultural origins, socioeconomic status, or psychological bent. This problem is, of course, not unique to quality-of-life studies but rather is a pervasive one as physicians develop information about patients in connection with the whole treatment process. However, if quality-of-life considerations are to be incorporated into clinical practice on a scientific basis, the issue is a core one in assessing the quality of life of the patient.

The Effects on Patients of Long-Term, Periodic Quality-of-Life Assessments

The long-term impact of periodic quality-of-life assessment upon patients in clinical care has not been systematically studied. While patients may initially agree to provide quality-of-life information on a regular basis over the years of treatment, some may eventually see this as a burden, an intrusion, or a stressful event. On the positive side are those benefits that come from the repeated assessment experience itself. As noted earlier, continued positive contact and support from the physician and associated staff may have some constructive effects on blood pressure control and adherence to the therapeutic regimen. As the systematic, long-term assessment of quality of life in clinical care is not yet widely practiced, there have been few opportunities to study these phenomena on a general basis.

Repeated Measures, The "Practice Effect," and Validity of Responses

If quality of life is to be assessed by instruments such as scales and indices at repeated intervals, the implications and consequences of such measurements must be considered. The "practice effect" in psychological testing is well-known. If assessments are done three times per year over a period of 10 years, what are the effects of completion of the same items in a questionnaire 30 times? Although the time interval can be lengthened, the same principle of possible influence of overfamiliarity with the items must be considered, even though its impact may vary among patients. The substance of the reports and their validity can be affected, but in addition, the prospect of patient boredom and resistance is a real one.

One alternative would be to employ equivalent but differing scales and instruments at differing time points. These would have to be carefully selected in order to ensure that they match in content, validity, and reliability. However, the array of tests and measures of quality of life currently available is characterized more by heterogeneity than by similarity or equivalence of measures, and the task of matching equivalent instruments is extremely difficult at present.

Problems in Quality of Life: Distinguishing the Treatment-Related Elements

Collecting information from hypertensive patients on the various dimensions of quality of life through systematic measurement will inevitably elicit a mass of data on life problems. Problems with children, unhappiness with a job because of unfriendly co-workers, or a sexually unsatisfactory marriage may all be part of the life pattern of the patient. Many such problems may appear to be beyond the sphere of professional responsibility of the clinician. At the same time, each of these could conceivably be subject to the influence of some antihypertensive medications, through increase in irritability, stimulation of paranoid feelings, and suppression of sexual interest. In addition, some of the quality-of-life-related problems that are reported may precede the therapy, along with concomitant physical ailments and conditions. Unfortunately, in the case of the hypertensive patient, the task of distinguishing between treatment-related and nontreatment-related conditions may not be a simple one, given the usual possibility of multiple factors in causation.

Periodic Presentation of Lists of Symptoms and Life Problems: Iatrogenic Effects?

The use of questionnaire instruments that inquire on a periodic basis and symptoms and problems may create attitudes and perceptions in susceptible patients which can interfere with the health care delivery process. Presenting patients with a list of symptoms or of problem life areas may have the effect of providing them with a cafeteria of complaints that they can identify as being possible consequences of the antihypertensive therapy. Consequently, they may consciously or unconsciously focus upon particular symptoms and report experiencing them. This may be seen particularly in patients with free-floating anxiety as well as those likely to somaticize.

Further, as studies have shown, the perception and reporting of symptoms may vary by such factors as cultural background, ethnic origins, socioeconomic status, and sex. This pattern of differential reporting may be further affected by the regular providing of symptom and problem lists to patients.

Quality of Life and Clinical Practice: Choices and Procedures for the Clinician

The application of quality-of-life assessments to clinical practice in a systematic manner is relatively new, going beyond their research usage in clinical trials and other studies. Considerations of quality of life were cited only as recently as 1988 in the Report of the Joint National Committee on Detection, Evaluation, and Treatment of High Blood Pressure. At this stage in the development of "quality of life" as a standard tool in treatment of the hypertensive patient, what kinds of options and choices are available to a clinician who wishes to employ the concept in the treatment of the individual hypertensive patient?

Assessing and Employing the Concept of Quality of Life

In clinical practice, the methods for assessing quality of life currently range from simply asking the patient "How are you feeling" and "How are things going?" to an intensive interview at each contact concerning all areas of quality of life. They range as well from requesting the patient to complete a short questionnaire concerning one limited dimension of quality of life such as well-being or symptoms, to collecting data through a self-administered questionnaire or a structured interview on a broad range of relevant dimensions of quality of life. Other alternatives include various combinations of these efforts and with varying degrees of emphasis. The amount of attention given to each may vary, ranging from occasional effort to routine collection of information at each clinical contact.

This array of alternatives in interviewing and questionnaire usage illustrates the broad scope of the choices for the clinican concerned with quality-of-life issues in the treatment of the hypertensive patient. Currently, physicians vary in their applications of quality-of-life considerations in their practice. Some physicians who have high interest in quality of life among their hypertensive patients may develop clinical studies with their patients as subjects, collecting data on a regular basis over an extended period of time through the use of comprehensive survey instruments in combination with interviews. Others with less concern for quality of life may follow a minimal course in collecting information through direct questioning about how the patient is feeling. Some simply expect that the patient will raise quality-of-life issues in the discussion if they are really salient.

Deciding on how the data on quality of life are derived, and by whom, can be important decisions for the physician who wishes to have the assessment accomplished effectively and with considerations of limited time and resources. In some instances, when minimal attention or only "lip service" is given to developing information on quality of life, the return may be minimal and even useless. For example, handing the

Quality of Life and the Patient • 235

patient a short, superficial questionnaire with the instruction, "Here, please fill this in, either in the office or at home," may produce a return of little value and validity, and may not be worth the time of the patient, the physician, or the office staff.

Contingencies Affecting Choice of Methods for Assessing Quality of Life in Clinical Practice

The participants in the clinical setting who may be involved in collecting the information on quality-of-life data range from the physician to various members of the staff or other professionals who may have an association with the clinician or office. The questionnaires may be in paper and pencil form or may be administered through a computer console. If questionnaires are used, there will be expenditures in terms of instruments, staff time for administration, scoring, record keeping and analyses, personnel expenses, space usage, and other costs. Depending on the scope of the effort to collect and manage the data, the costs can be considerable in the context of office practice with large numbers of patients over a period of years. The question of how this should be paid for and by whom has rarely been addressed in the literature on quality of life as a tool in clinical practice.

If the clinician is to assess quality of life only through a series of oral questions in the usual clinical interview, obviously the cost in resources can be minimal. However, making use of questionnaires, tests, scales—whether on paper or through the use of the computer—requires investment in the costs of the materials and the staff to administer, score instruments, evaluate, and file. Arrangements must be made for smooth processing of patients, providing time to complete the instruments without impeding the usual clinical work of the office. An increasing array of instruments and computer programs is likely to become available commercially over the next years. The costs of such materials and how they will be funded in the office practice will be another factor in affecting the use and diffusion of this type of quality-of-life measurement.

Whether in an interview or through use of self-completed questionnaires, the quality of information provided by the patient or other informants depends on such factors as the method by which it is collected, the setting, and by whom the information is being collected. The occupational identity of the person doing an interview can be important. For example, in interviews, patients may tell their physician about matters which they will not reveal to other office or professional personnel—

and conversely they may talk to the nurse or receptionist about matters on which they "don't wish to bother the doctor." Similarly, the amount and type of response by patients concerning symptoms, for example, can vary according to sex, cultural origin, as well as personality characteristics.

Selection of Instruments for Assessment: Criteria and Clinical Utility

One feature of the field of quality-of-life studies, as we have noted earlier, is the increasing proliferation of instruments to measure the construct. Hence, if the clinician decides to use scales and indices to measure quality of life over time in the hypertensive patient, he or she has a range of many instruments from which to choose. The clinician can make selections based on his or her conception of the scope and depth of quality-of-life areas desirable for measurement in the treatment of hypertensive patients.

It may be tempting in many instances simply to select scales and instruments that have been used to measure quality of life in clinical trials and other types of research efforts. However, the design and goals of research programs with larger populations are distinctive in many ways from those of private clinical care of hypertensive patients. The instruments which serve well for research purposes may not be suitable for clinical needs. It will be important to evaluate those which have been used in clinical trials and other types of research programs before assuming that they should be employed in clinical practice in the day-to-day treatment of hypertensive patient populations.

Given the state of flux in this field and the issues of conceptualization, measurement, validity, and reliability earlier noted, no general recommendations can be made concerning specific instruments appropriate for the special interest of each clinician. The process of selection can be aided by reference to the many review articles evaluating instruments that measure quality of life (see Suggested Reading list).

The clinician may wish to select indices that (a) assess particular subdimensions of quality of life, or (b) measure the global concept, or (c) a combination of both choices. In each instance, special consideration should be given to the nature of conceptualization of the construct to be measured, validity, reliability, standardization of the measure, and to the context in which the assessment is to occur.

If the clinician wishes to use an instrument designed to measure summary or global quality of life, particular attention should be given to validity of the instrument, given current ambiguities and lack of agreement about definition and delineated core nature of the construct. In the case of scales and indices measuring subdimensions of quality of life (such as well-being symptoms, emotional distress, cognitive function, or functional capacity), there are more choices available that meet criteria for validity, reliability, and standardization than is the case with global quality-of-life scales. Many of these focused scales were developed for psychometric measurement for other research purposes, but with due reservations, they can often be applied in quality-of-life assessment in clinical practice.

Prior to reliance on scales and indices as a method of assessing quality of life on a long-term basis, the physician should have a relatively clear idea of *what will be done with the data.* How will this body of information, the array of numerical scores, be employed in the treatment of the individual patient? Some sampling of the techniques through a preliminary try-out may be useful prior to establishing a commitment to one assessment system or another.

Using the Patient Focused Interview: An Example

Incorporating quality-of-life assessment into the focused, clinical interview constitutes a second method for choice. The focused interview can be adapted in length and intensity, depending on the clinician's judgment and the content of the report of the patient. It can be readily adapted to the particular characteristics and experience of the individual patient having more flexibility than standardized questionnaires, scales, and indices.

One example can be seen in the employment of a conceptual approach to quality of life which was developed by Sol Levine and me and which was employed in the first large multicenter clinical trial concerned with quality of life and the hypertensive patient. The clinical trial was concerned with measurement of health interventions—in this case the effects of the antihypertensive drugs—and we focused on a health-oriented conceptualization of the construct. Our view derives from the work of René Dubos, the eminent biologist. In defining health, as related to qualify of life, Dubos argued that "health," rather than being a state of being totally free of disease or disability, should instead refer to whether a person is able to do what he wants to do, is able to carry out the usual activities of day-to-day living, and has *joi de vivre* or enjoyment in doing so.

With this as our base, Levine and I defined quality of life in terms of the ability of the individual to carry out the activities or roles of daily life and the degree of satisfaction derived. The primary dimensions we selected for evaluation are shown in Figure 2: physical status, general well-being, emotional status, cognitive functioning, and performance of social roles.

We proceeded to a designation of key subareas of physical, social, and psychological functioning by which the construct can be assessed through questionnaires, rating scales, and psychometric tests. In general, where possible, we used generic, validated scales in the clinical trial—for example, the Rand General Well-Being Adjustment Scale, the Derogatis Brief Symptoms Inventory, the Halstead-Reitan and Wechsler tests of cognitive function and in other instances we constructed or adapted our own disease-specific and population-specific measures.

Patients did not receive a single total score for all these areas but rather they were rated on each one, using an assessment through the profile technique. Scores on individual patients on each of the generic, widely used measures can be compared with the work of others and

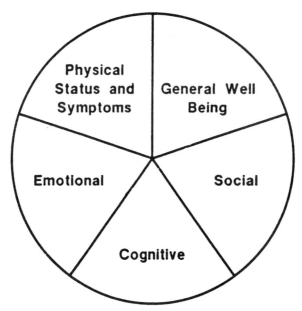

Figure 2. Areas for measurement in assessing quality of life.

Quality of Life and the Patient • 239

with norms reported with large samples of patients and with nonpatient populations.

This illustration offers only one way of conceptualizing and operationalizing the construct for a specific clinical trial, but the core notion and the measures we used may be adapted as an outline or checklist which could be employed in the clinical interview. As in the case of carrying out an interview for a general physical exminiation, the interview can follow a set of key areas for coverage. In doing so, the physician can proceed as with a physical examination in which questions are asked in a systematic manner concerning each organ system. It might follow an outline of major dimensions of quality of life, tapping a series of specific areas systematically. Through this, the physician will ask questions in the areas of emotional status, cognitive function, physical symptoms, sexual problems, work performance, feelings of well-being and life satisfaction, and other areas.

One listing of such areas is shown in Table 1. It is based in part on the dimensions assessed in the clinical trial, in part those suggested as domains of quality of life as outlined in a 1988 Workshop on Quality of Life and Cardiovascular Disease sponsored by the National Heart, Lung and Blood Institute. The list is not designed to be comprehensive, and its use should be adapted to the specific requirements of treating the individual patient.

The combination of the focused interview and the use of one or more standardized scales or indices is another option for selection. Thus, one device in clinical practice would be to employ a two-stage technique. The first would consist of the focused clinical interview, in whatever detail and scope is desirable at the particular stage of treatment. The second would be to require the patient to complete a short, well-validated generic instrument, one that can collect data in those limited, select areas which the physician wants especially to tap in a systematic manner. The information provided by the patient in the questionnaire can also serve as a guide to the physician in helping direct attention to particular problem areas and facilitating communication on these matters.

One widely tested instrument for such use could be the General Well-Being Adjustment Scale of the Rand Corporation. It is based on sophisticated application of principles of conceptualization and measurement, and it was employed with large samples in the National Health Insurance study and other research. The scale consists of 22 questions which form a series of subscales. These assess, in brief form, the areas of anxiety, depression, positive well-being, vitality, and gen-

Table 1.
Some Suggested Areas for Review in the Clinical Interview with Hypertensive Patients

Physical status
   Symptoms
   Sleep and rest
   Sexual functioning

Functional status
   Physical activity

Emotional status
   Anxiety
   Depression
   Irritability and anger
   Stress
   Spiritual well-being

Cognitive function
   Attention and concentration
   Clarity of thinking
   Psychomotor functioning

Performance of social roles
   Family membership roles
     (spouse, parent, sibling, etc.)
   Work performance
   Household management
   Community activities

General well-being
   Life satisfaction
   Energy and vitality

eral health. These subscales do not, of course, constitute an intensive assessment, and other longer, more directed instruments are available for such purposes. But scales such as the Rand measures are sufficiently sensitive for the purposes of this particular use in clinical practice and the need for a short, easily administered, and meaningful instrument. Other instruments may better suit the preferences of the individual clinician, and still others are being developed that can be considered as well in the future.

Such procedures can tap major areas of quality of life, as relevant to the situation of each patient. Supplementing the focused interview and the physical examination, the use of a standardized, self-completion instrument, one that is easily scored by office staff can provide an ongoing documentary record. The score can then be recorded by office personnel along with routine vital signs, weight, and other clinical information. It can be placed on a chronic disease flow chart, a functional problem checklist, or analogous record along with other clinical data to facilitate review and interpretation over time.

The procedures outlined do not, of course, constitute a comprehensive assessment of quality of life in terms of the global construct. Neither the Rand instrument nor the focused interview are designed to do that. The purpose is to collect in a relatively brief, effective, and adaptable way the kinds of information that can be most useful in monitoring antihypertensive therapy and the quality of life of the individual patient.

Conclusion

Clinical management of the hypertensive patient over the next decades will involve considerations of quality of life in selection of the appropriate antihypertensive therapy as well as in monitoring the impact of treatment over a period of years. As clinicians seek to transfer the findings from research programs into clinical practice, many challenging tasks remain. Fundamental among these are refinement of the conceptualization and definition of quality of life and the development of measures that are valid, reliable, and able to be integrated effectively into clinical practice. Beyond this, a major task is the translation of the meaning of scores from tests and scales in research programs into their clinical meanings, so that such information can be usefully employed in the initial screening and the treatment of the individual patient.

Although the achievement may be far in the future, comparative studies can help develop normative values for patient subgroups by age, sex, cultural background, and other relevant characteristics that can help the clinician in evaluating response of the individual patient. Along with the increasing proliferation of scales and questionnaires, various modes and techniques for evaluation of quality of life will become available through new developments in the technology of tests and measurements, including the use of the computer. The clinician will have many choices among means of assessing quality of life. In this chapter, we have reviewed some ways in which dimensions of quality of life can serve as a useful checklist in carrying out the clinical interview with the hypertensive patient.

Regardless of the approach to quality of life the clinician may choose to employ in treating the hypertensive patient, a prime consideration must be the effects on quality of care. Is the approach selected worth the effort and the cost? Is one method or another more effective in helping achieve blood pressure control, in maximizing compliance, in enabling systematic monitoring of change or stability in the patient's condition, in contributing to doctor-patient communication? Cost-benefit analyses need to be done, comparing alternative modes of assessing quality of life and employing it as a tool in clinical care. These should be comparative studies carried out in clinical settings, so that physicians can have a clear basis for deciding on how they should work with quality-of-life concepts in the treatment of the hypertensive patient and what types of resources should be committed. As part of such studies, the economics of assessing quality of life in clinical settings should be included. We need to know more as well about the implications of doing repeated measurement over a period of years in terms of their cost-benefit and utility in the health care process, and about the implications of the focus on quality of life for the role of the physician in primary care.

Acknowledgements: The author is grateful to Robert M. Baume, Ph.D., Sol Levine, Ph.D., Patrick J. O'Connor, M.D., Abraham Sudilovsky, M.D., and Peter A. Wyman, Ph.D. for comments and contributions to this chapter.

Selected References

Quality of Life: Issues in Conceptualization and Measurement

Bergner M: Quality of life, health status, and clinical research. Med Care 27(Suppl 3):S148–S156, 1989.
Bush, JW: Relative preferences versus relative frequencies in health-related quality of life evaluations. In: Wenger NK, et al (eds), Assessment of Quality of Life in Clinical Trials of Cardiovascular Therapies. New York, LeJacq, 1984, pp 118–139.
Croog SH, Levine S: Quality of life and health care interventions. In: Freeman

Quality of Life and the Patient • 243

HE, Levine S (eds), Handbook of Medical Sociology. Englewood Cliffs, New Jersey, Prentice Hall, 1989, pp 508-528.
Dupuis G: Quality of life: a new concept for an old problem. Perspect Cardiol 3:73-84, 1987.
Edlund M, Tancredi LR: Quality of life: an ideological critique. Perspect Biol Med 28:591-607, 1985.
Feinstein AR,, Josephy BR, Wells CK: Scientific and clinical problems in indexes of functional disability. Ann Intern Med 105:413-420, 1986.
Feinstein AR: Clinimetrics. New Haven, Yale University Press, 1987.
Guyatt GH, Bombardier C, Tugwell PX: Measuring disease-specific quality of life in clinical trials. Can Med Assoc J 134:889-894, 1986.
Kaplan RM: Quality of life measurement. In: Karoly P (ed), Measurement Strategies in Health Psychology. New York, John Wiley and Sons, 1985, pp 115-146.
Levine S, Croog SH: What constitutes quality of life? A conceptualization of the dimensions of life quality in healthy populations and patients with cardiovascular disease. In: Wenger NK, et al, (eds), Assessment of Quality of Life in Clinical Trials of Cardiovascular Therapies. New York, LeJacq, 1984, pp 46-58.
Schipper H, Levitt M: Measuring quality of life: risks and benefits. Cancer Treat Rep 69:1115-1123, 1985.
Shumaker SA, Furberg C: Research on quality of life and cardiovascular disease. Proceedings of the NHLBI Workshop on Quality of Life and Cardiovascular Disease, Winston-Salem, NC, 1988. Am J Prev Med 1989. In press.
Spitzer, WO: State of science 1986: quality of life and functional status as target variables for research. J Chron Dis 40:465-471, 1987.
Ware JE: The Assessment of Health Status. In: Aiken LH, Mechanic D (eds), Applications of Social Science to Clinical Medicine and Health Policy. New Brunswick, New Jersey, Rutgers University Press, 1986, pp 204-229.
Ware JE: Standards for validating health measures: definition and content. J Chron Dis 40:473-480, 1987.
Wenger NK, Mattson ME, Furberg CD, et al (eds): Assessment of Quality of Life in Clinical Trials of Cardiovascular Therapies. New York, LeJacq, 1984.

Reviews of Scales and Indices

Clark A, Fallowfield LJ: Quality of life measurements in patients with malignant disease: a review. J Royal Soc Med 79:165-169, 1986.
de Haes J, Van Knippenberg F: The quality of life of cancer patients: a review of the literature. Soc Sci Med 20:809-817, 1985.
Hollandsworth JG: Evaluating the impact of medical treatment on the quality of life. Soc Sci Med 26(4):425-434, 1988.
Hunt SM, McEwen J, McKenna SP: Measuring Health Status. London, Croom Helm, 1986.
Najman JM, Levine S: Evaluating the impact of medical care and technology on the quality of life: a review and critique. Soc Sci Med 15F:107-115, 1981.
McDowell I, Newell C: Measuring Health: A Guide to Rating Scales and Questionnaires. New York, Oxford University Press, 1987.

O'Connor PJ, Croog SH: Assessment of functional health status. In: Rakel RE (ed), Textbook of Family Medicine. Philadelphia, WB Saunders Co., 1989.

Patrick DL, Deyo RA: Generic and disease-specific measures in assessing health status and quality of life. Med Care 27(Suppl 3):S217–S232, 1989.

Read JL, Quinn RJ, Hoefer MA: Measuring overall health: an evaluation of three important approaches. J Chron Dis 40(Suppl 1):S7–S21, 1987.

Van Knippenberg FCE, de Haes JCJM: Measuring the quality of life of cancer patients: psychometric properties of instruments. J Clin Epidemiol 41:1043–1053, 1988.

Walker SR, Rosser RM (eds): Quality of Life: Assessment and Application. Lancaster, England, MTP Press Limited, 1988.

Wenger NK, Mattson ME, Furgerg CD, et al (eds): Assessment of Quality of Life in Clinical Trials of Cardiovascular Therapies. New York, LeJacq, 1984.

Measuring Aspects of Quality of Life: Scales and Indices

Bergner MB, Bobbitt RA, Carter WB, et al: The SIP: development and final revision of a health status measure. Med Care 19:787–807, 1981.

Bush JW: General health policy model: Quality of well-being (QWB) scale. In: Wenger NK, et al (eds): Assessment of Quality of Life. New York, LeJacq, 1984, pp 189–199.

Chambers LW: The McMaster Health Index Questionnaire: an update. In: Walker SR, Rosser RM (eds), Quality of Life: Assessment and Application. Lancaster, England, MTP Press, 1988, p 113.

Feeny DH, Torrance G: Incorporating utility-based quality of life assessment in measures of clinical trials: two examples. Med Care 27(Suppl 3):S190–S204, 1989.

Kaplan RM, Anderson JP, Wu AW, et al: The quality of well-being scale: applications in AIDS, cystic fibrosis, and arthritis. Med Care 27(Suppl 3):S27–S43, 1989.

Levine MN, Guyatt GH, Gent M, et al: Quality of life in stage II breast cancer: an instrument for clinical trials. J Clin Oncol 6:1798–1810, 1988.

McEwen J: The Nottingham Health Profile. In: Walker SR, Rosser RM (eds), Quality of Life: Assessment and Application. Lancaster, England, MTP Press, 1988, p 95.

Patrick DL, Danis M, Southerland LI, Hong G: Quality of life following intensive care. J Gen Intern Med 3:218–223, 1988.

Spitzer WO, Dobson AT, Hall J, et al: Measuring the quality of life of cancer patients: a concise quality of life index for use by physicians. J Chron Dis 14:585–597, 1981.

Stewart AL, Hays RD, Ware JE Jr: The MOS short-form general health survey: reliability and validity in a patient population. Med Care 26:724–735, 1988.

Ware JE, Jr, Brook RH, Davies-Avery A, et al: Conceptualization and Measurement of Health for Adults in the Health Insurance Study, Vol. I. Model of Health and Methodology. Santa Monica, Cal, Rand Corporation, 1980.

Quality of Life and the Patient • 245

Reports from Randomized Clinical Trials and Other Studies

Bulpitt CJ: Quality of life in hypertensive patients. In: Amery A, Fagard R, Lijnen P, Stassen J (eds), Hypertensive Cardiovascular Disease: Pathophysiology and Treatment. The Hague, Martinus Nijhoff, 1984, pp 929–948.

Croog SH, Levine S, Testa MA: The effect of antihypertensive therapy on the quality of life. N Engl J Med 314:1657–1664, 1986.

Croog SH, Levine S, Sudilovsky A, et al: Sexual symptoms in hypertensive patients: a clinical trial of antihypertensive medications. Arch Intern Med 148:788–794, 1988.

Croog SH, Sudilovsky A, Levine S, Testa MA: Work performance, absenteeism, and antihypertensive medications. J Hypertension 5(Suppl 1):S45–S54, 1987.

Guez D, Crocq L, Safarian A, Labardens P: Effects of indapamide on the quality of life of hypertensive patients. Am J Med 84(Suppl 1B):53–58, 1988.

Jachuck SJ, Brierley H, Jachuck S, et al: The effect of hypotensive drugs on the quality of life. J R Coll Gen Pract 32:103–105, 1982.

Jenkins CD, Stanton BA, Savageau J, Denlinger P, Klein M: Coronary artery bypass surgery: physical, psychological, social and economic outcomes six months later. JAMA 250:782–788, 1983.

Siegrist J: Impaired quality of life as a risk factor in cardiovascular disease. J Chron Dis 40:571–578, 1987.

Sudilovsky A, Croog SH, Crook T, et al: Differential effects of antihypertensive medications on cognitive functioning. Psychopharm Bull 25. In press.

Systolic Hypertension in the Elderly Program (SHEP) Cooperative Research Group: Rationale and design of a randomized clinical trial on prevention of stroke in isolated systolic hypertension. J Clin Epidemiol 41:1192–1208, 1988.

Wilhelmsen L: Trials in coronary heart disease and hypertension with special reference to the elderly. Eur Heart J 9:207–214, 1988.

Williams GH, Croog SH, Levine S, et al: Impact of antihypertensive therapy on quality of life: effect of hydrochlorthiazide. J Hypertension 5(Suppl 1):S29–S35, 1987.

Clinical Applications: Clinical Uses of Quality of Life Measures

Applegate WB: Use of assessment instruments in clinical settings. J Am Geriatr Soc 35:45–50, 1987.

Deyo RA, Patrick DL: Barriers to the use of health status measures in clinical investigation, patient care, and policy research. Med Care 27(Suppl 3):S254–S268, 1989.

Bergner M: Functional health assessments: are they ready for use in clinical practice? J Fam Pract 23:423–424, 1986.

Bulpitt CJ, Fletcher AE: The importance of well-being to hypertensive patients. Am J Med 84(1B):40–46, 1988.

Deyo RA, Centor RM: Assessing the responsiveness of functional scales to clinical change: an analogy to diagnostic test performance. J Chron Dis 39(11):897–906, 1986.

Elias MF, Robbins MA, Schultz NR, et al: Clinical significance of cognitive performance by hypertensive patients. Hypertension 9:192–197, 1987.

Epstein AM, Hall JA, Tognetti J, et al: Using proxies to evaluate quality of life: can they provide valid information about patients' health status and satisfaction with medical care? Med Care 27:S91–S98, 1989.

Joint National Committee: The 1988 Report of Joint National Committee on Detection, Evaluation and Treatment of High Blood Pressure. Arch Intern Med 148:1023–1038, 1988.

Kazis LE, Anderson JF, Meenan FM: Effect sizes for interpreting changes in health status. Med Care 27(Suppl 3):S178–189, 1989.

Nelson E, Wasson J, Kirk JW: Assessment of function in routine clinical practice: description of the COOP chart method and preliminary findings. J Chron Dis 40(Suppl 1):55S–63S, 1987.

Wenger NK: Quality of life issues in hypertension: consequences of diagnosis and considerations in management. Am Heart J 116:628–632, 1988.

Williams GH: Quality of life and its impact on hypertensive patients. Am J Med 82:98–105, 1987.

Chapter 13

Hypertension and Concomitant Diseases

Henry A. Punzi

Hypertension and Concomitant Diseases

In medical practice, the most frequent reason for office visits is hypertension. This arises from a heightened awareness of the disease process in the medical and lay communities. The last 30 years have proven that lowering elevated blood pressure decreases the incidence of stroke, heart failure, kidney failure, and premature death. In the early 1950s with the drugs available in our armamentarium (e.g., diuretics, reserpine, hydralazine), the treatment regimen for hypertension was less than desirable. The step-care approach was structured to educate physicians on the initial drug treatment of hypertension. During the last 15 years, pharmacological research has made available several new classes of antihypertensive agents. This, coupled with results from major clinical trials began to modify the prescribing habits of physicians. Over the years several recommendations were published, culminating in the 1988 Joint National Committee on the Detection and Evaluation of Hypertension guidelines. In this report, there is a specific effort made to promulgate the individualization of antihypertensive therapy.

Subsequent editorial comments have pointed out that the Joint National Committee did not venture far enough in breaking away from a regimented step-care approach. In contrast to the recommendations of the committee, many physicians believe that antihypertensive treatment should be tailored to fit the individual characteristics of the patient. The

---

From Punzi HA, Flamenbaum W (eds): *Hypertension*. Mount Kisco, NY, Futura Publishing Co., Inc., © 1989.

Table 1
Factors to Consider When Choosing an Antihypertensive Agent

Mechanisms of action
Antihypertensive effect
Antihypertensive safety
Patient compliance
Cost
Number of daily doses
Need for laboratory follow-up
Potential interaction with other drugs
Additional salutory effect on concomitant diseases

initial diagnosis of hypertension as well as the selection of the therapeutic agent will have a significant impact on the patients' life style and general well-being. Individualization of care is achieved by evaluating all aspects of the patient history and subsequent physical examination. The physician should utilize this information when considering appropriate first-step drugs. Factors affecting which antihypertensive agent is utilized for a particular patient are included in Table 1.

There are approximately 60,000,000 patients with hypertension in the United States. These hypertensive patients, especially the elderly, have a high frequency of concomitant diseases (Fig. 1). These diseases, which may or may not be hypertension related become important considerations when selecting antihypertensive therapy. Selection of antihypertensive agents for patients with concomitant diseases should be based not only on the hypotensive effect of the drug but on the effect the drug will have on the patient's concomitant disease.

The 1988 Report of the Joint National Committee on the Detection and Evaluation of High Blood Pressure recommends the use of diuretics, beta-blockers, angiotensin-converting enzyme (ACE) inhibitors, or calcium channel blockers as first-line therapy. A guideline of the steps set forth are illustrated in Figure 2. During the first office visit the clinician must take into consideration factors that will help in the selection of the best choice for initial therapy. Such clinical factors include the presence of co-existing left ventricular hypertrophy, coronary heart disease, heart failure, hyperlipidemia, etc. These co-existing medical conditions and their respective drug treatment will influence the choice of antihypertensive therapy. Medical management of hypertension in this select patient population is frequently difficult, and the patient is at higher risk

Hypertension and Concomitant Diseases • 249

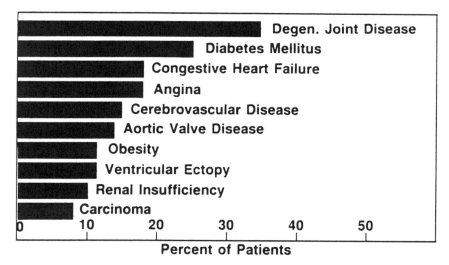

Figure 1. The number of concomitant diseases that are present in the elderly hypertensive patient population. (With permission from Anderson RJ, et al. Clin Ther 5:25, 1982.)

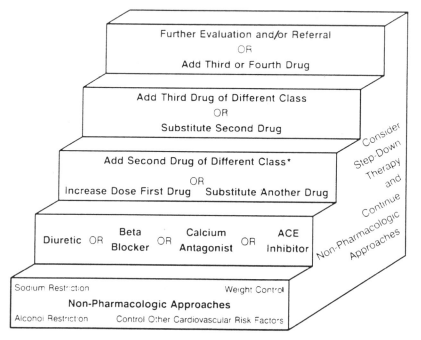

Figure 2. Modified step-care approach as presented by the 1988 Joint National Committee. (From 1988 Joint National Committee on the Detection and Evaluation of High Blood Pressure. Arch Int Med 148:1023, 1988.)

for increased morbidity and mortality. Each specific disease and its management are reviewed below.

Left Ventricular Hypertrophy

The use of echocardiography has detected left ventricular hypertrophy (LVH) in up to 50% of the hypertensive population. The presence of LVH is associated with a significant increase in morbidity and mortality from coronary events. LVH is a major independent risk factor for untoward cardiac events, including congestive heart failure, myocardial infarction, arrhythmias, and sudden death. Myocardial ischemia in patients with LVH is caused by an imbalance between oxygen supply and demand. Reversal of LVH may be related to factors such as the stability of blood pressure, the duration of antihypertensive therapy, the age of the patient, and the occurence of hemodynamic changes. LVH can no longer be considered a compensatory adaptation of the heart to increased afterload. In hypertensive patients the renin-angiotensin system as well as the sympathetic nervous system have an important role in LVH since norepinephrine and angiotensin II have been demonstrated to initiate myocyte hypertrophy.

Each class of antihypertensive agents, namely, diuretics, beta-blockers, vasodilators, calcium channel blockers, and ACE inhibitors, has a different mechanism of action and affects the course of LVH differently (Table 2). Adequate control of systolic and diastolic blood pressure with diuretics has failed to produce regression of LVH. Beta-blockers without intrinsic sympathomimetic activity (ISA) induce regression of LVH during treatment of hypertension. Vasodilators such as hydralazine do not decrease LVH and may increase left ventricular mass due to an increase in plasma norepinephrine levels and renin activity. Alpha-blockers have

---

Table 2
Therapy of Hypertension in Patients with LVH

A. Diuretics—high incidence of ventricular arrhythmias with low potassium and magnesiums levels.
B. Beta-adrenergic blocker—reduces LVH if not accompanied by ISA.
C. Calcium blockers and ACE inhibitors improve diastolic function and decrease the incidence of arrhythmias.

been associated with a decrease in LVH, despite the accompanying increase in plasma norepinephrine levels. Calcium channel blockers contribute to the regression of LVH, suppression of premature ventricular contractions, and improvement in ventricular diastolic function. The ACE inhibitors have been studied extensively in the regression of left ventricular hypertrophy. With an ACE inhibitor there is a decrease in sympathetic nervous system tone, with suppression of angiotensin II levels and regression of LVH. For example, left ventricular mass was shown to be progressively reduced to normal range when captopril was administered for six months. It was noted that the left ventricular systolic function was normal at rest. During isometric exercise, there was an improvement of the ventricular relaxation filling pattern resulting in improved diastolic function. In addition, the reduction in myocardial mass by ACE inhibitors may be beneficial in decreasing arrhythmias associated with LVH.

Coronary Heart Disease

Although the goal of treating hypertension is to reduce morbidity and mortality, the incidence of coronary heart disease in this population remains high. Epidemiological studies from nine randomized trials, including 43,000 patients for a total average follow-up of 5.6 years, netted a 8% reduction in fatal coronary heart disease (95% confidence interval [CI], −21 to 6%) and a 6% reduction of fatal myocardial infarction (95% CI, −22% to 14%). Despite a treatment-related reduction in the rate of fatal and nonfatal strokes by 39% (95% CI, −48% to −28%), the incidence of coronary heart disease was similar to comparison control groups. Explanations for the lack of effect on coronary events are speculative, but the issues of trial design and metabolic side effects of antihypertensive drugs, such as diuretics and beta-blockers, must be taken into consideration. It also has been postulated that significant lowering of blood pressure in patients with compromised myocardial perfusion causes an increased cardiac mortality ("J-shaped curve" hypothesis).

A recently published population-based case control study demonstrated that beta-blockers offer primary prevention from nonfatal myocardial infarctions in patients with hypertension. The presence of angina pectoris is a concomitant disease entity that results from a decrease in myocardial oxygen flow or increased myocardial oxygen demand. Beta-blockers and calcium channel blocking agents may be utilized to treat both hypertension and angina since beta-blockers reduce heart rate and decrease myocardial oxygen demand, while calcium channel blockers produce coronary artery vasodilatation. Diltiazem has specifically demonstrated favorable results in patients with non Q-wave myocardial infarctions. Alpha-diltiazem beta-blockers are another good choice in this setting because they decrease oxygen demand of the heart and produce peripheral vasodilatation thereby reducing anginal symptoms. ACE inhibitors have been shown to produce coronary vasodilatation and increase angina threshold in patients with coronary artery disease. Angiotensin II influences the coronary vascular tone, cardiac membrane stability, myocardial metabolism, and function. Reduction of angiotensin II levels with an ACE inhibitor results in favorable effects on the coronary circulation. It has been reported that captopril, a sulfhydryl containing ACE inhibitor, potentiates the vasodilatory effects of isosorbide dinitrate. Sulfhydryl containing ACE inhibitors may prevent further myocardial injury by the scavenging of free radicals generated during ischemia. A summary of these major points is highlighted in Table 3.

Congestive Heart Failure

Since there are approximately 400,000 cases of congestive heart failure diagnosed in the United States yearly, it is a frequently associated finding in patients with elevated blood pressure. When considering antihypertensive treatment, it is necessary to evaluate the patient's cardiac function. Elevated systemic arterial pressure exerts a higher stress on a dysfunctional left ventricle. In contrast to this, a reduction in blood pressure in the presence of a hypertrophic heart increases in coronary vascular resistance and decreases coronary flow reserve. Vasoconstriction, which is mediated by the renin-angiotensin and sympathetic nervous systems, maintains vital organ perfusion but can paradoxically decrease cardiac output.

Diuretics are the mainstay of heart failure therapy. Loop diuretics induce a rapid diuresis that is of great importance in the presence of acute pulmonary edema. Their use is accompanied by an afterload reduction with a decrease in diastolic and mean arterial pressures. Vasoconstriction is present with further activation of the renin-angiotensin aldosterone system begetting an increase in systemic vascular resistance.

The vasodilating drugs prazosin, terazosin, and hydralazine have been useful in the treatment of patients with congestive heart failure. The initial hemodynamic effects of prazosin in patients with congestive

Table 3
Therapy of Hypertension in Patients with Coronary Heart Disease

A. Diuretics
   Avoid hypokalemia due to increased incidence of arrhythmias
B. Beta-adrenergic blockers
   1. Helpful in patients with angina by decreasing heart rate and decreasing myocardial oxygen demand, particularly in an exercise state
   2. Offers prevention of nonfatal myocardial infarcts
   3. Blood flow to subendocardial area is redistributed despite a small change in coronary blood supply to ischemic myocardial tissue
C. Alpha-beta-blockers
   May be used in patients presenting with associated peripheral vascular disease
D. Calcium channel blockers
   Produces coronary vasodilatation, thus is useful in patients with angina
E. ACE inhibitors
   1. By blocking angiotensin II formation and preventing aldosterone induced loss of potassium, the incidence of arrhythmias is reduced
   2. Angina thresholds are also increased
   3. Captopril is associated with scavenging free radicals that promote myocardial injury

---

heart failure include reductions in systemic and pulmonary vascular resistance and a decrease in left ventricular filling pressures. However, the long-term efficacy of these agents has not be maintained due to the development of tolerance. Beta-blockers and certain calcium channel blockers should be avoided in this patient population because of their negative inotropic effects on the heart.

The ACE inhibitors captopril, enalapril, and lisinopril have been used successfully in the treatment of heart failure, although the most extensive experience has been with captopril. A significant improvement in exercise tolerance time and ejection fraction was demonstrated in a multicenter trial of 92 patients with moderate to severe heart failure. Symptoms, exercise tolerance, as well as New York Heart Association (NYHA) class were significantly improved in the captopril treated patients, with 80% of patients demonstrating a clinical improvement. In the placebo group only a 20% improvement during the three-month study was shown. Deaths were significantly higher in the placebo-treated group (21%) when compared to the captopril group (4%). During long-term treatment, 124 NYHA Class III–IV patients on captopril showed improved exercise tolerance and ejection fraction and significantly reduced heart size and symptomatology of the disease. In patients with mild-to-moderate heart failure (NYHA II–III), captopril has been shown to improve exercise performance, NYHA class, and reduce ventricular arrhythmias compared to patients treated with digoxin. Thus, captopril is a suitable alternative to digoxin in patients on maintenance diuretics.

Frank heart failure may be preceded by asymptomatic left ventricular dysfunction or occur following myocardial infarction. When captopril was given to patients with anterior wall infarction, an attenuation of progressive left ventricular enlargement was demonstrated when compared to the placebo group. The long-term implications of these findings and effects of ACE inhibitors on survival post myocardial infarction currently are being evaluated. Clinical response to captopril when compared to prazosin, hydralazine, and nifedipine has been superior. The combination of hydralazine and nitrates in heart failure has been shown to be effective and may improve the prognosis of these patients. The ACE inhibitors have also been shown to improve survival of heart failure patients.

Consideration must also be given to tachycardia that may be caused by nonspecific vasodilators. Tachycardia caused by these agents could increase oxygen consumption and subsequently worsen heart failure. However, clonidine and other centrally acting agents may decrease tachycardia induced by nonspecific vasodilators. A highlight of management is summarized in Table 4.

Arrhythmias

Sudden death due to arrhythmias presents most frequently in patients with underlying coronary heart disease. Etiologic factors that link cardiac arrhythmias with LVH include subendocardial ischemia, myocyte hypertrophy, and small areas of fibrin deposits. Specific antihypertensive therapy may influence the appearance or suppression of cardiac arrhythmias. For instance, diuretics have a potassium- and magnesium-depleting effect, which may exert a proarrhythmogenic stimulus on the myocardium. A subgroup analysis of the Multiple Risk Factor Intervention Trial demonstrates that patients in the special in-

Table 4
Management of Patients with Hypertension and Congestive Heart Failure

A. Achieve blood pressure control
B. If normotensive, reduce afterload (decreasing peripheral vascular resistance)
C. Diuresis is essential to relieve pulmonary congestion and edema; compensatory peripheral vasoconstriction may result. Avoid incipient hypokalemia
D. Beta-adrenergic inhibitors should be avoided because of negative inotropic effects; however, an agent improving cardiac function may be used in conjunction
E. Alpha-1 blockers (e.g., prazosin and terazosin) may be beneficial in heart failure. Pseudotolerance is seen frequently
F. Vasodilators (e.g., hydralazine) decrease elevated vascular resistance and increase cardiac output
G. Calcium channel blockers have negative inotropic effects and are contraindicated in patients having left ventricular systolic dysfunction and ejection fracture <30%
H. ACE inhibitors (e.g., captopril, enalapril) reduce both preload and afterload, lower heart-rate blood pressure product, and reduce coronary blood flow and myocardial oxygen consumption, resulting in decreased pulmonary capillary wedge pressure and increased cardiac output. Other characteristics:
  1. sodium and water retention is not produced
  2. blocks aldosterone-mediated potassium loss
  3. may improve renal blood flow
  4. captopril has less of a hypotensive effect than enalapril

tervention group with abnormal electrocardiographic findings had a higher incidence of sudden death. These patients were taking high doses of diuretics as specified by the protocol. The resultant hypokalemia has been postulated as a possible mechanism of this arrhythmia induction. Beta-blockers exhibit an antiarrhythmic effect in the presence of myocardial ischemia. Calcium entry blockers decrease peripheral vascular resistance and contribute to the regression of LVH. This leads to a reduction of the prevalence of ventricular ectopic beats and more complex arrhythmias. Intravenous calcium entry blockers, such as verapamil, have been utilized in the termination of paroxysmal supraventricular tachycardia; oral formulations are then used to avoid reccurrences.

Peripheral Vascular Disease

Peripheral vascular disease is a result of segmental deposits of atherosclerotic plaque that cause a partial or complete occlusion of the arteries. The lower extremities are more frequently involved causing the most classical clinical symptoms of intermittent claudication—pain at rest, and severe trophic changes. Drugs that increase peripheral resistance are not suitable for use in these patients. Diuretic therapy may be accompanied by leg cramping secondary to an increase in blood viscosity and a reduction in muscle blood flow. Nonspecific beta-blockers are known to worsen peripheral vascular disease. Beta-blockers with intrinsic sympathomimetic activity and alpha- beta-blockers may be utilized with caution. Adrenergic blockers and centrally acting agents may be useful in this group of patients. If using centrally acting agents, it is important to note that impotence is a major clinical finding in patients with peripheral vascular disease, which may be worsened with the use of these agents. Calcium channel blockers and ACE inhibitors are a logical choice in this patient group. Their primary mechanism of action is a decrease in peripheral vascular resistance and maintenance of collateral circulation, thus enhancing blood flow distal to the atherosclerotic lesions. As a result, the occurrence of impotence may be decreased. They also have a neutral lipid effect avoiding further cholesterol elevation. Animal studies have demonstrated that calcium blockers and ACE inhibitors can avoid vascular calcium overload and subsequent sclerotic vascular injury. These findings will need further clinical correlation, but they do give a potential indication for their use.

Renal Impairment

The relationship between the kidney and hypertension has long been an important one. Primary hypertension may be related to a defect in renal function, and at the same time, chronic renal failure is a predominant cause of secondary hypertension. Elevated serum creatinine levels are associated with an increased risk of mortality in hypertensive patients. A two-year survival rate of 45% is achieved in dialysis patients with concomitant hypertension, while that of normotensives is 81%. In renal failure there is a critical mass of nephrons below progression to end-stage disease occurs. Progressive destruction of these renal nephrons may be attributed to mechanisms independent of the original renal ailment. The surviving nephrons adapt to this loss by increasing the glomerular filtration rate to maintain water and electrolyte homeostasis. Decreased preglomerular resistance present in chronic renal failure transmits systemic pressures through the glomerular capillaries. The intrarenal renin-angiotensin systems plays an important role in blood pressure control through the local intrarenal generation of angiotensin. Angiotensin II causes an increase in both glomerulocapillary and systemic pressures.

To arrest progression of renal impairment, it is critical to control elevated blood pressures. Diuretics are an important part of the armamentarium in treating patients with renal impairment. Thiazide diuretics may be used in patients with mild renal failure, but when renal function has declined to levels less than 40 mL/min, loop diuretics are the drug of choice. Potassium-sparing diuretics and potassium supplements are to be avoided in patients with renal insufficiency since these can cause hyperkalemia. ACE inhibitors stabilize and improve renal parameters in these patients. This is not merely a function of lowering systemic blood pressure but also a decrease in angiotensin II levels followed by a decrease in intraglomerular pressures.

Minoxidil has been utilized safely in patients with severe renal impairment, often with significant improvement of renal function. If not contraindicated, beta-blockers and loop diuretics should be used in combination to blunt the very potent sodium-retaining properties and tachycardia of minoxidil. Beta-blockers produce varied effects on renal function and the alpha- beta-blockers such as labetalol appear to result in little change in renal blood flow or function. Centrally acting agents do not affect renal blood flow. Calcium blockers do not significantly affect, or may in fact improve, renal hemodynamic parameters in certain patients.

It is important to remember that there may be a worsening of azotemia when blood pressure is reduced. These patients need to be followed by frequent serum creatinine measurements while bringing blood pressure to normal levels. If there is a precipitous rise in serum creatinine concentration, then antihypertensives should be tapered but not necessarily discontinued. Once creatinine levels have stabilized, drug therapy may again be increased to bring blood pressure down to normal levels. Table 5 lists important guidelines in the management of renal failure.

Hypertension and Diabetes

More than 2,500,000 people in the United States have both hypertension and diabetes. Epidemiologic studies reveal that hypertension is

Table 5
Therapy of Hypertension in Patients with Renal Failure

A. Foremost, achieve blood pressure control, regardless of etiology
B. Failure to control the blood pressure is ensued by inevitable severe renal failure
C. Remember, renal function may paradoxically temporarily worsen in the period shortly after attainment of blood pressure control
D. Thiazide diuretics may be used in mild cases; however, once serum creatinine exceeds 2 mg/dL or if the creatinine clearance is less than 40 mL/min, loop diuretics (e.g., furosemide, bumetanide, or metazolone) may be used in the face of declining renal function. Metalozone may be combined with furosemide if the dose is greater than 400 mg/d. Response is assessed by body weight. Avoid hyponatremia and hypokalemia
E. Beta-adrenergic blockers present with variations independent of cardioselectivity or partial agonist activity
F. Vasodilators (e.g., hydralyzine, minoxidil), alpha-1 blockers (e.g., terazosin, prazosin), calcium blockers, and central alpha agonists (e.g., clonidine, methyldopa) do not decrease renal blood flow. Minoxidil may actually improve renal function. Must be used with a beta-blocker and diuretic combination
G. ACE inhibitors may maintain or increase renal blood flow. Furthermore, they decrease proteinuria and decrease intraglomerular pressures. If renal function deteriorates rapidly, suspect bilateral renal artery stenosis

twice as common among diabetic as nondiabetic patients. Hypertension and diabetes are independent risk factors that increase morbidity and mortality from serious cardiovascular events. Co-existence of both diseases makes their management more complex. A common precursor to both illnesses is obesity mediated through certain pathophysiological mechanisms including increased intravascular volume, cardiac output, stroke volume, insulin resistance, and increased catecholamine levels. Hyperglycemia and hypertension increase glomerular ultrafiltration by increasing the hydrostatic pressure and osmolar load. Glomerular hyperperfusion causes protein deposition in the basement membrane with subsequent glomerulosclerosis. The presence of proteinuria (protein excretion >0.5 g/d) is an indication that a progressive and rapid decline in renal function will follow. The blood pressure should be optimally maintained at <140/90 mmHg or below.

In the United States, diuretics are by far the most frequently pre-

Hypertension and Concomitant Diseases • 259

scribed drug by physicians for the treatment of hypertension. Biochemical changes associated with diuretics have been observed and include hypokalemia, hyponatremia, hypomagnesemia, hyperuricemia, and hyperlipidemia (Fig. 3). Hypokalemia in these patients induces insulin resistance either precipitating overt diabetes in patients with glucose intolerance or worsening hyperglycemia. Diuretic-induced elevation of total cholesterol and LDL cholesterol levels may adversely affect the patient by increasing the risk of coronary heart disease.

Beta-blockers should be avoided in patients with insulin-dependent diabetes who rely on epinephrine secretion during the recovery from hypoglycemic episodes. Nonselective beta-blockers will block these epinephrine-mediated recovery mechanisms and may increase the risk of prolonged hypoglycemia. Since the sensation of hunger and tachycardia are masked with beta-blockers, increased sweating may be the only clinical sign of hypoglycemia in these patients. Cardioselective beta-blockers may be utilized but may also promote hyperglycemia in these patients. In patients with borderline cardiac reserve, overt failure may be precipitated by using beta-blockers. These drugs may also raise triglycerides and lower HDL cholesterol, possibly contributing to an increased risk of coronary heart disease.

Alpha-adrenergic blockers may be a good choice for the treatment of hypertension in the diabetic patient because they do not interfere with carbohydrate or lipid metabolism. First-dose orthostatic hypotension, which is a potential side effect, can be avoided by stopping the concurrent administration of other antihypertensive drugs, such as diuretics, two days prior and two days after initiating prazosin therapy. In addition to withholding additional medications, the first dose of an alpha-blocker should be taken in the evening and the patient should remain supine for several hours. Some patients may experience protracted orthostatic hypotension. Centrally acting agents such as methyldopa, clonidine, guanfacine, and guanabenz do not interfere with glucose homeostasis, and they are an acceptable choice in hypertensive patients with diabetes. However, a high incidence of adverse side effects with centrally acting agents such as sedation, dryness of mouth, and impotence may result in noncompliance. Nonspecific vasodilators, such as hydralazine and minoxidil, decrease peripheral vascular resistance but will cause an increase in cardiac output accompanied by fluid retention and reflex tachycardia. The utilization of calcium entry blockers reduces peripheral vascular resistance and does not appear to have an effect in insulin secretion or carbohydrate metabolism.

ACE inhibitors have become the drug of choice in treating the hy-

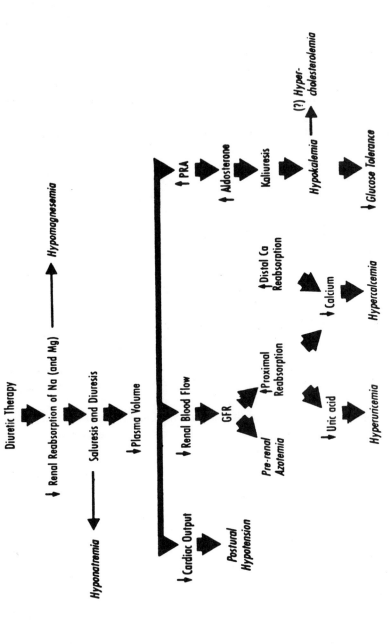

Figure 3. Diuretic therapy and possible mechanisms of action that lead to the various metabolic complications. (With permission from Punzi HA, Kaplan NM: Therapy for hypertension in the diabetic patient: pharmacologic intervention. Cardiovasc Rev Rep 8:37–40, 1987.)

pertensive diabetic patient. Glomerulocapillary hyperperfusion and intraglomerular hypertension may cause glomerulostructural injury. The ACE inhibitors reduce intraglomerular pressures by selectively reducing efferent arteriolar resistance thereby decreasing glomerulostructural injury. Strict blood pressure control is of greater importance in the preservation of renal function than strict metabolic controls in the hypertensive diabetic patient (Fig. 4). In patients with severe diabetic nephropathy, the reduction in severe proteinuria during captopril therapy did not correlate with the fall in systemic blood pressure. Long-term studies utilizing captopril demonstrate a decrease in the progression of renal dysfunction in hypertensive diabetic patients. The presence of microalbuminuria in these patients is a marker of impending renal compromise. The prevalence of micro- and macroalbuminuria is significantly higher in patients whose diabetes developed prior to 20 years of age. The prevalence of hypertension as well as retinopathy increases with the appearance of albuminuria. A six-month study in diabetics with mild nephropathy and persistent microalbuminuria demonstrated that ACE inhibitors reduced albuminuria with little change in systemic blood pressure. ACE inhibitors may improve renal function in normotensive diabetic patients with nephropathy. Glucose control may improve in patients taking captopril since it enhances insulin sensitivity as demonstrated by muscle glucose uptake. Finally, ACE inhibitors are not associated with adverse effects on lipids or sexual function. The use of ACE inhibitors must be monitored carefully to avoid hyperkalemia, since diabetic hypertensive patients may have hyporeninemic hypoaldosteronism.

Postural hypotension may be severe in patients with autonomic neuropathy. A low dose of an antihypertensive agent that will not interfere with the homeostatic mechanisms of blood pressure regulation should be utilized. In addition to a lower dose of medication, elastic support hose and elevating the head of the bed are mechanical maneuvers that can minimize symptoms. A synopsis of the medical management of patients with diabetes mellitus is found in Table 6.

Uric Acid Metabolism

Hyperuricemia is a common finding in patients with hypertension. The risk of gout increases with the degree of increase in uric acid levels. Diuretics cause hyperuricemia due to sodium and fluid loss and subsequent volume constriction and avid reabsorption of solutes in the prox-

262 • HYPERTENSION

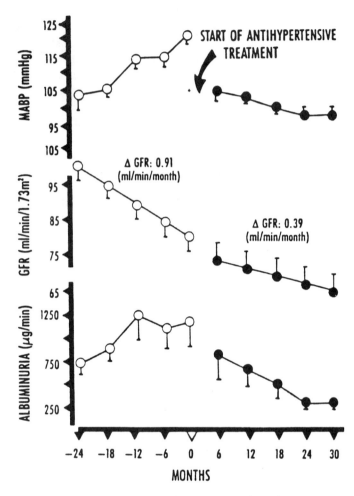

Figure 4. Aggressive antihypertensive therapy with triple-drug therapy reduces the rate of renal failure and proteinuria. (With permission from Punzi HA, Kaplan NM: Therapy for hypertension in the diabetic patient: nonpharmacologic intervention. Cardiovasc Rev Rep 8:61–63, 1987.)

imal tubule of the kidney. Attacks of gout may be precipitated by the use of diuretics, such as hydrochlorothiazide and furosemide. The concomitant use of uricosuric agents or colchicine may prevent diuretic-induced gout. Beta-blockers, alpha-blockers, centrally acting agents, ACE inhibitors, and calcium blockers do not affect uric acid metabolism making them suitable drugs for use in this situation. Indeed, the con-

Table 6
Therapy of Hypertension in Patients with Diabetes Mellitus

A. Thiazide diuretics
 1. increases the risk of developing diabetes in patients with poor pancreatic β cell function
 2. exacerbates hyperglycemia by depleting potassium and interfering with insulin release
 3. lipid abnormalities aggravated by increasing LDL cholesterol and the LDL/HDL ratio
 4. in conjunction with ACE inhibitors, serum potassium levels may be normalized and prove effective
 5. avoid potassium supplements and potassium-sparing diuretics; the presence of hyporeninemic hypoaldosteronism may induce hyperkalemia
B. Potassium-sparing diuretics (amiloride, triamterene, spironalactone)
 1. usual doses do not interfere with glucose tolerance
 2. effect limited by low hypertensive efficacy of recommended dosages
 3. increases the risks of hyperkalemia
C. Beta-adrenergic inhibitors
 1. cardioselective agents are preferred when used in lowest effective doses
 2. noncardioselective agents increase plasma glucose levels and decrease serum insulin levels. Hyperglycemia may be worsened. Signs of hypoglycemia other than sweating may be obscured: anxiety, tachycardia, and palpitations. In addition, the duration of hypoglycemia may be increased. Lipid profiles may be worsened and rarely nonketotic hyperosmolar coma may be induced secondary to poor diabetic control. In rare instances, paradoxical hypertension, significant bradycardia, peripheral vasoconstriction, and cyanosis may occur
D. Alpha-blockers, centrally acting agents, and calcium channel blockers do not alter glucose metabolism nor do they alter lipid metabolism
E. ACE inhibitors
 1. the preferred therapy for hypertension and diabetes mellitus since insulin release and glucose metabolism are not affected. Diabetic control is not compromised and may be enhanced
 2. diabetic nephropathy is neither initiated nor promoted. However, caution should be exercised since patients predisposed to hyperkalemia may develop this state
 3. lipid metabolism is not affected
 4. offers favorable intrarenal dynamics

Table 7
Therapy of Hypertension in Patients with Chronic Pulmonary Disease

A. Control of hypertension of vital importance because of propensity of developing left and right congestive heart failure
B. Exercise caution: avoid agents increasing workload of the heart
C. Avoid medications inducing bronchospasm
D. ACE inhibitors, calcium channel blockers, alpha-1 blockers, and centrally acting sympatholytics do not induce bronchospasm

comitant use of ACE inhibitors appears to minimize hydrochlorothiazide-associated increases in uric acid concentration.

Chronic Obstructive Pulmonary Disease

It is very important to evaluate the effects of antihypertensive agents and their potential interactions in patients with chronic obstructive pulmonary disease. Diuretics have no direct effect on airway reactivity, but may cause metabolic derangements such as sodium and chloride depletion and severe dehydration, causing hyperchloremic alkalosis as well as aggravating asthma. Hyperglycemia may also be present or be exacerbated by epinephrine used in the treatment of asthmatic patients. Cardiac arrhythmias may be precipitated by diuretic-induced potassium and magnesium efficiency. Caution must be taken when there is concomitant utilization of corticosteroids in this patient group. Beta-blockers should not be used in the asthmatic patient population. Even though cardioselective agents are less likely to produce bronchoconstriction, cardioselectivity is relative and diminishes as dosage is increased. Alpha-blockers such as prazosin as well as calcium blockers and ACE inhibitors do not adversely affect COPD or pulmonary function. Studies have demonstrated that ACE inhibitors may increase vital capacity and reduce hypoxic pulmonary vasoconstriction, thus avoiding pulmonary hypertension and right ventricular hypertrophy. This may be an important factor since the major of deaths from chronic obstructive pulmonary disease occur after 65 years of age. (See Table 7.)

Arthritis

Degenerative joint disease is more prevalent as the population ages. The disease process itself does not interfere with antihypertensive ther-

Table 8
Other Concomitant Medical Conditions and Antihypertensive Drug Therapy

Conditions	Drugs
Insomnia	Central agonist
Migrane headaches	Lipid soluble beta-blockers
	Calcium channel blockers
Esophageal dysfunction	Calcium channel blockers
Sexual dysfunction	Converting enzyme inhibitors
	Calcium channel blockers
Nephrolithiasis	Thiazide diuretics
Osteoporosis	Thiazide diuretics

apy, but the drugs used to treat this condition may have a bearing on therapy. Nonsteroidal anti-inflammatory agents have been implicated in the inhibition of prostaglandin synthesis, blunting the antihypertensive effect of many drugs. There may be an increase in volume expansion secondary to sodium retention from the nonsteroidal anti-inflammatory agents that could also blunt the effects of antihypertensive agents. Inhibition of the renal cyclo-oxygenase synthesis by nonsteroidal anti-inflammatory agents could precipitate acute or worsen chronic renal failure. Calcium blockers may be useful since they do not directly rely on the prostaglandin cascade for their antihypertensive effect.

Table 8 summarizes the preferred treatment for other concomitant miscellaneous conditions.

Summary

The presence of concomitant diseases will have an impact on the initial choice of antihypertensive drugs. As new information becomes available regarding mechanisms of action, side effects, and potential benefits of newer antihypertensive drugs, physicians must evaluate this information in order to choose a treatment regimen that will not have a deleterious effect on concomitant diseases. The ACE inhibitors as well as calcium channel blockers are excellent first-choice drugs in the treatment of hypertensive patients with concomitant illnesses. These drugs not only decrease systemic blood pressures but also prevent further target organ deterioration. They may also be effective in halting progression or even reversal of atherosclerotic plaque formation in the vascular wall. Clinical judgment should always prevail over the utilization of technically advanced hemodynamic testing when treating the majority of patients with hypertension.

Acknowledgments: I would like to thank my staff for all their efforts in preparing this manuscript, especially, Reneé Benedict and Janith Mills, PA-C. I would also like to thank Karen Porrini, Pharm D., and Carmen Bell, R.N. for their editorial assistance.

Selected References

Anderson S, Meyer TW, Remke HG, et al: Control of glomerular hypertension limits glomerular injury in rats with reduced renal mass. J Clin Invest 76:612–619, 1985.
Bergman SM, Wallin DJ: Antihypertensive therapy in the patient with other chronic diseases. Geriatr Med Today 8:38–38, 1989.
Bertoli L, Fusco M, Lo Cicero S, et al: Influence of ACE inhibitors on pulmonary hemodynamics and function in patients in whom beta-blockers are contraindicated. Post Grad Med J 62:47–51, 1986.
Brest AN: Antihypertensive therapy in perspective, Part II. Mod Cardiovasc Dis 58:1–5, 1989.
Captopril Multicenter Research Group: Comparative effects of therapy with captopril and digoxin in patients with mild to moderate heart failure. JAMA 259:539–544, 1988.
Captopril Multicenter Research Group I: A cooperative multicenter study of captopril in congestive heart failure: hemodynamic effects and long term response. Am Heart J 110:439–447, 1985.
Case DB: Patient population as consideration for antihypertensive therapy. In: Hollenberg NK (ed), Management of Hypertension: A Multifactorial Approach. Boston, Scientific Therapeutics Information, Inc., pp 101–120, 1987.
Devereux RB: Echocardiographic insights into the pathophysiology and prognostic significance of hypertensive cardiac hypertrophy. Am J Hypertens 2:(Suppl)186–195.
Dzau VJ, Colucci WS, William GH, et al: Sustained effectiveness of converting enzyme inhibition in patients with severe congestive heart failure. N Engl J Med 302:1373–1379, 1980.
Faubert PF, Porush JG: Managing hypertension in chronic renal disease. Geriatrics 42:49–58, 1987.
Flekenstein A, Flekenstein-Grun G, Frey M, et al: Calcium antagonism and ACE inhibition. Two outstandingly effective means of interference with cardiovascular calcium overload, high blood pressure and arteriosclerosis in spontaneously hypertensive rats. J Hypertens 2:194–204, 1989.
Frishman WH, Charlap S: Alpha adrenergic blockers—Cardiovascular pharmacotherapy II. Med Clin North Am. 72:427–440, 1988.
Kaplan NM: Importance of coronary heart disease risk factors in the management of hypertension. An overview. Am J Med 86:1–4, 1989.

Hypertension and Concomitant Diseases • 267

Kaplan NM: Renal parenchymal hypertension. In: Kaplan NM (ed), Clinical Hypertension. Baltimore, William and Wilkins Co, pp 292-316, 1986.

Levy D, Anderson KM, Savage DD, et al: Echocardiographically detected left ventricular hypertrophy: prevalence and risk factors. Ann Int Med 108:7-13, 1988.

Levy D, Garrison RJ, Savage DD, et al: Left ventricular mass and incidence of coronary heart disease in an elderly cohort. Ann Int Med 110:101-107, 1989.

McLenachan JM, Henderson E, Morris KI, et al: Ventricular arrhythmias in patients with hypertensive left ventricular hypertrophy. N Engl J Med 317:787-792, 1987.

Messerli FH, Nunez BD, Nunez MM, et al: Hypertension and sudden death. Disparate effects of calcium entry blockers and diuretic therapy on cardiac dysrhythmias. Arch Intern Med 149:1263-1268, 1989.

Muiesan ML, Agabiti-Rosei E, Romanelli G, et al: Beneficial effects of one year's treatment with captopril on left ventricular anatomy and function in hypertensive patients with left ventricular hypertrophy. Am J Med 84(Suppl 3A):129-132, 1988.

Noth RH: Diabetic nephropathy: hemodynamic basis and implications for disease management. Ann Intern Med 110:795-813, 1989.

O'Kelly BF, Massie BM, Tubau JF, et al: Coronary morbidity and mortality, preexisting silent coronary artery disease, and mild hypertension. Ann Int Med 110:1017-1026, 1989.

Papademetriou V: Can diuretic therapy cause arrhythmias in systemic hypertension. Cardiovas Board Rev 6:23-30, 1989.

Parving HH, Anderson AR, Smidtum, et al: Early aggressive antihypertensive treatment reduces rate of decline in kidney function in diabetic nephropathy. Lancet 2:1175-1179, 1983.

Psaty BM, Koepsell TD, Logerfo JF, et al: β-Blockers and primary prevention of coronary heart disease in patients with high blood pressure. JAMA 261:2087-2094, 1989.

Puddy IB, Bielin R, Vandongen R, et al: Differential effects of sulindac and indomethacin on blood pressure in treated essential hypertensive subjects. Clin Sci 69:327-336, 1985.

Punzi HA, Kaplan NM: Therapy of hypertension in the diabetic patient: nonpharmacologic intervention. Cardiovasc Rev Rep 8:61-63, 1987.

Punzi HA, Kaplan NM: Therapy of hypertension in the diabetic patient: pharmacologic intervention. Cardiovasc Rev Rep 8:37-41, 1987.

Roberts DH, Tsao Y, McLoughlin GA, et al: Placebo-controlled comparison of captopril, atenolol, labetalol and pindolol in hypertension complicated by intermittent claudication. Lancet 650-653, 1987.

Ruilope LM, Miranda B, Morales JM, et al: Converting enzyme inhibition in chronic renal failure. Am J Kidney Dis 13:120-126, 1989.

Sheiban I, Arcaro G, Coui G, et al: Regression of cardiac hypertrophy after antihypertensive therapy with nifedipine and captopril. J Cardiol Pharmacol 10(Suppl 10):S187-S191, 1987.

Stamler J, Wentworth D, Neaton JD, et al: Is the relationship between serum cholesterol and risk of premature death from coronary heart disease continuous and graded? Findings in 356,222 primary screenees of the multiple risk factor intervention trial (MRFIT). JAMA 256:2823-2828, 1986.

Ventura HO, Frohlich ED, Messerli FH, et al: Cardiovascular effects and regional blood flow distribution associated with angiotensin converting enzyme inhibition (captopril) in essential hypertension. Am J Cardiol 55:1023–1026, 1985.

Weber JR: Left ventricular hypertrophy: its prime importance as a controllable risk factor. Am Heart J 116:272–279, 1988.

Wenger NK, O'Rourke R, Marcus FI: The care of elderly patients with cardiovascular disease. Ann Int Med 109:425–425, 1988.

Zusman RM: Left ventricular function in hypertension: relevance to the selection of antihypertensive therapy. Am J Hypertens 2:200S–206S, 1989.

Chapter 14

Hypertension in the Elderly: Impact, Pathophysiology and Treatment

Myron H. Weinberger

Introduction

In recent decades, life span has increased in most societies. Blood pressure is known to increase with age, at least in cultures where sodium intake is abundant. Thus, it is not surprising to observe that the prevalence of hypertension increases with advancing life span. Indeed, recent observations from the NHANES survey indicate that about 50% of the 45- to 54-year-old American population have an increased blood pressure (>140/90 mmHg). By age 65, this figure increases to over 65% of the population with an additional 10% or so having an isolated elevation of systolic pressure (>160/<90 mmHg). More important than the frequent occurrence of elevated blood pressure in the older population is its well-documented and dramatic impact on cardiovascular morbidity and mortality. In general, elderly individuals with hypertension have a death rate twice that of their normotensive counterparts and a rate of cardiovascular events that is tripled by elevated blood pressure. Regardless of the nature of the blood pressure elevation in the elderly, systolic, diastolic, or both, an increase in left ventricular hypertrophy, congestive heart failure, coronary artery disease, peripheral vascular

From Punzi HA, Flamenbaum W (eds): *Hypertension*. Mount Kisco, NY, Futura Publishing Co., Inc., © 1989.

disease, vascular aneurysms, cardiac arrhythmias, cerebrovascular disease, renal failure, and senile dementia have been shown to be more frequent when blood pressure is elevated.

These cardiovascular events contribute enormously to the costs of health care, an area of mounting concern. The elderly population consume a disproportionately greater share of medical care costs in medication, professional visits, laboratory testing, and hospital charges than do younger individuals. The expenses of rehabilitative and supportive care for those suffering chronic and debilitating diseases, often related to cardiovascular catastrophes, are enormous. In view of the direct relationship between elevated blood pressure and most, if not all, of these major and devastating cardiovascular events, it is clear that uncontrolled hypertension and its consequences are too expensive to be ignored. Furthermore, accumulating evidence suggesting that effective antihypertensive therapy can reduce cardiovascular morbidity and mortality emphasizes the benefit to be derived from effective antihypertensive therapy, particularly if carefully chosen to minimize other potentially adverse effects.

Until recently, there was little direct evidence that reduction of elevated blood pressure in elderly individuals was beneficial. Indeed, because of the "natural" sclerosis of the vascular tree, many experts considered an increase in pressure to be necessary (essential) in order to maintain organ and tissue perfusion. Faced with overwhelming data from epidemiological studies indicating a relationship between elevation of diastolic and/or systolic pressure and every form of cardiovascular disease, a number of studies were designed and conducted over the past two decades to determine whether reduction of elevated pressure was beneficial.

Background

The first major study focusing on the benefits of treating hypertension in the older population was the European Working Party on Hypertension in the Elderly (EWPHE). This was a double-blind, randomized, placebo-controlled trial in over 800 hypertensives above age 59 with blood pressure above 160/90 mmHg who were assigned to receive hydrochlorothiazide plus triamterene or placebo. Active treatment reduced overall cardiovascular mortality by 38% and fatal myocardial infarction by 60%. In addition, nonfatal strokes were reduced by 52% and congestive heart failure by 63% with active treatment.

In the Hypertension Detection and Follow-up Program (HDFP), the benefits of intensive stepped-care (SC) therapy were compared to less rigid referred care (RC) blood pressure management. Mean arterial pressure was reduced approximately 5 mmHg more in the SC group than in the RC group. Among individuals in the 60–69 age range participating in the SC group, a 16% reduction in all-cause mortality was observed. Furthermore, the oldest subjects, those who were 65–74 years old at the end of the study, had a greater reduction in fatal and nonfatal strokes (-45%) than did their younger counterparts. These benefits from treating systolic-diastolic hypertension in elderly individuals were also evident in the Veterans Administration Cooperative Study and in a placebo-controlled trial of Australian hypertensives.

While the benefit of treating established systolic-diastolic hypertension is now unequivocal in older individuals, controversy exists regarding the optimal levels of blood pressure reduction and of intervention in isolated systolic hypertension (ISH). Recent meta-analyses of several studies has suggested the presence of a "J-shaped" curve relating diastolic pressure to mortality in treated hypertensives. This observation has suggested the possibility that excessive reduction or diastolic pressure below a critical level (about 80–85 mmHg) could contribute to an *increased* risk of cardiovascular disease, presumably by decreasing coronary artery blood flow as a result of decreased coronary filling during diastole. Although this possibility has not been proven, it would seem prudent, particularly in older hypertensives in whom the likelihood of unrecognized coronary artery disease is high, to avoid excessive reduction in diastolic pressure.

The benefit of treating ISH (systolic >160 mmHg, diastolic <90 mmHg) is less well established. The presence of ISH significantly increases the risk for stroke, myocardial infarction, congestive heart failure, and death. Ample evidence indicates that systolic pressure is a better predictor of cardiovascular morbidity and mortality than diastolic pressure. However, at present, only indirect evidence is available to demonstrate the benefit of treating isolated increases in systolic pressure. A definitive, prospective trial, Systolic Hypertension in the Elderly Program, is currently in progress to test the benefit of reducing an isolated elevation of systolic pressure. A pilot study has been launched to examine the efficacy of diuretic against placebo in this population. Chlorthalidone reduced blood pressure significantly more ($p < 0.05$) than did placebo. Complete results in terms of benefit of reducing elevated systolic pressure on cardiovascular morbidity and mortality await completion of the study in 1992.

272 • HYPERTENSION

The effective and safe treatment of hypertension in the elderly requires consideration of the alterations in physiology that occur with aging, particularly in hypertensives, as well as pharmacokinetic alterations that may modify their responses to drug therapy. The most consistent pathophysiological change contributing to blood pressure elevation in the elderly is an increased peripheral resistance due to vascular sclerosis. These changes occur primarily by thickening of the arterial intima and increased deposition of connective tissue and calcium in vascular smooth muscle cells. There is also an increase in the number of cells and in their lipid content. These changes reduce vascular elasticity and compliance. At the level of the microcirculation, these changes increase resistance and decrease blood flow, thus compromising tissue perfusion. Intravascular volume generally is reduced in elderly hypertensives owing to the decreased vascular capacitance. With this diminished blood volume there is a decrease in cardiac output, accentuated by cardiac changes associated with aging. In normal individuals, cardiac output decreases at a rate of about 1% per year after age 20. With advancing age, the heart rate responses to stress and exercise and stroke volume also decrease while resistance to left ventricular emptying increases. With age, left ventricular mass also increases and, because of collagen deposition, compliance decreases. Beta-adrenergic responsiveness is also diminished in the aging myocardium, further reducing hemodynamic function despite increased circulating catecholamine levels. Baroreceptor sensitivity also decreases with age. Thus, a major mechanism for preventing marked alterations in hemodynamic stability in the face of acute changes in volume or pressure is often relatively ineffective in older individuals. For this reason, exaggerated hypotensive responses to antihypertensive agents and potential harm is more apt to occur in older than in younger individuals. Interactions of these unique alterations in the aging with specific drug treatment for hypertension is discussed later in this chapter.

The heart is not the only organ in which age-related changes occur. Renal function also declines with age as a result of microvascular alterations and a decrease in renal blood flow in conjunction with loss of filtering nephrons associated with aging. This results in a decreased excretory capacity and sodium retention. This, in turn, coupled with decreased beta-adrenergic responsiveness, appears to account for the decreased renin response seen with age. In addition to a decrease in the major stimulus for aldosterone production (angiotensin II via renin secretion) the adrenal appears to have a generalized decrease in responsiveness in the aged. Aldosterone production is also found to be

Hypertension in the Elderly • 273

significantly reduced in the elderly. These changes appear to contribute to the increase in sodium sensitivity of blood pressure seen in the older population. The therapeutic implications of these observations are discussed subsequently.

Alterations in gastrointestinal function and mesenteric blood flow, frequent in the aging, can modify absorption of medication as well as its systemic distribution, similar changes in renal and hepatic blood flow and function can also modify the bioavailability and metabolism of drugs that are processed by these organs. The elderly hypertensive is more likely to have other medical problems than younger individuals. Frequent associated disorders include diabetes mellitus, dyslipidemia, angina, congestive heart failure, pulmonary disease, peripheral vascular disease, arthritis or gout, depression, renal disease, and sexual dysfunction. Interactions may exist between medications used to treat these disorders and blood pressure regulation. As examples, nonsteroidal anti-inflammatory agents, often used by older individuals, can impair renal function, promote salt and water retention, raise blood pressure, or blunt the efficacy of diuretics and other antihypertensive agents. Tricyclic antidepressants and estrogens often raise blood pressure. These associated problems may be influenced, favorably or adversely by specific antihypertensive drugs. Beta-adrenergic blocking agents can have adverse effects in insulin-treated diabetics by masking the symptoms of hypoglycemia and amplifying the vascular effects of consequent catecholamine stimulation. These agents can raise triglyceride levels and reduce high density lipoproteins. Beta-blockers can precipitate or worsen congestive heart failure by reducing cardiac output. They may induce bronchospasm and exacerbate asthma or obstructive pulmonary disease. Beta-blockers may increase peripheral resistance and decrease blood flow leading to peripheral vascular symptoms. Their renal vascular effects may reduce renal function by altering hemodynamics. Depression and sexual dysfunction are not uncommon with beta-adrenergic blocking agents and, if present, can be exacerbated by their initiation. Such problems and the potential for drug interactions mandate careful consideration in the selection of antihypertensive therapy for the elderly.

Therapy

In approaching selection of a specific drug to reduce blood pressure in any hypertensive subject, assessment of the probable pathophysiology is often helpful. Segregation of agents into those acting primarily by reducing extracellular fluid volume (diuretics), decreasing sympathetic activity (central antisympathetic drugs, beta-adrenergic blockers, ganglioplegic agents) and those that reduce peripheral resistance (direct- and indirect-acting vasodilators) provides a categorical basis for choosing antihypertensive therapy.

Diuretics

When blood pressure is elevated because of salt sensitivity, diuretics are often an effective therapeutic choice. Despite the increase in salt sensitivity of blood pressure with age, diuretics may not be ideal antihypertensive agents for the elderly. These agents lower blood pressure primarily by reducing extracellular fluid volume, a component that is already contracted in the older hypertensive. Further reduction in volume may reduce tissue perfusion and induce renal, coronary, or cerebral ischemia. Another effect of volume depletion is an increase in blood viscosity that may contribute to thrombosis. Moreover, the diminution of baroreceptor sensitivity and adrenergic sensitivity commonly associated with aging may impair the ability of the diuretic-treated elderly hypertensive to protect against orthostatic hypotension, syncope, and even cardiovascular collapse. Recent reports of an exaggerated postprandial decrease in blood pressure with an inadequate heart rate response in untreated, normotensive, well elderly subjects compared to younger subjects provide a more compelling rationale for avoiding volume depletion in the elderly hypertensive.

Diuretics have other consequences that are of particular concern in the elderly hypertensive. Hyponatremia is more common and more symptomatic in elderly diuretic-treated subjects than in their younger cohorts. This may reflect a diminished level of renal function, vasopressin sensitivity or responsiveness, or a manifestation of the decreased aldosterone production associated with aging. Hypokalemia is a common occurrence in diuretic-treated subjects. This may be exacerbated by a potassium-poor diet engendered by economic considerations. Hypokalemia may contribute to the asthenia, cramps, and weakness often observed in diuretic-treated elderly individuals. However, the most life-threatening consequence of diuretic therapy resides in its arrhythmogenic propensity. Cardiac arrhythmias, including sudden death, have been reported to be increased in diuretic-treated hypertensives. In the presence of coronary artery disease and/or left ventricular hypertrophy or dysfunction, both more likely in older hypertensives, the risk of a life-threatening arrhythmia is increased.

Diuretics are also commonly associated with elevations in blood sugar and decreased insulin sensitivity. This may result from several factors including hypokalemia, a direct effect of diuretics in pancreatic insulin release, alterations in membrane transport, or glucose metabolism. Since insulin resistance recently has been reported to occur frequently in untreated essential hypertensives, it would seem prudent to avoid exacerbation of insulin-glucose dynamics by antihypertensive therapy. Hyperuricemia is another frequent result of diuretic therapy and may lead to symptomatic joint disease. Finally, the adverse and persistent effects of diuretics to raise cholesterol, triglycerides, and low density lipoproteins have provided another reason to seek alternative therapeutic agents in patients in whom atherogenesis, coronary artery disease, and peripheral vascular disease frequently are present or for whom an increased risk is recognized. Another consideration regarding antihypertensive therapy relates to the "J" mortality curve related to diastolic pressure. Diuretics cause a proportionate reduction in systolic and diastolic pressures. In the elderly, in whom a disproportionate increase in systolic pressure is often seen, marked reduction in diastolic pressure with diuretics may not be desirable.

These concerns have reduced enthusiasm for the use of diuretics as initial therapeutic agents in hypertensives in general and in elderly individuals in particular. When diuretics are used, safety and efficacy can be enhanced by choosing them as adjunctive therapy when another antihypertensive drug is not adequate for blood pressure control and by employing low doses. In the uncomplicated elderly hypertensive, diuretic dosage of hydrochlorothiazide (or its equivalent) should begin with no more than 25 mg/d. If marked orthostatic blood pressure alterations are present before diuretics are used, 12.5 or even 6.25 mg/d are appropriate when it is deemed necessary to add diuretic therapy to an initial agent. This reduced dosage schedule of diuretic adjunctive therapy is likely to produce satisfactory blood pressure reduction and minimize adverse effects.

Sympatholytics

Drugs that decrease sympathetic nervous system activity (central alpha-agonists and antisympathetic agents) or block peripheral sympathetic stimulation (ganglioplegics, beta-adrenergic blockers) have been used extensively in the treatment of hypertension. In general, they are not attractive choices in elderly hypertensives. The centrally acting and antisympathetic as well as the ganglionic blocking agents may precipitate orthostatic hypotension in all subjects and especially in elderly individuals in whom such changes are more common. These agents may also produce depression, lethargy, central nervous system changes and interfere with sexual function. All of these are endemic problems in the elderly population. The beta-adrenergic blocking drugs have been used extensively in the treatment of hypertension. From a theoretical viewpoint, the reduced cardiac output and decreased beta-adrenergic sensitivity characteristic of the elderly hypertensive make these agents appear to be poor therapeutic choices. The decreased sensitivity should reduce the efficacy of beta-blockers in the elderly or, at least, require higher doses. The impact of such effective beta-blockade on an already decreased cardiac output may increase the risk of cardiac decompensation and symptomatic bradycardia or more serious cardiac conduction disturbances. The potential adverse effects of beta-blockers on lipids, insulin sensitivity, the peripheral circulation, the central nervous system, pulmonary function, and behavior and sexual function have already been discussed. These are the factors that have diminished the enthusiasm for using beta-blocking agents in the elderly hypertensive.

Vasodilators

Two classes of vasodilators provide an approach to dealing with the most likely aberration in the elderly hypertensive, an increased peripheral resistance. The direct-acting vasodilators (hydralazine, minoxidil) generally are not chosen as first-step agents because of their myriad adverse effects and inevitable need for other agents to combat many of these effects. The marked activation of the renin-angiotension-aldosterone and sympathetic nervous systems when these agents are used accounts for many of their adverse effects. Salt and water retention is notable, and the consequent expansion of extracellular fluid volume may attenuate their blood pressure-lowering effects (pseudotolerance) unless a potent diuretic is administered. Peripheral edema may also be observed. The marked sympathetic activation is most immediately reflected by the increase in pulse rate and manifestations of tachycardia, pounding of the heart, as well as headache and flushing, which are frequent patient complaints. This sympathetic stimulation of the heart is also associated with increased myocardial oxygen consumption, wors-

Hypertension in the Elderly • 277

ening or provocation of angina and, in rare instances, acute myocardial infarction. For these reasons, agents such as hydralazine and minoxidil usually are reserved for third or fourth drug consideration in severe and refractory hypertensives.

The indirect-acting vasodilators, however, can reduce resistance and pressure without these adverse effects. Included in this class are the peripheral alpha-1-adrenergic antagonists, the angiotensin-converting enzyme inhibitors (ACEI), and the calcium channel entry blockers (CCB). Alpha-adrenergic blocking drugs (prazosin, terazosin) reduce resistance and pressure without promoting salt and water retention and the volume expansion associated with direct-acting vasodilators. They usually do not promote reflex sympathetic activation and tachycardia on a chronic basis and, thus, generally are safe to use in patients with coronary disease. Unlike diuretics, alpha-blockers have no adverse metabolic effects and, in fact, have been shown to have a beneficial effect on lipid profile and insulin sensitivity. Their beneficial hemodynamic actions makes them useful in the treatment of congestive heart failure and left ventricular hypertrophy although development of tolerance may limit their long-term efficacy. Because they block alpha-1 receptor-mediated responses, they may not be desirable agents in patients with existent sympathetic dysfunction or orthostatic hypotension.

The calcium channel entry blockers (nifedipine, nicardipine, verapamil, and diltiazem) represent the newest group of antihypertensive agents approved for routine use. These agents appear to lower blood pressure in two distinct ways. They are vasodilators with varying, dose-dependent effects on the peripheral vasculature. In addition, these agents have been shown to have diuretic and natriuretic actions, which may explain their effectiveness in salt-sensitive hypertensives as well as salt-resistant subjects. The major differences among these agents are doses for antihypertensive efficacy and side effect profiles. Nifedipine appears to be the most potent antihypertensive agent of the group requiring 30-60 mg/d for efficacy. At present, the long-acting preparation is not yet available, and thus 3-4 times-a-day dosing is required for smooth blood pressure control. The shortness of duration and need for frequent dosing probably account for many of the annoying side effects such as flushing, headache, tachycardia, and occasionally, dependent edema. Verapamil and diltiazem are available in sustained release preparations. Therapeutic doses of verapamil are generally 240-480 mg/d, and twice daily dosing is sometimes required. The most common complaint with this agent is severe constipation, a side effect that occurs more frequently in the older population. The negative inotropic effect of therapeutic doses of verapamil have decreased enthusiasm for this agent in patients with cardiac conduction abnormalities, in congestive heart failure, or in patients receiving beta-adrenergic blocking agents. Diltiazem requires doses of 300 mg/d or higher for antihypertensive efficacy despite antianginal benefit at much lower doses. The recent introductin of the sustained release, twice-a-day formulation has made effective dosing easier. The major side effects have been skin rash, headache, dependent edema, and similar negative inotropic effects to those observed with therapeutic doses of verapamil. In general, the calcium channel entry blockers have not been observed to have adverse metabolic effects. They are particularly useful in hypertensives with angina.

The angiotensin-converting enzyme inhibitors (ACEI) have emerged as one of the most surprisingly efficacious and safe groups of available antihypertensive agents. Initially developed specifically to attack renin-dependent forms of hypertension, these agents were predicted to have a narrow spectrum of efficacy. Extensive studies in virtually all physiological and demographic categories of hypertension have demonstrated the broad range of blood pressure responses to ACEI. While these agents have been very effective in such high renin states as malignant hypertension and renal vascular hypertension, they are also effective in salt-sensitive, traditionally low renin forms of hypertension. This is particularly true when combined with diuretic therapy. While initially recommended primarily for young or white hypertensives, numerous studies have demonstrated impressive efficacy when ACEIs are used alone in black or older individuals. These agents are also largely devoid of adverse metabolic effects and may even have positive effects in these parameters. When combined with diuretic therapy, ACEI, by decreasing the stimulation of the renin-angiotensin-aldosterone system resulting from volume depletion, these agents actually can prevent or blunt some of the typical metabolic effects of diuretic therapy, including hypokalemia, hyperglycemia, hyperuricemia, and hypercholesterolemia. Recent studies indicate that ACEIs, like some alpha-1 blockers, may improve the abnormal insulin resistance characteristic of many essential hypertensives. The major side effects of ACE inhibition appear to be annoying, but not life-threatening problems such as cough, skin rash, or alterations in taste perception. The skin rash and taste changes appear to be self-limiting and frequently remit with long-term treatment. The cough may be prevented or diminished by changing from one agent of this class to another or by administration of mild nonsteroidal anti-inflammatory agents. The broad patient acceptance of ACEIs reflects their documented ability to improve a variety of objective and subjective components comprising the "quality of life." Such aspects as intellectual and cognitive capacity, feeling of well-being, work performance, social function, and physical capacity were shown to be more beneficially influenced with captopril than with propranolol or methyldopa.

A recent postmarketing study with captopril conducted in a large primary care population has confirmed these findings. In addition, this population provided confirmation of the impressive antihypertensive efficacy of captopril in the elderly hypertensive population, black, white, and Hispanic. Included in this study were a substantial number of subjects with isolated systolic hypertension in whom captopril significantly reduced systolic pressure without lowering diastolic pressure. Thus, captopril may be uniquely beneficial in this group with isolated systolic hypertension since it can reduce systolic elevation without compromising coronary perfusion by excessive lowering of diastolic pressure.

ACEIs have also been found to be efficacious in the treatment of congestive heart failure. This apparently results from the marked reduction in afterload resulting from interruption of hyperreninemia and increased angiotensin II and catecholamine levels often observed in such patients. In addition, a beneficial effect of captopril in ventricular function after acute myocardial infarction has suggested a cardioprotective effect for these agents. This would be an attractive benefit for elderly hypertensives, many of whom have decreased cardiac output, left ventricular hypertrophy and dysfunction, and coronary artery disease.

Summary

In summary, elevated blood pressure is a common and life-threatening concomitant of aging. All forms of cardiovascular disease are increased in the presence of an increase in diastolic and/or systolic pressure. Direct and indirect evidence indicates that careful and effective reduction of elevated blood pressure in the elderly hypertensive can decrease cardiovascular morbidity and mortality. The selection of antihypertensive therapy should consider the unique pathophysiology as well as the adverse effects of specific agents in elderly hypertensives. As a group, the indirect-acting vasodilators, alpha-1-blockers, calcium channel entry blockers, and particularly, angiotensin-converting enzyme inhibitors appear to be sufficiently safe and effective to be preferred initial therapeutic considerations.

Acknowledgments: The author wishes to thank Mrs. Cassandra Brown for expert secretarial assistance in the preparation of this manuscript.

Selected References

Amery A, Birkenhager W, Bogaert M et al: Antihypertensive therapy in patients above 60 with systolic hypertension. Clin Exp Hypertens A4:1151–1176, 1982.

Amery A, Birkenhager W, Brixho P, et al: Mortality and morbidity results from the European Working Party on High Blood Pressure in the Elderly Trial. Lancet i:1349–1354, 1985.

Bauer JH, Reams G: Short and long-term effects of calcium entry blockers in the kidney. Am J Cardiol 59:66A–71A, 1987.

Brandfonbrenner M, Landowne M, Shock NW: Changes in cardiac output with age. Circulation 12:557–566, 1955.

Chait A: Effects of antihypertensive agents on serum lipids and lipoproteins. Am J Med 86:5–7, 1989.

Corea L, Bentivoglio M, et al: Converting enzyme inhibition versus diuretic therapy as first therapeutic approach to the elderly hypertensive patient. Curr Ther Res 36:347–351, 1984.

Cornoni-Huntley J, LaCroix AZ, Havlik RJ: Race and sex differentials in the impact of hypertension in the United States. Arch Intern Med 149:780–788, 1989.

Croog SH, Levine S, Testa MA, et al: The effects of antihypertensive therapy on the quality of life. N Engl J Med 314:1657–1664, 1986.

Cruickshank JM, Thorp JM, Zacharias FJ: Benefits and potential harm of lowering high blood pressure. Lancet i:581–584, 1987.

Curb JD, Borhani NO, Entwistle G, et al: Isolated systolic hypertension in 14 communities. Am J Epidemiol 121:362–370, 1985.

Drayer J, Weber M: Monotherapy of essential hypertension with a converting enzyme inhibitor. Hypertension 5(Suppl III):108–113, 1983.

Ferrannini, Buzzigoli G, et al: Insulin resistance in essential hypertension. N Engl J Med 317:350–357, 1987.

Forette F, de la Fuente X, Golmard JF, et al: The prognostic significance of isolated systolic hypertension in the elderly. Results of a ten-year longitudinal study. Clin Exp Hypertens A4:1177–1191, 1982.

Garland L, Barrett-Connor E, Suarez L, et al: Isolated systolic hypertension and mortality after 60 years. Am J Epidemiol 118:365–376, 1983.

Gerstenblith G, Fredericksen J, Yin FCP, et al: Echocardiographic assessment of a normal aging population. Circulation 56:273–278, 1977.

Gifford RW Jr: Isolated systolic hypertension in the elderly: Some controversial issues. JAMA 247:781–785, 1982.

Gribbin B, Pickering TG, Sleight P, et al: Effect of age and high blood pressure on baroreflex sensitivity in man. Circ Res 29:424–431, 1971.

Hypertension Detection and Follow-up Program Cooperative Group: Five-year findings of the Hypertension Detection and Follow-up Program: II Mortality by race-sex and age. JAMA 242:2572–2577, 1979.

Hulley SB, Furberg CD, Gurland B, et al: Systolic hypertension in the elderly

program. Antihypertensive efficacy of chlorthalidone. Am J Cardiol 56:913–920, 1985.
Kannel WB: Prevalence, incidence and hazards of hypertension in the elderly. Am Heart J 112:1362–1363, 1986.
Kannel WB, Dawber TR, McGee DL: Perspectives on systolic hypertension. The Framingham Study. Circulation 61:1179–1182, 1980.
Kannel WB, Gordon T, Schwartz MJ: Systolic versus diastolic pressure and risk of coronary heart disease: The Framingham Study. Am J Cardiol 27:335–346, 1971.
Kannel WB, Wolf PA, McGee DL, et al: Systolic blood pressure, arterial rigidity, and the risk of stroke: The Framingham Study. JAMA 245:1225–1229, 1981.
Leenen FHH: Left ventricular hypertrophy in hypertensive patients. Am J Med 86:63–65, 1989.
Luft FC, Aronoff GR, Sloan RS, et al: Calcium channel blockade with nitrendipine: Effects on sodium homeostasis, the renin-angiotensin system, and the sympathetic nervous system in humans. Hypertension 7:438–442, 1985.
Luft FC, Weinberger MH, Fineberg NS, et al: Effects of age on renal sodium homeostasis and its relevance to sodium sensitivity. Am J Med 82(Suppl 1B):9–15, 1987.
Management Committee: Australian Therapeutic Trial in Mild Hypertension. Lancet i:1261–1267, 1980.
Messerli FH, Ventura HO, Glade LB, et al: Essential hypertension in the elderly: Hemodynamics, intravascular volume, plasma renin activity and circulating catecholamine levels. Lancet ii:983–986, 1983.
O'Malley K, Docherty JR, Kelly JG: Adrenoceptor status and cardiovascular function in aging. J Hypertension 6(Suppl 1):S59–S62, 1988.
Packer M, Lee WH, Yushak M, et al: Comparison of captopril and enalapril in patients with severe chronic heart failure. N Engl J Med 315:847–853, 1986.
Peitzman SJ, Berger SR: Postprandial blood pressure decrease in well elderly persons. Arch Intern Med 149:286–288, 1989.
Pollare T, Lithell H: Increased insulin sensitivity during captopril treatment. (abstract) Circulation 78(4 part II):II268, 1988.
Pollare T, Lithell M, Selinas I, et al: Application of prazosin is associated with an increase of insulin sensitivity in obese patients with hypertension. Diabetol 31:415–420, 1988.
Rowe JW: Systolic hypertension in the elderly. N Engl J Med 309:1246–1247, 1983.
Rutan G, Kuller LH, Neaton JD, et al: Mortality associated with diastolic hypertension and isolated systolic hypertension among men screened for the Multiple Risk Factor Intervention Trial. Circulation 77:504–514, 1988.
Schoenberger JA: Quality of life assessment study. Arch Int Med, in press.
Sharpe N, Smith H, Murphy J, et al: Treatment of patients with symptomless left ventricular dysfunction after myocardial infarction. Lancet i:255–259, 1988.
Shen DC, Shieh SM, Fuh MM, et al: Resistance to insulin-stimulated glucose uptake in patients with hypertension. J Clin Endocrinol Metab 66:580–583, 1988.
Tuck ML, Katz LA, Kirkendall WM, et al: Low dose captopril in mild to moderate geriatric hypertension. J Am Ger Soc 34:693–696, 1986.
Veterans Administration Cooperative Study Group on Antihypertensive Agents:

Effects of treatment on morbidity in hypertension. III. Influence of age, diastolic pressure and prior cardiovascular disease. Circulation 45:991–1004, 1972.

Weidmann P, DeMyttenaere-Burzstein S, Maxwell MH, et al: Effect of aging on plasma renin and aldosterone in normal man. Kidney Int 8:325–333, 1975.

Weinberger MH: Antihypertensive therapy and lipids: Paradoxical influences on cardiovascular disease risk. Am J Med 80:64–70, 1986.

Weinberger MH: Blood pressure and metabolic responses to hydrochlorothiazide, captopril and the combination in black and white mild-to-moderate hypertensive patients. J Cardiovasc Pharm 7:S52–S55, 1985.

Weinberger MH: Diuretics and their side effects: Dilemma in the treatment of hypertension. Hypertension 11(Suppl II):II16–II20, 1988.

Weinberger MH: The influence of an angiotensin converting enzyme inhibitor, captopril, on diuretic-induced metabolic effects in hypertension. Hypertension 5:III132–III138, 1983.

Weinberger MH, Miller JZ, Luft FC, et al: Definitions and characteristics of sodium sensitivity and blood pressure resistance. Hypertension 8:II27–II34, 1986.

Chapter 15

Hypertension in the Perioperative Period

Thomas G. Pickering

Introduction

As many as 10% of the 2 million people with hypertension may have surgery in any given year, and of all patients admitted to hospital for surgery, about 10% have hypertension. The potential hazards of surgery in hypertensive patients are surprisingly high: in one prospective survey of nonemergency surgery 10.7% of hypertensive patients developed major complications postoperatively, which included myocardial infarction, pulmonary edema, cerebrovascular accidents, and acute renal failure. The complication rate for normotensive subjects was 3.9%.

Reasons for the Increased Risk in Hypertensive Patients

The main reason why hypertensive patients are at such high risk can probably be related to the extreme fluctuations of blood pressure that occur during anesthesia and surgery and the fact that many hypertensive patients have coronary and cerebrovascular disease. Anesthetic agents mostly produce a dose-related depression of myocardial contractility with a fall of cardiac output and a decreased blood flow to the brain and kidneys. Autoregulation, by which organ blood flow can

---

From Punzi HA, Flamenbaum W (eds): *Hypertension*. Mount Kisco, NY, Futura Publishing Co., Inc., © 1989.

remain more or less constant despite fluctuations of blood pressure, may also be impaired, thus increasing the susceptibility of the brain and kidney to sudden changes in pressure. Thus, in hypertensive patients, autoregulation of cerebral blood flow is reset to a higher range than normal, which, while it may protect the brain against sudden increases of pressure and hypertensive encephalopathy, may at the same time make it more vulnerable to sudden episodes of hypotension. What this means in practice is that when blood pressure is lowered acutely, hypertensive patients will show signs of cerebral ischemia at a higher level of blood pressure than normotensive patients. The same may also be true for the coronary circulation. Thus, hypotensive episodes during which the mean arterial pressure falls to half its waking level have been correlated with postoperative cardiac complications.

Transient myocardial ischemia can be demonstrated by ECG monitoring during anesthesia, and although only a small proportion of patients who show such ischemic changes go on to develop a myocardial infarction, it has been demonstrated that there is a relationship between the two. Until a few years ago, it was thought that blood pressure should be lowered as much as possible in hypertensive patients, but there is increasing evidence from clinical trials of the efficacy of treatment that, while this may be appropriate for the prevention of stroke, excessive reduction of diastolic pressure may result in a paradoxical increase of myocardial ischemia and infarction. The relationship between coronary heart disease and morbidity may thus be J-shaped. There is some disagreement as to whether this is a function of the absolute level of pressure achieved as opposed to the extent to which it is reduced by treatment. The phenomenon can be explained on the basis of impaired coronary artery perfusion at lower levels of diastolic pressure when there is a fixed coronary artery stenosis, which has been demonstrated experimentally in animals.

Intraoperative hypertension may also be more common in hypertensive than in normotensive patients, and may be associated with electrocardiographic changes of myocardial ischemia. The type of surgery does not seem to be a major factor in causing these episodes of hyper- and hypotension: they can occur whether the surgery is intrathoracic, abdominal, or peripheral vascular surgery.

Hemodynamic Changes Occurring During Surgery

Characteristic hemodynamic changes and circulatory instability may be expected to occur during three different phases of the operation: induction; intubation; and on awakening. These are summarized below.

Induction

All the commonly used inducing agents, including the short-acting barbiturates and neuroleptoanalgesics, cause a sudden transient hypotension as a result of depression of myocardial contractility and peripheral vasodilation (both venous and arterial). The fall of blood pressure may be greater in patients with untreated hypertension due to a greater degree of vasodilatation. Blood pressure following induction is not any lower as a result of treatment.

Intubation

The process of intubation stimulates laryngeal and tracheal receptors that produces a marked increase in sympathetic nervous activity and hence tachycardia and a rise of blood pressure (Fig. 1). Plasma catecholamines are also increased. In normotensives the increase of pressure is approximately 20–25 mmHg, but may be much greater in hypertensives. The rate of increase of pressure may also be greater in hypertensive patients because of the previously lower pressures occurring during induction. Such changes presumably cause a large increase of myocardial oxygen demand and hence are likely to induce myocardial ischemia in susceptible patients. This increase of pressure occurs as a result of adrenergic vasoconstriction and is attenuated in hypertensive patients taking beta-blockers, but not in normotensive patients. There is a profound decrease of left ventricular ejection fraction at this time, which is particularly marked in patients with coronary artery disease. The increase of pressure may be less with neuroleptoanesthesia than with other agents in hypertensive patients and can be reduced by sodium nitroprusside. It can also be blunted by administering esmolol, a short-acting beta-blocker, immediately prior to intubation. However, no agent has been found to be completely effective in abolishing this sympathetic response.

Maintenance

All the inhalation anesthetics have major effects on the heart, brain, and kidneys. Thus, myocardial contractility is uniformly depressed, and in hypertensive patients, cardiac output falls by about 30%. Blood pressure falls more in hypertensive than in normotensive patients, because

HYPERTENSION

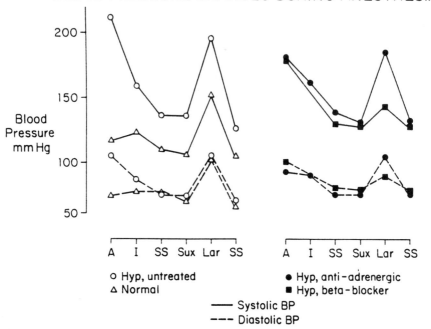

Figure 1. Blood pressure changes during anesthesia in normal and hypertensive patients. Left: untreated patients; right: effects of treatment by antiadrenergic drugs (e.g., guanethidine) or beta-blockers. A = awake; I = induction; SS = steady state; Sux = suxamethanium; Lar = laryngoscopy. (Data from Slogoff S, Keats AJ, Anesthesiol 62:107–114, 1985; Cruikshank JM, Br J Med 297:1227–1230, 1989; Harrison DG, Florentine MS, Brooks LA, et al, Circulation 77:1108–1115, 1988.)

there is a greater fall of peripheral resistance. When mean pressure falls below 80 mmHg, there is a significant risk of myocardial ischemia in hypertensive patients. Normotensive patients can tolerate lower pressures than this without ischemic changes. Traction on viscera or other noxious maneuvers during surgery may cause a sudden tachycardia and hypertension due to vasoconstriction. Vasoconstriction may also be induced by hypocapnia during mechanical ventilation, which without any attendant increase of cardiac output, may cause a further decrease of blood pressure.

Cerebral blood flow is normally held constant by autoregulation, but this property is significantly impaired by inhalation anesthetics such as halothane, which may actually increase cerebral blood flow. Although there is scant information about what happens to cerebral blood flow in hypertensive patients during surgery, the facts that cerebral blood flow autoregulation is reset to a higher level and may also be impaired in elderly patients suggest that cerebral hypoperfusion may be a significant hazard.

Renal blood flow normally falls by about 40% during surgery, with an increased renal vascular resistance and decreased urine flow. As in the brain, the autoregulation that normally protects the kidney against sudden swings of pressure is impaired by anesthetics, and there is a redistribution of blood flow from the cortex to the medulla, as occurs in acute renal failure. The exact mechanism of these changes is unclear, although the increases of plasma renin activity and antidiuretic hormone probably contribute. These changes of renal hemodynamics are usually not seen until mean arterial pressure falls to below 80 mmHg. There is little information about changes in renal hemodynamics in hypertensive patients during surgery, but since renal flow may already be reduced in these patients, it is likely that further decreases occur.

Recovery Period

As with induction of intubation, the immediate postoperative period is one of great circulatory instability. There is an abrupt increase of cardiac output, heart rate, peripheral resistance, and blood pressure, which may lead to complications such as acute left ventricular failure, myocardial ischemia, or hemorrhage. These changes are more marked in hypertensive patients, and are commonly associated with arrhythmias. They may be treated effectively with intravenous beta-blockers such as dilavalol or labetalol.

Perioperative Myocardial Infarction

One of the major hazards facing patients with hypertension or other types of cardiovascular disease is perioperative myocardial infarction. This is most likely to occur not, as might be expected, so much during the surgery, but within the first two or three days following it. Preoperative hypertension has been reported to be a predictor of myocardial infarction in some studies, but not all. Hypotensive episodes during surgery may increase the risk by as much as five times. One remarkable feature of such infarcts is that a high proportion of them, perhaps 50%,

Table 1a
Factors Predicting Perioperative Cardiac Complications*

	Points
History: (a) Age >70 years	5
(b) MI in previous 6 months	10
Physical exam: (a) S_3 gallop of JVD	11
(b) Aortic stenosis	3
Electrocardiogram: (a) not sinus rhythm	7
(b) PVCs >5/min	7
General: (a) Hypoxia, hypercapnia, hypokalemia, uremia, liver disease, or bedridden	3
Operation: (a) Intraperitoneal, intrathoracic, or aortic	3
(b) Emergency surgery	4

* Adapted from: Goldman L, Caldera DL, Nussbaum, SR, et al: Multifactorial index of cardiac risk in noncardiac surgical procedures. New Engl J Med 297:845–850, 1977.

are silent, presumably because the pain is masked by postoperative analgesics. The mortality is surprisingly high, with figures of 50% and 60% being quoted. Although some of the series were published before the widespread use of beta-blockers and calcium antagonists, even the most recent series, published in 1987, reported a mortality of 43%.

Factors Predicting Cardiovascular Risk in Patients Undergoing Noncardiac Surgery

The risk of a myocardial infarction or stroke following surgery in a hypertensive patient is a matter of potential concern because of the frequent coexistence of hypertension with coronary or cerebrovascular disease. Nevertheless, one large survey of risk factors in patients undergoing general (mostly abdominal) surgery did not find hypertension itself to be an important risk factor. The factors that were found to predict the risk of postoperative cardiac complications were mostly cardiac (Table 1a). Estimated risk is shown in Table 1b.

Another common problem is the finding of an asymptomatic carotid bruit. Although the incidence of stroke is increased in such patients, the type of stroke is not necessarily thrombotic or related to the carotid artery in which the bruit was heard. They are thus general predictors of vascular disease. It might be expected that such bruits might be predictors of perioperative strokes, because of the intraoperative hypotension. In fact, this risk is relatively small (Table 2).

Hypertension in the Perioperative Period • 289

Table 1b Estimation of Risk	
Total Points	Life-Threatening or Fatal Complication (%)
0–5	1
6–12	7
13–25	13
>26	78

Hypertension and Cardiac Surgery

Hypertension is a common problem in patients undergoing cardiac surgery. Preoperatively, it has been reported in 15% of patients before coronary artery bypass surgery when it may be associated with ECG signs of ischemia. It is also common during sternotomy. During cardiopulmonary bypass, blood pressure usually is maintained, but hypertensive episodes may occur as a result of vasoconstriction. Of greater consequence is the paroxysmal hypertension in the immediate postoperative period, which may occur in nearly 50% of patients following coronary bypass surgery and somewhat less frequently following valve replacement. Such increases of blood pressure may occur regardless of whether the patient was hypertensive preoperatively. Hemodynamically, the hypertension is associated with a mild tachycardia and increased peripheral resistance. It has been suggested that it is caused by the activation of pressor reflexes from the heart, leading to increased sympathetic nervous activity. This possibility received support from the finding that it can be prevented by unilateral stellate block. Activation of the renin-angiotensin system is also involved, and the administration of converting enzyme inhibitors may control the hypertension.

Table 2 Asymptomatic Bruits and Risk of Perioperative Stroke		
	% Stroke	
Type pf Surgery	With Bruit	Without Bruit
Peripheral vascular	1	1
Coronary bypass	5	2
General	3	—

Postoperative hypertension is also common after repair of coarctation of the aorta and may develop months after replacement of a regurgitant aortic valve by a homograft.

Management of Hypertensive Patients Undergoing Surgery

Unless the patient is undergoing emergency surgery, there are a number of criteria that should be satisfied before the hypertensive patient can be cleared for operation. First, the diagnosis as to the underlying cause of the hypertension should be accurate. Surgical mortality is relatively high in patients with renovascular hypertension, and failure to diagnose a pheochromocytoma preoperatively may prove fatal because anesthetic agents often precipitate a crisis in such patients. Second, the metabolic state of the patient should be optimal. Hypokalemia and hypomagnesemia are common in diuretic-treated patients and may increase the risk of arrhythmias occurring during surgery. Third, the possibility of ischemic heart disease or cerebrovascular disease should be evaluated. A full 12-lead ECG is essential.

There is still some controversy as to whether antihypertensive medications should be discontinued preoperatively, largely because relatively few studies have been performed to answer this question. It was traditionally recommended that medication be discontinued on the grounds that its continuation would interfere with the ability of the autonomic nervous system to maintain circulatory homeostasis. Current opinion generally favors continuation of medications right up to the time of surgery. Nevertheless, it has been shown that inadequate blood pressure control preoperatively did not result in any detectable increased risk of cardiovascular complications provided that the preoperative diastolic pressure was less than 110 mmHg. Studies in patients taking reserpine suggested that the risks were greater if it was discontinued, and the same is probably true for propranolol, where there is concern about precipitation of ischemic myocardial events following abrupt discontinuation of medication. Beta-blockade does not impair the hemodynamic response to hemorrhage unless trichlorethylene anesthesia is used, which results in a profound fall of cardiac output. It also has no adverse effects on the response to hypoxia. In a prospective study of 128 mildly hypertensive patients who were untreated preoperatively, Stone and co-workers randomly allocated the patients to receive no treatment or to be administered a beta-blocker immediately before the operation. All patients had continuous ECG monitoring to detect changes of myocardial ischemia. All ischemic episodes occurred during periods of stimulation, such as intubation, or emergence from anesthesia. They were seen in 28% of the untreated patients, but only 2% of the treated ones, a highly significant difference. In patients undergoing coronary artery bypass, the increase of pulmonary artery wedge pressure and heart rate that accompany noxious stimuli such as rib retraction are reduced by beta-blockade. Beta-blockers may diminish the large increase of blood pressure that occurs during laryngoscopy, the incidence of arrhythmias, and episodes of myocardial ischemia. Not only do beta-blockers have beneficial effects during surgery, but their abrupt discontinuation may actually precipitate myocardial ischemic events. This withdrawal syndrome is characterized by an enhanced sensitivity to sympathetic stimulation and has been attributed to various factors, including sympathetic nervous overactivity, increased triodothyronine levels, but most probably occurring as a result of increased beta-receptor density. It may be seen with any beta-blockers except those that possess intrinsic sympathomimetic activity, such as pindolol and oxprenolol.

Despite their effectiveness as antianginal agents, calcium antagonists do not appear to prevent intraoperative ischemia. In a series of 803 patients undergoing coronary artery bypass grafting, Tuman and co-workers found the lowest incidence of postoperative myocardial infarction in patients treated with both beta-blockers and calcium antagonists.

A problem may arise postoperatively in patients who require gastrointestinal suction, and who therefore cannot take their medications by mouth. Many antihypertensive drugs (e.g., prazosin) cannot be given systemically, but usually a substitute can be found. For patients taking beta-blockers, propranolol or metoprolol can be given by intravenous infusion. Methyldopa has the advantage of being relatively long acting when given intravenously, so that the problems of regulating a continuous infusion can be avoided.

Another useful agent is labetalol, which has been found to be effective in this regard when given as an intravenous infusion in a dose of 0.15 mg/kg/hr. Patients on converting enzyme inhibitors can be treated with intravenous enalaprilat (1.25 mg q6h). For patients taking clonidine, it may be possible to use the transdermal preparation instead of pills.

Since the greatest hazard to hypertensive patients occurs during episodes of hyper- and hypotension, intra-arterial blood pressure monitoring is advised in patients undergoing major surgery, together with

292 • HYPERTENSION

electrocardiographic monitoring that includes a V5 lead to detect lateral myocardial ischemia.

Arrhythmias are common, particularly junctional rhythms and Mobitz II atrioventricular block. Such arrhythmias may cause a dramatic fall of cardiac output and arterial pressure, and may be prevented to some extent by atropine.

Selected References

Becker RC, Underwood DA: Myocardial infarction in patients undergoing noncardiac surgery. Cleve Clin J Med 54:25–28, 1987.
Estafanous FG, Tarazi RC: Systemic arterial hypertension associated with cardiac surgery. Am J Cardiol 46:685–694, 1980.
Foex P, Prys-Roberts C: Anesthesia and the hypertensive patient. Br J Anaesth 46:575–588, 1974.
Gal T, Cooperman LH: Hypertension in the immediate postoperative period. Br J Anaesth 47:70–74, 1971.
Goldman L, Caldera DL: Risks of general anesthesia and elective operation in the hypertensive patient. Anesthesiol 50:285–292, 1979.
Goldman L, Caldera DL, Nussbaum SR, et al: Multifactorial index of cardiac risk in noncardiac surgical procedures. New Engl J Med 297:845–850, 1977.
Goldman L, Caldera DL, Southwick FS et al: Cardiac risk factors and complications in non-cardiac surgery. Medicine 57:357–370, 1978.
Ngai SH: Current concepts in anesthesiology effects of anesthetics on various organs. New Engl J Med 302:564–566, 1980.
Prys-Roberts C, Foex P, Biro GP: Studies of anesthesia in relation to hypertension—beta adrenergic blockade. Br J Anaesth 45:671–681, 1973.
Prys-Roberts C, Foex P, Biro GP, et al: Studies of anaesthesia in relation to hypertension V: adrenergic beta receptor blockade. Br J Anaesth 45:671–680, 1973.
Prys-Roberts C, Greene LT, Meloche R, et al: Studies of anesthesia in relation to hypertension. Hemodynamic consequences of induction and endotracheal intubation. Br J Anaesth 43:531–546, 1971.
Prys-Roberts C, Meloche R, Foex P: Studies of anesthesia in relation to hypertension—cardiovascular response of treated and untreated patients. Br J Anaesth 43:122–137, 1971.
Stone JG, Foex P, Sear JW, et al: Myocardial ischemia in untreated hypertensive patients: effect of a single small oral dose of a beta-adrenergic blocking agent. Anesthesiol 68:495–500, 1988.
Strandgaard S, Olsen J, Skinhof E, et al: Autoregulation of brain circulation in severe arterial hypertension. Br Med J 1:507–510, 1973.
Tuman KJ, McCarthy JR, Spiess BD, et al: Post-operative myocardial infarction: importance of calcium entry and beta adrenergic blocking drugs. Anesth Analg 68:S294, 1989.
Yatsu FM, Hart RG: Asymptomatic carotid bruit and stenosis: a reappraisal. Curr Conc Cerebrovascular Dis 17:21–25, 1982.

Chapter 16

Hypertension and Pregnancy

Mark S. Paller

Introduction

Hypertension is one of the most frequent medical complications of pregnancy. An increase in maternal and fetal morbidity associated with hypertension during pregnancy demands attention to this problem. However, considerable controversy exists regarding both the diagnosis and treatment of hypertension in pregnant women. In this chapter, accepted data regarding pregnancy and hypertension will be presented, controversial data will be discussed, and suggestions will be made as to what additional studies are needed and how their results might change our therapeutic approach in the future. In order to fully appreciate this condition, a brief discussion of the normal changes in circulatory physiology during pregnancy is useful.

Cardiac output increases in the first trimester of pregnancy and reaches a maximum value of 30%–40% above the nonpregnant level by the 24th week of gestation. Initially, an increase in stroke volume mediates this increase in cardiac volume. Later, heart rate increases while stroke volume decreases to nonpregnant levels. Expansion of the plasma volume is the likely cause for the increase in stroke volume. In single pregnancies, plasma volume increases by approximately 50% whereas plasma volume expansion is even greater in women with multiple pregnancies. Despite an increase in plasma volume, elevated cardiac filling pressures have not been detected during any phase of pregnancy.

From Punzi HA, Flamenbaum W (eds): *Hypertension*. Mount Kisco, NY, Futura Publishing Co., Inc., © 1989.

A striking decrease in peripheral vascular resistance also occurs early in pregnancy. The early increase in cardiac output is undoubtedly the product of this decrease in cardiac afterload. Late in pregnancy, when uterine blood flow has risen dramatically, a portion of the decrease in peripheral vascular resistance may be due to arteriovenous shunting through the uterine vascular bed. However, earlier in pregnancy, the decrease in peripheral vascular resistance is secondary to systemic vasodilatation.

Systemic vasodilatation is best explained as the result of alterations in the balance between vasodilator and vasoconstrictor hormones and autocoids. Plasma levels of prostaglandin E and prostacyclin have been found to be elevated in pregnant women by a number of investigators. Vasodilator prostaglandins may originate in vascular sites but probably also enter the venous circulation from the uterus and the kidney, sites of increased prostaglandin production during pregnancy. A reproducible alteration in hemodynamics in pregnant women and experimental animals is a diminished pressor responsiveness to vasoconstrictor agents such as angiotensin II, norepinephrine, and arginine vasopressin. In many studies, pressor responsiveness to these agents has been restored to nonpregnant levels by inhibiting prostaglandin synthesis. These findings are interpreted to suggest that increased levels and effects of prostaglandins and prostacyclin directly vasodilate and also antagonize agonist-induced vasoconstriction during pregnancy. The net result of these prostaglandin effects is to decrease peripheral vascular resistance.

Clinically, a decrease in peripheral vascular resistance translates into a decrease in blood pressure. Figure 1 shows data obtained from the Collaborative Perinatal Project in which 58,800 women were studied. The curve for women in the 50th percentile shows that systolic blood pressure remained less than 120 mmHg and diastolic blood pressure was less than 75 mmHg. The curves for the 90th and 99th percentile are instructive in demonstrating an often observed decrease in blood pressure in the second trimester followed by an increase in blood pressure, particularly diastolic pressure, to nonpregnant levels in the third trimester. Women with chronic hypertension also show a decrease in blood pressure in the second trimester. If a pregnant woman is not first examined until the second trimester and has normal blood pressure which then increases to abnormally high levels in the third trimester, a diagnosis of pregnancy-induced hypertension would usually be entertained. Thus, to detect "pseudo-normalization" of blood pressure in the second trimester in women with pre-existing hypertension, it is important to

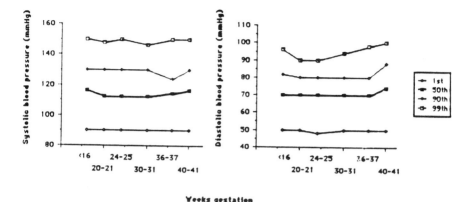

Figure 1. Effect of gestational stage on systolic and diastolic blood pressure. Adapted from data obtained in the Collaborative Perinatal Project. Data plotted are median (50th percentile) and extreme (1st, 90th, and 99th percentile) results.

obtain accurate blood pressure determination as early in pregnancy as possible.

Hypertension in Pregnancy

Hypertension complicating pregnancy may be due to a pre-existent disease or arise de novo in pregnancy. Pre-existent diseases include essential hypertension, chronic renal disease, or any other secondary cause of hypertension such as hyperaldosteronism, renal artery stenosis, and pheochromocytoma. Pregnancy-induced hypertension or pre-eclampsia usually develops spontaneously but may be superimposed upon pre-existent hypertensive disease. As will be discussed, accurate differentiation between pregnancy-induced hypertension or hypertension due to an underlying cause may be difficult or impossible. Furthermore, it is not clear whether pregnancy outcomes are different depending on the cause of hypertension if analysis is controlled for the severity of hypertension. It has been argued that morbidity and mortality due to hypertension in pre-eclampsia is less frequent than in women with other causes of hypertension. Until better data are available in this regard, therapeutic approaches to the pregnant woman with hypertension are best predicated upon an assessment of individual risk and benefit.

Even the definition of hypertension in pregnant women has been debated. The American College of Obstetricians and Gynecologists has recommended that 130/80 mmHg be considered the upper limit of normal for blood pressure during pregnancy. As shown in Figure 1, approximately 90% of women will have blood pressures lower than this level, except in the last 4 weeks of gestation when blood pressure rises 3–5 mmHg. An additional criteria for the diagnosis of hypertension is a rise in systolic blood pressure greater than 30 mmHg or a rise in diastolic blood pressure greater than 15 mmHg at any time during gestation. This definition adjusts for the expected fall in blood pressure in the second trimester and the subsequent rise in the third trimester and takes into account the baseline blood pressure which can be highly variable (Fig. 1). As discussed in greater detail below, adverse pregnancy outcomes are associated with a mean arterial pressure greater than 90 mmHg in mid-trimester or 95 mmHg in late pregnancy. A diastolic blood pressure greater than 84 mmHg has also been associated with an increased risk of perinatal mortality. Of greatest importance is recognition of the mid-trimester decrease in blood pressure. It has been claimed that in women with pre-existent essential hypertension, this mid-trimester fall in blood pressure is accentuated such that blood pressure in the mid-trimester truly appears "normal." With the late trimester increase in blood pressure, hypertension will again be clearly manifest.

Essential Hypertension

Essential hypertension is a ubiquitous disease in the United States and women of childbearing age are not exempt. It is not uncommon for essential hypertension to first be diagnosed during or following pregnancy. Because pregnancy often represents the first occasion of intensified medical observation for adult women, nonpregnant blood pressure measurements may not be available and a diagnosis of essential hypertension, therefore, may not have been made prepartum. Essential hypertension can present as elevated blood pressures throughout pregnancy. However, essential hypertension may also present as elevated blood pressure only in the third trimester and, therefore, may be confused with pre-eclampsia (Table 1). Unlike women with pre-eclampsia, women with essential hypertension will either have sustained hypertension following pregnancy or less commonly, blood pressure will decrease to near-normal values following pregnancy only to rise again in later years. Only in retrospect will the diagnosis be unambiguous. When

Table 1.
Clinical Features in Pre-Eclampsia, Essential Hypertension, and Renal Disease in Pregnancy

	Pre-Eclampsia	Essential Hypertension	Renal Disease
First 20 Weeks			
Hypertension	−	+/−	+/−
Proteinuria	−	−	+
Microscopic hematuria	−	−	+/−
Increased creatinine	−	−	+/−
Last 20 Weeks			
Hypertension	+	+	+
Proteinuria	+	−	+
Microscopic hematuria	−	−	+/−
Increased creatinine	+/−	−	+/−
Increased uric acid	+	−	+/−
Coagulation abnormalities	+/−	−	−
Neurologic abnormalities	+/−	−	−

+ = usually present; −/+ = may be present; − = usually absent

essential hypertension complicates pregnancy, renal function is normal and, unlike pre-eclampsia, proteinuria is absent. However, women with essential hypertension are also more susceptible to develop superimposed pre-eclampsia. Otherwise, pregnancy has no additional implications for these patients.

Chronic Renal Disease

The most prominent manifestation of underlying renal disease in women with pregnancy is the development of hypertension, which is often severe. Because renal disease is often silent, hypertension during pregnancy may be the first clue to a serious kidney condition. Although hypertension may be the presenting sign of renal disease, a careful search will usually reveal additional evidence for renal disease, including proteinuria and occasionally microscopic hematuria or elevated serum creatinine (Table 1). Women with chronic renal disease are also at risk of developing superimposed pre-eclampsia. The risk of superimposed pre-eclampsia occurring in women with underlying renal disease is between 20% and 40%. In the absence of renal insufficiency or high-grade proteinuria, pregnancy outcome may be no different than for women with comparable degrees of hypertension due to other causes. However, in women with co-existent severe renal insufficiency, fetal mortality may be as high as 60%–80%.

Hypertension may also have adverse consequences for the kidney. Recent evidence suggests that hyperfiltration and increased intraglomerular pressure accelerate the progression of chronic renal disease. A normal consequence of pregnancy is afferent glomerular arteriolar dilatation. This afferent arteriolar dilatation would permit a greater portion of systemic blood pressure to be transmitted into the glomerulus. Therefore, when hypertension co-exists with pregnancy, intraglomerular pressures might rise dramatically compared to the nonpregnant state. Although experimental data to support this hypothesis do not yet exist, approximately one-third of women with moderate renal insufficiency (creatinine 1.5 to 2.5 mg/dL) will experience a more rapid decline in renal function during pregnancy than expected. It is likely that systemic hypertension is a contributor to the more rapid deterioration of renal function in this subset of women. Pregnancy does not appear to adversely affect renal function in women with renal disease and normal renal function.

Pre-Eclampsia

Pre-eclampsia, or pregnancy-induced hypertension, is an incompletely understood disease specific to pregnancy. The incidence of pre-eclampsia varies from 5% to 22% of all pregnancies. Pre-eclampsia characteristically manifests in the second half of pregnancy, most commonly after 32 weeks of gestation and may appear for the first time as late as 48 hours postpartum. However, careful retrospective analysis has suggested that pre-eclampsia pregnancies have higher blood pressure than normal pregnancies as early as the first trimester although there is marked overlap between these groups. Pre-eclampsia is a disease that affects nulliparous women at the extremes of reproductive age (teenagers <16 years and women older than 35 years). Other conditions that have been associated with pre-eclampsia include multiple pregnancies, Rh incompatibility, hydatidiform mole, and pre-existing hypertension, renal disease, or vascular disease. When pre-eclampsia is associated with another condition, multiparous as well as nulliparous women are affected and the disease may be manifest earlier than 32 weeks. In one study, 25% of all cases of pre-eclampsia had onset before 37 weeks of gestation. Ninety percent of these women had chronic renal disease or essential hypertension. Pre-eclampsia can be differentiated from other hypertensive disorders of pregnancy (except renal disease) by the presence of proteinuria in excess of 300 mg/24 h (Table 1). When seizures complicate pre-eclampsia, the disorder is called eclampsia.

Pathophysiology of Pre-Eclampsia

Because there is no entirely suitable animal model of pre-eclampsia and because clinical investigation of pregnant women has been understandably cautious, the etiology of pre-eclampsia is still not clear. Two pathophysiologic alterations occur during pregnancy which may or may not be the primary events in the disease. Uteroplacental blood flow is clearly diminished in pre-eclampsia. Recent studies using Doppler ultrasound evaluation of uterine blood flow have demonstrated markedly diminished flow in severe pre-eclampsia. Lesser reductions in uterine blood flow are also observed in essential hypertension and in idiopathic intrauterine growth retardation. Additional evidence of inadequate blood supply is retarded placental growth and placental infarcts. However, placental infarcts and hemorrhage may be consequences of ischemia and hypertension rather than causes. Trophoblastic invasion of maternal blood vessels is abnormal in pre-eclampsia and stops at the decidual level leaving the placental arteries with excessive numbers of smooth muscle cells and inadequate vasodilatation. Normal placentation is thought to be a prostacyclin-dependent phenomena. One popular theory for the pathogenesis of pre-eclampsia is that prostacyclin production is deficient. In the uterus and placenta, this would produce the observed abnormalities.

Uteroplacental ischemia may directly cause generalized vasoconstriction and hypertension through release of vasoconstrictor substances such as angiotensin II or thromboxanes or may be a secondary manifestation of generalized vasoconstriction. The latter possibility is favored since the kidney also undergoes extensive changes in pre-eclampsia. Kidneys in patients with severe pre-eclampsia show glomerular endotheliosis, a swelling of both endothelial and mesangial cells that obliterates the capillary lumen. Involved glomeruli appear large and bloodless. Transmission electron microscopy shows extensive swelling as well as vacuolization of capillary endothelial cells. These renal lesions are completely reversible, usually within 2 to 3 weeks. Because pre-eclampsia can complicate chronic renal disease, biopsies have occasionally shown other lesions such as arteriolar nephrosclerosis with focal glomerulosclerosis. Patients with these findings on kidney biopsy are more likely to have progressive renal involvement. Such patients, however, should not be classified as having primary pre-eclampsia but rather chronic renal disease with superimposed pre-eclampsia.

Hypertension in pre-eclampsia is due to increased systemic vascular resistance. A reduction in vasodilatory prostaglandins such as prostacyclin may play a role in this development. Normally in pregnancy, the vasculature develops an insensitivity to the pressor effects of angiotensin II and other vasoconstrictor substances. As noted earlier, this pressor insensitivity to angiotensin II appears to be prostaglandin-mediated. Normotensive women who eventually develop pre-eclampsia have been found to lose this insensitivity to angiotensin II as early as 18 to 20 weeks of gestation. Decreased levels of vasodilatory prostaglandins in maternal umbilical and placental vessels, plasma, and urine, as well as an increase in placental and platelet-derived thromboxane, have been observed in pre-eclampsia and suggest an imbalance between vasodilator and vasoconstrictor influences in this condition. Because the loss of insensitivity to angiotensin II precedes the development of hypertension, some investigators believe that a primary abnormality in prostaglandin production is a crucial step in the development of pre-eclampsia.

Recently there have been two interesting clinical trials of low dose aspirin in women to prevent the development of pre-eclampsia. Beaufils and colleagues treated 102 women at high risk of developing pre-eclampsia because of previous complicated pregnancies or underlying essential hypertension with either aspirin, 150 mg daily, and dipyridamole, 300 mg, or no treatment starting in the second trimester. Most authorities feel that sufficient antiplatelet effects can be produced by aspirin alone and that dipyridimole was not necessary. Pre-eclampsia developed in six of 50 patients receiving no therapy, but in none of 52 patients receiving aspirin. Fetal death or severe growth retardation occurred in nine control patients, but in no aspirin-treated patients. Interestingly, although aspirin prevented the development of pre-eclampsia (hypertension with proteinuria), it did not prevent the development of hypertension. Nevertheless, aspirin appeared to prevent the complications of hypertension: pre-eclampsia, fetal death, and fetal growth retardation. Wallenburg and colleagues gave 60 mg of aspirin daily or placebo to 46 normotensive women who were at risk of developing pre-eclampsia because they had an increased angiotensin II blood pressure response at 28 weeks of gestation. Two of 23 aspirin-treated women developed hypertension without proteinuria whereas four placebo-treated patients developed hypertension and an additional seven developed hypertension and proteinuria (pre-eclampsia). Fetal outcome was similar in both groups although there was a tendency for fewer low birth weight infants in the aspirin-treated group. Although these two studies combined comprised a small number of women, they do suggest that low dose aspirin protects against the development of pre-eclampsia. A potential explanation for this beneficial effect of aspirin is that when given in low doses, aspirin inhibits platelet and vascular thromboxane production but does not inhibit vascular prostacyclin production. These findings, therefore, support the hypothesis that an imbalance in vasodilatory and vasoconstrictor prostaglandins causes pre-eclampsia. These initial trials also give hope that effective prophylaxis against pre-eclampsia in high-risk women is possible.

Abnormalities in sodium metabolism have also been implicated as causative factors in the development of pre-eclampsia. Although extensive generalized edema is often present when hypertension appears, approximately one-third of women with uncomplicated pregnancies also have edema at some time during their pregnancy. Thus, edema is not a useful clinical discriminator for pre-eclampsia. Total body exchangeable sodium is increased in women with pre-eclampsia compared to nonpregnant women and normal pregnant women. Furthermore, postpartum sodium losses are greater in pre-eclamptic than in normal pregnant women. When pre-eclamptic women are given a sodium chloride infusion, they excrete less of the sodium load than do normal pregnant subjects. These observations all suggest an abnormality in renal sodium handling. Despite the increase in total body sodium, plasma volume is frequently diminished in pre-eclampsia compared to normal pregnancy. In one study, although plasma volume was decreased, total extracellular volume was not. A pattern of early volume expansion followed by a late contraction of the plasma volume has been observed in pre-eclampsia. These findings are consistent with the hypothesis that vasoconstriction causes a shift of fluid from the intravascular to extravascular space. Such a shift has also been recognized in nonpregnant patients with severe hypertension.

Clinical Features of Pre-Eclampsia

The clinical manifestations of pre-eclampsia are primarily neurological in origin. These symptoms include headache, visual changes, apprehension, and epigastric discomfort. Physical findings include segmental arteriolar narrowing and rarely congestive heart failure, both consequences of hypertension. Increased nervous system irritability is manifested by hyperactive deep tendon reflexes. Although rapid weight gain and generalized edema are common, these findings are not specific.

One of the most useful laboratory markers for pre-eclampsia is an increase in the serum uric acid level. Serum urate rises as glomerular filtration rate and renal plasma flow fall in pre-eclampsia. In normal pregnancy, serum uric acid levels decrease by 25% because of increased renal clearance. Thus, the expected serum uric acid is 2.5 to 4 mg/dL and a "normal" nonpregnant value for serum uric acid is suspicious. If renal disease and diuretic-induced volume depletion can be ruled out, an increased serum uric acid is a useful marker for pre-eclampsia. Serum uric acid does not increase in pregnant women with essential hypertension. A consumptive coagulopathy with thrombocytopenia may also occur in pre-eclampsia and shares features with thrombocytopenic purpura although severe thrombocytopenia is relatively rare in pre-eclampsia. These changes are thought to be manifestations of endothelial cell injury. Hepatocellular injury also occurs and may mimic hepatitis or acute fatty liver of pregnancy.

Differential Diagnosis

It is often difficult to differentiate early pre-eclampsia from chronic hypertension or from new onset hypertension during pregnancy due to an underlying cause such as essential hypertension since women with renal disease or chronic hypertension have an increased risk of developing pre-eclampsia. Therefore, in addition to the three categories of illness shown in Table 1, a fourth category, chronic hypertension with superimposed pre-eclampsia, is also required. Often, a specific diagnosis can only be made retrospectively after prolonged postpartum follow-up. Classic pre-eclampsia does not recur in subsequent pregnancies and does not cause chronic hypertension. Mild essential hypertension or renal disease will usually declare themselves with time. The difficulty in establishing a specific etiologic diagnosis in hypertensive women during pregnancy has hampered interpretation of therapeutic trials of antihypertensive agents.

Antihypertensive Therapy

General Considerations

Therapy of hypertension in pregnant women is an extraordinarily controversial area. Regardless of the cause of hypertension, two fun-

Hypertension and Pregnancy • 303

damental questions can be asked. Should the hypertension be treated? What therapeutic agents should be employed? Because of the limited amount of data regarding risks and benefits, particularly for the fetus, the first question is sometimes difficult to answer. Numerous case reports have documented adverse fetal effects of antihypertensive agents, although in some cases these agents have been inappropriately employed. Unfortunately, there are very few studies examining fetal outcome at a time period more distant than the immediate peripartum period. Thus, it is nearly impossible to say whether strict control of maternal hypertension during pregnancy is beneficial or harmful for a child's long-term intellectual and physical development. Without solid data to answer this question, disagreement will continue to arise.

Substantial data exist to establish the short-term risks of hypertension during pregnancy. There is a direct correlation between maternal blood pressure and fetal morbidity and mortality. Data from the Collaborative Perinatal Project show that in women with pre-eclampsia, the perinatal death rate was 6% to 10%, accounting for twice as many perinatal deaths as abruptio placenta and five times as many perinatal deaths as cord prelapse or birth trauma. Pre-eclampsia was associated with a 30% prematurity rate and neurological or developmental defects in 10% to 25% of these premature infants. Perinatal mortality was increased when diastolic blood pressure was greater than 84 mmHg at any time during pregnancy. Infant birth weight was also low if diastolic blood pressure was greater than 84 mmHg. The association between elevated diastolic blood pressure and increased mortality existed regardless of whether infants were delivered prematurely or at term. Perhaps not surprisingly, women who also had proteinuria as well as hypertension had even greater rates of fetal mortality. For example, when maternal diastolic blood pressure was between 95 and 104 mmHg and 2+ proteinuria was present, there was a ninefold increase in fetal mortality. In a study of nearly 15,000 women, perinatal mortality rose progressively as a function of the increase in mean arterial pressure. A mean arterial pressure in the second trimester of 90 mmHg or greater (if blood pressure is 120/80 mmHg, then mean arterial pressure is approximately 93 mmHg) was associated with an increased risk of stillbirth, fetal growth retardation, and eventual development of pre-eclampsia.

In a limited number of studies, therapy of hypertension has been shown to favorably affect fetal outcome. In studies comparing placebo versus methyldopa, actively treated patients experienced a decrease in midpregnancy abortion and perinatal death rate as well as heavier infant birth weight. At one year of age, infants of mothers with hypertension who had been actively treated had a lower incidence of abnormal neurological examinations and developmental screening tests compared with babies of untreated hypertensive mothers. However, longer term evaluation of neurological development has not been performed and the screening tests employed in the study cited have been criticized as being nonspecific.

Pre-eclampsia also carries some risk of maternal mortality, particularly in women over 35 years of age. Although pre-eclampsia is a disease primarily of primiparas, death due to pre-eclampsia is a problem of multiparas. Mortality rates vary from 0% to 15% and are due primarily to cerebral hemorrhage. In one study, when systolic blood pressure exceeded 200 mmHg, the maternal mortality rate was 22%.

Despite the obvious risks to mother and fetus, there is continued reticence by some physicians to treat hypertension during pregnancy. In general, British and European obstetricians treat hypertension more aggressively than do their American counterparts. Internists and nephrologists recommend more vigorous therapy than do obstetricians. This conservative approach by American obstetricians is based on concerns regarding uteroplacental blood flow in pregnancy. Pregnant sheep are not able to autoregulate uterine blood flow because of fixed vasodilatation of uterine vessels so that when blood pressure is lowered, uteroplacental blood flow falls. On the other hand, pregnant rabbits are able to autoregulate uterine blood flow over a wide range of perfusion pressures. Data in pregnant women are mixed. The metabolic clearance of dehydroepiandrosterone (DHEA) has been used as an index of fetal-placental function. Normotensive women given diuretics or hydralazine had a decrease in DHEA clearance which was assumed to represent a decrease in uteroplacental blood flow. However, these women became frankly hypotensive. Since the goal of therapy in hypertension patients is to lower blood pressure to normal, not subnormal levels, their findings may not be clinically applicable. Furthermore, when normotensive women were infused with angiotensin II to raise blood pressure, DHEA clearance also fell, suggesting that neither hypertension or hypotension are optimal for fetal-placental function. There are also major concerns that DHEA clearance is not an accurate marker for placental blood flow. Because there are several prospective control studies of antihypertensive therapy in hypertensive women demonstrating fetal survival at least as good as in untreated women (usually improved fetal outcome), these theoretical concerns regarding fetal-placental blood flow do not appear relevant to clincal practice.

The choice of antihypertensive agent in pregnancy is also controversial, particularly regarding the use of diuretics. Published controlled

Table 2
Controlled Trials of Antihypertensive Therapy in Pregnancy

Authors, Year	No. of Patients Randomized	Treatment	Relative Risk of Fetal Death, Active versus no Therapy*
Leather et al., 1968	100	methyldopa + thiazide vs. none	0.61
Redman et al., 1976	247	methyldopa vs. none	0.13
Rubin et al., 1983	120	atenolol vs. placebo	0.5
Wichman et al., 1984	52	metoprolol vs. placebo	0

* With permission from Fletcher AE, Bulpitt CJ: A review of clinical trials in pregnancy hypertension. In: Rubin PC (ed), Handbook of Hypertension. Vol. 10: Hy in Pregnancy. Amsterdam, Elsevier, 1988, pp 186–201.

trials of antihypertensive therapy provide little guidance as to the choice of antihypertensive agent because of the limited number of patients studied. Table 2 summarizes the results of five of these studies. Leather and colleagues treated 52 women with methyldopa and bendrofluazide, a thiazide diuretic, and compared the results with 48 patients receiving no therapy. When hypertension developed early in pregnancy (<20 weeks' gestation), antihypertensive therapy resulted in longer gestation, heavier infant birth weight, and lower perinatal mortality (0/23 versus 2/24). When therapy was begun later in pregnancy, the gestational period was only extended in those patients without proteinura. In this study, proteinuria was a worse prognostic indicator than the level of diastolic blood pressure.

Redman treated 247 patients with either methyldopa or no therapy. Patients with early hypertension were defined as those with a blood pressure greater than 140/90 mmHg before 28 weeks, whereas those with late hypertension were defined as patients with blood pressure >150/95 mmHg after 28 weeks. No patients were entered into the study beyond 36 weeks' of gestation and women with blood pressure >170/110 mmHg were excluded. Actively treated patients could also have hydralazine or clonidine added to methyldopa if blood pressure remained elevated. In the early hypertension group, therapy reduced midpregnancy abortions from 4 of 107 to 0 of 106. The control group had two perinatal deaths, whereas the therapy group had only one. In the patients with late hypertension, therapy was associated with a prolongation of gestation by 8 days. Perinatal deaths occurred in 0 of 16 cases in the treated group versus 3 of 18 cases in the control group. Overall, therapy was associated with only one fetal loss in 122 pregnancies compared to nine fetal losses in 125 untreated pregnancies ($p < 0.013$).

Rubin and associates randomized 120 women with hypertension in the last trimester to receive either atenolol or a placebo. These women had diastolic blood pressure between 90 and 110 mmHg. A large number of patients were withdrawn from the study primarily because of an increase in blood pressure to greater than 170/110 mmHg. Eighty-five patients completed the study (46 in the active therapy group, 39 in the placebo group). There was a decreased incidence of new proteinuria in patients receiving active therapy (3 of 32 versus 10 of 35). Fetal loss was low in both groups: one in the active therapy group, two in the placebo group. Of note, infants whose mothers received atenolol had an increased incidence of perinatal bradycardia which was not felt to be clinically important and a decreased incidence of hypoglycemia and respiratory distress. Wichman et al. compared metoprolol to placebo in 52 women with mild to moderate hypertension. One fetal death was reported in the placebo group, and both groups experienced relatively small decreases in blood pressure. Proteinuria and an increase in uric acid developed in six women in each group.

These studies are all hampered by a small number of subjects. Only in Redman's group was the difference in mortality between active therapy and no therapy statistically significant. Combining the results of these studies, Fletcher and Bulpitt calculated a relative risk of fetal death of 0.37 for active therapy versus no therapy. Although large numbers of patients would be necessary to ascertain any beneficial or harmful effect of therapy on fetal mortality rates, other parameters of fetal well-being are also important. Overall these trials showed no difference in birth weight between infants born of treated or untreated mothers. Redman's group re-evaluated the infants at one year of age. Infants whose mothers received methyldopa were born with small head size for gestational age but at one year head size was normal. All infants of treated mothers had normal Denver Development Screening Tests, whereas 13 of 55 children of placebo-treated mothers had borderline or overtly abnormal examinations due to delayed gross motor function and abnormal tone on neurological examination. Thus, taken as a whole, these studies suggest benefits of therapy in terms of perinatal mortality and perhaps a benefit in long-term sensory-motor development in infants of treated mothers without any evidence of long-term adverse effects on infants of treated mothers. It is apparent, however, that data on a large number of children of treated mothers is woefully scarce and additional carefully planned studies are needed.

A limited number of studies comparing different antihypertensive agents have also been performed. In a study of 100 women given either methyldopa or oxprenolol because of a diastolic blood pressure >95 mmHg, both drugs controlled blood pressure and fetal mortality was low in both groups of patients. Fetal bradycardia was more common in the beta-blocker-treated group. Gallery et al. also compared these two agents in 169 women with a diastolic blood pressure >90 mmHg. Hypertensive control was similar in both groups, but infants of oxprenolol-treated mothers had higher birth weights and a lower incidence of fetal distress during fetal heart rate monitoring. Four perinatal deaths were seen in the methyldopa group and none in the oxprenolol group. Based on the perceived advantage of oxprenolol over methyldopa, these authors recommended use of the beta-blocker if there was no contraindication. Horvath and colleagues treated 100 women with either methyldopa or clonidine. Both drugs effectively lowered blood pressure and there was one fetal death in each group in patients with severe hypertension (blood pressure >170/110 mmHg). There were no apparent differences in fetal outcome. The authors concluded that the two antihypertensive agents were similar.

Diuretics have also been extensively employed as antihypertensive agents in nonpregnant patients. As the data will suggest, dogmatic statements regarding their use or prohibition in pregnancy are inappropriate. Table 3 summarizes eight studies of the prophylactic use of diuretics to prevent pre-eclampsia. These studies were undertaken based on the perhaps faulty assumption that pre-eclampsia was the result of excessive sodium retention. Several studies showed a reduction in the incidence of pre-eclampsia when diuretics were given whereas others did not. When data from all these studies were combined in a meta-analysis, it was found that the prophylactic diuretics significantly reduced the incidence of pre-eclampsia by about 35%. There was also a trend towards a reduction in the incidence of stillbirths. More important, however, is the often ignored conclusion stemming from these studies that diuretics did not appear to be more harmful than no therapy even if a benefit of diuretic use was not established. In light of this evidence to suggest that diuretics are safe and impose no threat to fetal well-being, diuretics can be recommended for use as antihypertensive agents in the appropriate

Table 3
Prophylactic Use of Diuretics in Toxemia

Author	Number of Patients	Incidence of Pre-Eclampsia (%)		Fetal Mortality (%)	
		Diuretics	No Diuretics	Diuretics	No Diuretics
Flowers et al.	519	2.4	6.4	1.8	2.7
Weseley and Douglass	267	10.7	10.3	0	0.7
Fallis et al.	80	16	45	2.6	7.5
Cuadros and Tatum	1771	1.2	4	1.4	1.7
Landesman et al.	2706	10.1	13.1	6	5
Finnerty et al.	3083	4.5	15.5	0.7	3.7
Kraus et al.	1030	3	3.8	2.7	3.0
Campbell and MacGillivray	102	35	42	—	—
COMBINED		7.7	10.8		

With permission from Paller MS, Ferris TF: Use (of diuretics) in pregency. In: Eknoyan G, Martinez-Maldonado M (eds): The Physiological Basis of Diuretic Therapy in Clinical Medicine. Orlando, Grune and Stratton Inc., 1986, pp. 267–276.

setting. Diuretics are clearly not appropriate as initial therapy for pre-eclampsia hypertension except in the setting of severe fluid overload and pulmonary edema. Because the primary abnormality in pre-eclampsia is an increase in peripheral vascular resistance, initial antihypertensive therapy should involve drugs that will decrease vascular resistance. A consquence of vasodilatation may be a shift of excess sodium and water back into the intravascular space from the interstitial space. Vasodilators may, therefore, produce an inadequate antihypertensive response because of this secondary expansion of intravascular space. It is at this time that judicious use of diuretics is appropriate and desirable. In this manner, diuretics prevent the rebound sodium retention that occurs with vasodilatation whether induced by methyldopa, beta-blockers, hydralazine, or diazoxide.

In acute severe hypertension, intravascular volume may be decreased secondary to intense vasoconstriction. In complicated patients with pre-eclampsia, placement of a Swan-Ganz pulmonary artery catheter may be necessary to characterize the hemodynamic status. In severe hypertension, systemic vascular resistance is normal or high but left

Hypertension and Pregnancy • 309

ventricular filling pressure can be decreased, normal, or increased. Only in the latter situation should diuretics be given. Plasma volume expansion has also been advocated as therapy for pre-eclampsia. This approach is only rational for the very small subset of patients with impaired cardiac output secondary to low left ventricular and diastolic volume (or pressure). Swan-Ganz monitoring is necessary to detect and monitor these rare patients.

Pre-Eclampsia

The definitive treatment of pre-eclampsia is delivery. Acute antihypertensive therapy has as its goal the prevention of maternal death, particularly due to intracerebral hemorrhage. To avoid a reduction in uteroplacental blood flow, maternal blood pressure should not be lowered excessively. However, recommendations for a diastolic blood pressure goal have ranged from as low as 90 mmHg to as high as 110 mmHg. Using ^{113}Indium to measure uteroplacental blood flow, investigators have shown that although baseline uteroplacental blood flow was markedly diminished in women with pre-eclampsia, lowering mean arterial pressure from 114 to 98 mmHg by administration of the beta-blocker labetalol resulted in no additional decrease in uteroplacental blood flow. Similarly, intravenous dihydralazine caused a nonsignificant decrease in uteroplacental blood flow while effectively lowering maternal blood pressure. These limited studies suggest that in women with pre-eclampsia and acutely elevated blood pressure, maternal risk can be lessened with antihypertensive therapy without adversely affecting the fetus. We look forward to similar trials employing Doppler ultrasound to measure placental and fetal blood flow before and after emergent therapy or chronic therapy of hypertension in pregnant women.

Most studies have examined the effects of therapy in pregnancy-induced hypertension. Underlying essential hypertension was not usually rigorously excluded in most studies, however. Pregnant women with hypertension due to essential hypertension or renal disease should also have their blood pressure lowered to protect both the fetus and the mother. Women previously taking antihypertensive medication should continue taking their medication although dosage adjustments may be required. Diuretics should be continued in those patients taking them prior to pregnancy since diuretic administration does not adversely affect intrauterine fetal growth. Diuretics can be added to the antihypertensive regimen of women not already taking them if blood pressure control is not adequate when other agents are used or if evidence of excessive weight gain and marked edema occurs. Because pregnant women with renal disease are at great risk to develop sodium retention and edema, diuretic therapy is often necessary in these patients. Guidelines for treatment should be similar to those employed for nonpregnant women with renal disease.

Specific Antihypertensive Agents

Vasodilators

Hydralazine is used frequently for both chronic oral therapy and for acute parenteral therapy. Use of a vasodilator as the initial antihypertensive drug is quite appropriate based on our understanding of the pathophysiology of pre-eclampsia and hypertension. Extensive experience with hydralazine suggests that it is generally safe. The alpha-adrenergic antagonist prazosin is usually better tolerated than hydralazine for chronic use in nonpregnant patients, but it has not been extensively studied for use in pregnancy.

For emergency use, both diazoxide and sodium nitroprusside have also been employed. Diazoxide is effective but unpredictable in its efficacy and occasionally causes severe hypotension, an undesirable effect in terms of fetal well-being. Diazoxide also causes uterine relaxation and cessation of labor. Sodium nitroprusside is easy to employ and can be titrated to attain the desired blood pressure. However, prolonged use of sodium nitroprusside is contraindicated in pregnancy because of potential fetal cyanide toxicity. Therefore, sodium nitroprusside should be used only for very short periods of time as a temporizing measure. Its most frequent application is to be employed while emergent delivery by caesarean section, the definitive therapy for pre-eclampsia, is being planned.

Centrally Acting Agents

For chronic oral administration, methyldopa probably has attained the widest usage, particularly in the United States. As noted above, beneficial effects in terms of fetal well-being have been ascribed to treatment of hypertension using methyldopa. Unfortunately, most studies of the therapy of hypertension in pregnant women have neglected to focus on maternal side effects due to therapy. In nonpregnant subjects, methyldopa has a high incidence of undesirable side effects, particularly lethargy, fatigue, and orthostatic hypotension which has largely resulted in methyldopa being supplanted by other classes of antihypertensive agents. Beta-adrenergic antagonists (beta-blockers) have also been used in pregnancy with acceptable results. Propranolol, labetolol, oxprenolol, atenolol, and metoprolol have all been employed and are generally considered to be as safe and effective as either methyldopa or hydralazine. In nonpregnant subjects, beta-blockers have a lower incidence of side effects than methyldopa, particularly the longer-acting β_1-selective blockers. Experience with other centrally acting agents such as clonidine is limited but suggests that this agent is also useful in pregnancy.

Other Antihypertensive Agents

Angiotensin-converting enzyme inhibitors effectively lower blood pressure in pregnant women. However, studies in pregnant rabbits and sheep using captopril detected increased fetal loss, probably because angiotensin II is important in uteroplacental blood flow autoregulation. In addition, both captopril and enalapril have been reported to cause reversible acute renal failure in neonates. Therefore, angiotensin-converting enzyme inhibitors are relatively contraindicated in pregnancy.

Calcium channel blockers might be ideal antihypertensive agents for use in pregnancy. These vasodilators are very well accepted in nonpregnant hypertensive subjects, and in limited usage have been well tolerated by pregnant women. They have the potential to interfere with uterine contraction and should be avoided during active labor. In nonpregnant patients with urgent severe hypertension, sublingual nifedipine has proven to be such a simple and effective means of treating hypertension that the emergency use of nitroprusside and diazoxide has greatly diminished. Similar use of nifedipine in acutely, severely hypertensive pregnant women should be evaluated. Magnesium sulfate is frequently administered to women with pre-eclampsia to prevent seizures. Magnesium is a weak vasodilator and an unreliable antihypertensive agent. Benzodiazepines are alternative anticonvulsants.

Breast Feeding

A related concern is the choice of antihypertensive agent for use in women with chronic hypertension in the postpartum period when breast feeding is desired. White has summarized the available pharmacokinetic data for a number of antihypertensive agents with particular emphasis on transfer into breast milk. The accumulated data is sparse but show that the beta-blockers other than propranolol accumulate in the breast milk and should probably be avoided. In addition, captopril appears in low concentrations in the milk although effects on infants have not been reported. Data from many of the most commonly employed antihypertensive agents are, unfortunately, not available.

Selected References

Beaufils M, Uzan S, Donsimoni R, et al: Prevention of pre-eclampsia by early antiplatelet therapy. Lancet i:840–842, 1985.

Collins R, Yusuf S, Peto R: Overview of randomized trials of diuretics in pregnancy. Br Med J 290:17–23, 1985.

Evans S, Frigoletto FD Jr, Jewett JF: Mortality of eclampsia: A case report and the experience of the Massachusetts Maternal Mortality Study, 1954–1982. N Engl J Med 309:1644–1647, 1983.

Ferris TF: Toxemia and hypertension. In: Burrow GN, Ferris TF (eds): Medical Complications During Pregnancy. Philadelphia, W.B. Saunders Co, 1988, pp 1–33.

Fidler J, Smith V, Fayers P, et al: Randomized controlled comparative study of methyldopa and oxprenolol in treatment of hypertension in pregnancy. Br Med J 286:1927–1930, 1983.

Fletcher AE, Bulpitt CJ: A review of clinical trials in pregnancy hypertension. In: Rubin PC (ed), Handbook of Hypertension. Vol. 10: Hypertension in Pregnancy. Amsterdam, Elsevier, 1988, pp 186–201.

Friedman EA, Neff RK: Pregnancy Hypertension: A Systemic Evaluation of Clinical Diagnostic Criteria. Littleton, Mass, PSG Publishing Co, 1977.

Gallery EDM, Ross MR, Gyorgy AZ: Antihypertensive therapy in pregnancy: Analysis of different responses to oxprenolol and methyldopa. Br Med J 291:563–566, 1985.

Gant NF, Whalley PJ, Everett RB, et al: Control of vascular reactivity in pregnancy. Am J Kidney Dis 9:303–307, 1987.

Horvath JS, Phippard A, Korda A, et al: Clonidine hydrochloride: A safe and effective antihypertensive agent in pregnancy. Obstet Gynecol 66:634, 1985.

Ihle BU, Long P, Oats J: Early onset pre-eclampsia: Recognition of underlying renal disease. Br Med J 294:79–81, 1987.

Leather HM, Humphreys DM, Baker P, et al: A controlled trial of hypotensive agents in hypertension in pregnancy. Lancet 2:488–490, 1968.

Lindheimer MD, Katz AI: Hypertension in pregnancy. N Engl J Med 313:675–680, 1985.

Mutch LMM, Moar VA, Ounsted MK, et al: Hypertension during pregnancy, with and without specific hypotensive treatment. II. The growth and development of the infant in the first year of life. Early Human Dev 1:59–67, 1977.

Page EW, Christianson R: The impact of mean arterial pressure in the middle trimester upon the outcome of pregnancy. Am J Obstet Gynecol 125:740–745, 1976.

Paller MS: Decreased pressor responsiveness in pregnancy: Studies in experimental animals. Am J Kidney Dis 9:308–311, 1987.

Paller MS, Ferris TF: Use (of diuretics) in pregnancy. In: Eknoyan G, Martinez-Maldonado M (eds): The Physiological Basis of Diuretic Therapy in Clinical Medicine. Orlando, Grune and Stratton Inc., 1986, pp 267–276.

Redman CWG, Beilin LJ, Bonnar J, et al: Fetal outcome in trial of antihypertensive treatment in pregnancy. Lancet 2:753–756, 1976.

Rubin PC (ed): Handbook of Hypertension. Vol. 10: Hypertension in Pregnancy. Amsterdam, Elsevier, 1988.

Rubin PC, Butters L, Clark DM, et al: Placebo-controlled trial of atenolol in treatment of pregnancy-associated hypertension. Lancet i:431–434, 1983.

Wallenburg HCS, Dekker GA, Makoritz JW, et al: Low dose aspirin prevents pregnancy-induced hypertension and pre-eclampsia in angiotensin-sensitive primigravidae. Lancet i:1–3, 1986.

White WB: Management of hypertension during lactation. Hypertension 6:297–300, 1984.

Wichman K, Ryden G, Karlberg BE: A placebo controlled trial of metoprolol in the treatment of hypertension in pregnancy. Scand J Clin Lab Invest 44 (suppl 169):90–95, 1984.

Chapter 17

Urgent, Emergent, and Refractory Hypertension

Donald G. Vidt

Introduction

The development of new classes of antihypertensive agents over the past three decades has provided tremendous advances in the efficacious treatment of arterial hypertension, regardless of severity. It is now possible to reduce blood pressure through interference with or inhibition of virtually every recognized pressor mechanism underlying hypertensive disease. A nationwide education program focusing on detection and evaluation of the patient with hypertension as well as application of sound principles of aggressive nonpharmacological and pharmacological therapy have resulted in a dramatic increase in the numbers of hypertensive patients recognized and treated. We have also seen significant improvement in the numbers of patients with effectively controlled hypertension.

Extensive clinical trials have documented effective control and reduced cardiovascular morbidity and mortality with every available class of agents, whether used alone or in combination therapy.

This chapter addresses the problem of resistant hypertension first, since the failure to provide suitable long-term control of mild to moderate hypertension clearly contributes to later accelerated or malignant hypertension and may represent a pivotal contribution to a hypertensive urgency or emergency.

To define resistant hypertension, we must consider both current

From Punzi HA, Flamenbaum W (eds): *Hypertension*. Mount Kisco, NY, Futura Publishing Co., Inc., © 1989.

recommendations for adequate treatment and the currently available pharmacological agents.

The Joint Committee on Detection, Evaluation, and Treatment of High Blood Pressure offers practical guidelines for nonpharmacological and pharmacological therapies based on current definitions of hypertension. There is general agreement that patients with persistent diastolic blood pressures greater than 94 mmHg whose disease does not respond to nonpharmacological efforts should benefit from drug therapy. Patients with diastolic blood pressures between 90 and 94 mmHg and otherwise at low risk of developing cardiovascular disease should be treated with nonpharmacological measures. Many experts recommend that drug treatment should be initiated in essentially all patients whose diastolic blood pressures remain greater than 90 mmHg despite vigorous nonpharmacological therapy. The goal of therapy should be maintenance of blood pressure less than 140/90 mmHg with minimal or no adverse effects. Although individual patients may respond better to selected agents, clinical experience has shown that mild hypertension will be controlled by initial therapy with recommended doses of any agent (regardless of class) in almost one half of patients. The options for subsequent therapy are many, and when appropriately individualized or tailored to the patient, the vast majority of hypertensives will attain goal blood pressure reductions.

Resistant Hypertension

In arriving at a definition of resistant hypertension, we must take into consideration current recommendations for treatment and currently available pharmacological agents. Resistant hypertension can be arbitrarily defined as persistent blood pressure greater than 150/100 mmHg despite an adequate three-drug regimen. An adequate regimen can be considered as one that includes maximal, recommended, or tolerated doses of a natriuretic diuretic, a beta-adrenergic blocker or other antiadrenergic agent, and a vasodilator, calcium-entry blocker, or angiotension-converting enzyme (ACE) inhibitor.

Apparent resistance to therapy necessitates a thorough, stepwise re-evaluation of the patient and regimen. Table 1 outlines the most common reasons for inadequate blood pressure control. This checklist is helpful in undertaking a systematic evaluation of your patient.

Is the patient compliant? The most common reason for inadequate blood pressure control relates to poor patient adherence (patient resis-

Table 1
Reasons for Resistant Hypertension

1. Nonadherence with therapy (patient resistance)
2. Inappropriate regimens (physician resistance)
3. Inadequate patient education and understanding
4. Pseudoresistance (sodium/volume)
5. Office hypertension
6. Secondary hypertension

tance) to nonpharmacological treatment, prescribed drugs, or recommended follow-up. Keep in mind that adverse drug effects continue to be a barrier to effective control and represent a major reason that patients discontinue treatment.

Is the treatment regimen appropriate? It may be the physician who is resistant if poor control results from an inadequate or inappropriate drug regimen. A reluctance to use diuretics in view of current concerns about these agents may contribute to drug resistance. It is the responsibility of the physician to forewarn patients regarding potential interfering drugs; a thorough understanding of a patient's other disease conditions, related symptoms, and therapies is critical to appropriate drug selection. The interaction between tricyclic antidepressants and guanethidine is often cited as a classic drug interaction, despite the fact that guanethidine rarely is used in today's practice. Far more common is the potential interaction between nonsteroidal anti-inflammatory agents and diuretics to produce blunted natriuresis.

Does the patient understand the disease and its risks? Physicians must assume the responsibility for providing sufficient education regarding hypertension and its risks, the chronic nature of the disease and the need for lifetime therapy. For treatment to be successful, patients must understand the risks and must accept the responsibility of active partnership in their own care, including adherence with therapy and regular follow-up.

Is the patient ingesting excessive sodium? Sodium and fluid volume play a role in resistant hypertension. Ingestion of excessive sodium may negate the antihypertensive effect of both diuretic and nondiuretic agents. Genetic salt sensitivity in humans appears to represent at least one factor determining individual susceptibility to variable salt intakes. In the patient with progressive renal parenchymal disease, retention of salt and water occurs early and contributes to the establishment of hypertension. As the disease progresses, other hemodynamic and humoral factors, as well as changes in adrenergic responses, may contribute to the persistence of hypertension. Careful adherence to an appropriate, sodium-restricted diet can enhance the effectiveness of the antihypertensive drug regimen.

Does the patient have office hypertension? An excessive pressor response to office visits may give the appearance of resistant hypertension and can represent a perplexing factor in patient treatment. Ambulatory blood pressure recording techniques can help identify the patient with office hypertension; the absence of significant target organ involvement despite apparent significant elevations of blood pressure in the office setting provides a valuable clue to this diagnosis.

Is the diagnosis erroneous? Careful attention to the initial office evaluation of the hypertensive patient should provide clues to the presence of most secondary causes of hypertension. On occasion, resistant hypertension may be due to secondary hypertension that has been overlooked. It is well recognized that pheochromocytoma responds poorly, or even paradoxically, to antihypertensive therapy. The onset of renovascular hypertension can be new or associated with recent worsening of previously controlled blood pressure, and the hypervolemia associated with primary hyperaldosteronism can lead to resistant hypertension with or without evident hypokalemia. When hypertension cannot be controlled adequately and the above questions have been appropriately addressed, further diagnostic evaluation is indicated to rule out a secondary and potentially reversible cause of hypertension. Further study may also be appropriate to identify the underlying hemodynamic and/or humoral mechanisms responsible for the resistance in an effort to alter the treatment regimen appropriately.

Progression to accelerated or malignant hypertension may occur in patients untreated or in those treated inadequately, for established hypertension. Truly resistant hypertension, if not controlled, may cause the constellation of symptoms and target organ dysfunction currently associated with the accelerated or malignant phase of hypertensive disease.

Accelerated hypertension represents severe hypertension ($\geq 180/120$ mmHg) with evidence of central nervous system, cardiac, and renal damage, with grade III hypertensive retinopathy (characterized by hemorrhages and exudates, but without papilledema). Malignant hypertension presents the features of accelerated hypertension and is associated with necrotizing arteriolitis, retinal hemorrhages, exudates, and papilledema (grade IV fundoscopic changes). This severity of hypertension, while most commonly seen in the course of untreated or inadequately controlled essential hypertension, may occur as a complication of renovascular hypertension, acute or chronic glomerulonephritis, preeclampsia of pregnancy, and pheochromocytoma. Collagen vascular illnesses such as scleroderma, polyarteritis, or systemic lupus erythematosus, particularly when associated with progressive renal impairment, may be associated with rapid progression to accelerated or malignant hypertension. While less common, hypertension associated with atheroembolic renal disease, primary aldosteronism, or Cushing's disease, if inadequately controlled, carry a similar risk of progression.

With progression of target organ damage, the risk of encephalopathy, intracranial hemorrhage, left ventricular failure, and renal failure is significant, and if left untreated the mortality from accelerated or malignant hypertension approaches 100% within one year.

There is no universally accepted definition of malignant hypertension. The histologic hallmark, fibrinoid necrosis of arterioles, may be seen in patients with hypertension and renal disease who do not demonstrate the ophthalmological features of hemorrhagic and exudative retinopathy. The World Health Organization tends to classify patients with bilateral hemorrhages and exudates, with or without papilledema, together. Earlier definitions were based in part on observations that patients with Keith-Wagener grades III and IV retinopathy have different survival rates over time. More recent studies have suggested that there are no overall differences in survival in these groupings and that accelerated and malignant hypertension represent the same disease.

It is clear that patients with resistant hypertension (with or without target organ damage), as well as those with accelerated or malignant hypertension and significant target organ damage, need aggressive treatment and optimal long-term control of blood pressure.

Management of Resistant, Accelerated, and Malignant Hypertension

For patients with these conditions, a tailored approach to therapy is appropriate: three or more drugs will usually be required for control. Resistant hypertension that has not yet led to progressive target organ damage can be managed appropriately on an outpatient basis. For the patient with accelerated or malignant hypertension, aggressive outpatient management can be considered providing that rapid deterioration in target organ function is not evident. Keep in mind that sudden deterioration in target organ function may precipitate a hypertensive urgency or emergency, requiring immediate hospitalization and meticulous monitoring until blood pressure is adequately controlled.

The clinical pharmacology of available classes of antihypertensive agents has been reviewed elsewhere in this volume and will not be covered here. Table 2 outlines a recommended approach for individualized drug selection for the patient with refractory, accelerated, or malignant hypertension. Sodium and fluid volume play a major role in refractory hypertension, and retention of both may contribute to refractoriness to many antihypertensive agents, particularly when renal function is impaired. For this reason, an oral diuretic in maximal recommended doses would seem appropriate in essentially all cases. Significant renal insufficiency (serum creatinine greater than 3.0 mg/dL)

Table 2
Therapy for Refractory, Accelerated, or Malignant Hypertension

1. *Oral Diuretic**
   Hydrochlorothiazide OR Furosemide
   Chlorthalidone   Bumetanide

2. *Antiadrenergic Agent*   *ACE Inhibitor*** *Calcium Channel Blocker***
   Beta blocker   Captopril   Verapamil
   Alpha-beta blocker   OR   Enalapril   OR Diltiazem
   Alpha agonist   Lisinopril   Nifedipine
   Alpha blocker   Nicardipine

                              PLUS

3. *Direct Vasodilator*
   Hydralazine
   Prazosin+   OR   Minoxidil++
   Terazosin

4. Additional Drugs†

* If serum creatinine >3.0 mg/dl, substitute furosemide or bumetanide.
** ACE inhibitor or calcium channel blocker can also be used as an alternative Step-3 agent.
+ If not utilized in Step 2, may be added as Step 3 agent.
++ If minoxidil added, will usually require co-administration of a loop diuretic and beta-blocker or alpha-beta blocker.
† Guanethidine or guandrel usually relegated to Step 4; ACE inhibitor or calcium channel blocker can also be added here.

will necessitate substitution of a loop diuretic such as furosemide or bumetanide.

A regimen consisting of an oral diuretic plus a beta-blocker or other adrenergic inhibitor and a vasodilating agent such as hydralazine has proved effective in severe hypertension. The alpha-adrenergic blockers, prazosin or terazosin, may be substituted for hydralazine. For more resistant cases, the potent vasodilator minoxidil can be added. Historically, minoxidil has been recognized as a potent vasodilator but its use usually necessitates a loop diuretic to overcome intense fluid retention and a potent beta-blocker to negate significant reflex tachycardia. Hypertrichosis may represent a cosmetically unacceptable adverse effect with prolonged usage in females or children. The addition or substitution of guanethidine or guanadrel may also be considered. A propensity for postural hypotension may occur with these potent sympathetic inhibitors and can be exaggerated with activity.

Several new classes of antihypertensive agents have demonstrated efficacy in the treatment of refractory, accelerated, or malignant hypertension.

Combined Alpha- and Beta-Adrenergic Blockers

Labetalol is the prototype of a new class of agents with both alpha- and beta-adrenergic receptor-blocking properties. While the nonselective beta-adrenergic blocking effects are comparable to those observed with propranolol, potent alpha blockade reduces peripheral vascular resistance. As a consequence, cardiac output is well maintained and heart rate is only minimally suppressed. Unlike most beta-adrenergic blockers, antihypertensive effects are seen within two hours of administration, and the prolonged duration of action enables twice-daily dosing. Postural hypotension is the most common adverse effect due to the drug's alpha-adrenergic blocking properties, whereas side effects relating to beta-adrenergic blockade are similar to those observed with other beta-adrenergic blocking agents.

Dilevalol, the R-R isomer of labetalol, is currently under development. Unlike its parent compound, dilevalol demonstrates potent and selective beta-2 agonist effects, as well as nonselective beta antagonism. No beta-1 agonist or alpha-1 antagonist effects are observed. Dilevalol lowers blood pressure by reducing peripheral vascular resistance without suppressing cardiac output and does not induce postural hypotension. Dilevalol can be administered once daily and preliminary studies show it to be effective in all degrees of hypertension, including hypertension associated with renal impairment. Dilevalol is promptly effective when given intravenously in the management of hypertensive urgencies or emergencies.

Two other agents, medroxolol and celiprolol, appear to have properties similar to labetalol. They have not yet been approved for clinical use by the FDA. Carteolol and penbutolol are new nonselective beta-1, beta-2 antagonists with intrinsic sympathomimetic activity (ISA). The antihypertensive effects of these compounds appear due to reduction in cardiac output and heart rate but without significant changes in peripheral vascular resistance.

Calcium Channel Blockers

The list of calcium channel blockers continues to grow with the addition of nicardipine and nitrendipine to the previously available agents, verapamil, diltiazem, and nifedipine. As potent vascular smooth muscle dilators, these agents have proved useful in the management of severe hypertension. Negative inotropic effects, when present, are offset by vasodilation so that adverse effects on left ventricular function are infrequent. In clinical practice, the combination of a beta-adrenergic blocker with a negative inotropic calcium channel blocker (verapamil or diltiazem) has been well tolerated and effective, providing left ventricular function is adequate.

Nifedipine in particular has been widely used in managing severe hypertension. Maximal reductions of blood pressure are seen within one hour following oral administration. Unfortunately, the short duration of action of this agent may necessitate frequent dosing if utilized alone to control severe hypertension. By administering nifedipine in combination with a loop diuretic and an antiadrenergic agent, the effective dosing interval can often be prolonged. Hypotension has rarely been observed when nifedipine is administered alone, but appropriate caution should be observed in patients receiving concurrent therapy with other agents, particularly diuretics. The selectivity of nifedipine for vascular smooth muscle is shared by other dihydropyridine derivatives, nicardipine and nitrendipine, which offer the potential advantage of longer durations of action. They do, however, share a propensity for flushing, headache, and tachycardia when used as monotherapy; these symptoms are effectively blocked by administration of an antiadrenergic agent.

Angiotensin-Converting Enzyme (ACE) Inhibitors

Captopril, the prototype of the ACE inhibitors, was approved initially for therapy of severe or refractory hypertension. Subsequent agents, enalapril and lisinopril, offer a longer duration of action with a similar mechanism of action. All ACE inhibitors inhibit the generation of angiotensin II and secondarily suppress aldosterone secretion. A precipitous response to the first dose may occur in patients with high angiotensin II levels. Particular caution must be exerted in considering ACE inhibitors for patients with severe hypertension in whom renal artery stenosis and angiotensin II-dependent hypertension are suspected. Acute renal failure has been well documented in patients with bilateral renal artery stenosis or high-grade stenosis to a solitary functioning kidney. Like the calcium channel blockers, ACE inhibitors exert their major hemodynamic effect on peripheral vascular resistance, and as such these agents may be substituted for or added to other agents in the regimen. If not utilized as a second agent, they represent appropriate additional considerations when treating the patient with refractory or severe hypertension. ACE inhibitors may be particularly appropriate choices in patients with severe hypertension complicated by congestive heart failure.

Careful and individualized treatment with available agents will control blood pressure in most patients with refractory, accelerated, or malignant hypertension. For the occasional patient in whom hypertension persists despite an appropriate three- or four-drug regimen, selectively increasing the dose of one or more agents beyond recommended levels may be effective. Recognize that achieving control of blood pressure under these circumstances may require toleration of more adverse effects, which can represent a major barrier to compliance. Further restriction of dietary sodium intake to less than 2 g daily may be tried, and substitution of a loop diuretic may be considered if it is not already part of the regimen. Keep in mind that there is little pharmacological advantage in combining two agents of the same class, such as two beta-adrenergic blocking drugs or two ACE inhibitors.

The Hypertensive Urgency or Emergency

A clear distinction between moderate uncomplicated hypertension and a hypertensive urgency or emergency cannot be made solely on the basis of the level of blood pressure. The determination of a hypertensive urgency or emergency is based on the degree of associated target organ damage and the perceived immediate risk of a morbid cardiovascular event. It is helpful to consider hypertensive emergencies as those clinical situations in which blood pressure should be lowered to a safer level within one hour, while in a hypertensive urgency, the immediate risk is less, but prompt institution of oral drug therapy is desirable to reduce blood pressure over several hours to 24 hours (Table 3). As an example, the patient who presents to the emergency room with a blood pressure of 220/130 mmHg but without other symptoms and no clinical evidence

Table 3
Conditions Presenting as Hypertensive Urgencies and Emergencies

Urgencies

Accelerated or malignant hypertension
Acute glomerulonephritis with severe hypertension
Scleroderma crisis
Acute vasculitis with severe hypertension
Surgical emergencies with severe hypertension
Acute postoperative hypertension
Severe epistaxis
Rebound (overshoot) hypertension following sudden withdrawal of antihypertensives
Severe hypertension associated with spinal cord injury
Selected drug interactions

Emergencies

Hypertensive encephalopathy
Malignant hypertension (some cases)
Hypertension in association with acute complications:
A. Cerebral hemorrhage
   Subarachnoid hemorrhage
   Acute atherothrombotic infarct
B. Aortic dissection
   Pulmonary edema
   Acute myocardial infarction
   Unstable angina pectoris
Eclampsia of pregnancy
Pheochromocytoma/acute catecholamine crisis
Head trauma
Postcoronary artery bypass hypertension
Postoperative bleeding at vascular suture lines

of target organ damage may require little more than initial observation, subsequent appropriate evaluation, and individualized drug therapy. However, if the same patient has grade III hypertensive retinopathy, with hemorrhages and exudates, significant left ventricular hypertrophy on the electrocardiogram, severe hypertensive headaches, and increasing dyspnea upon exertion, the patient may benefit from appropriate treatment as a hypertensive urgency with efforts made to reduce the blood pressure over a period of hours. Finally, should this patient present with grade III or IV retinopathy, clinical evidence of pulmonary edema, and recent changes in mentation consistent with hypertensive encephalopathy, this would justify management as a hypertensive emergency. Blood pressure should be lowered to a safer level within minutes to one hour by the parenteral administration of one or more appropriate agents. Both the hypertensive urgency and emergency are justifiably managed in-hospital, where appropriate monitoring and supervision are immediately available.

Management Guidelines for the Hypertensive Urgency or Emergency

Admission to the hospital is strongly urged for the patient with a hypertensive urgency or emergency. For initial management, an intensive care unit or alternative nursing unit where continuous blood pressure monitoring can be made available is advised. A thorough history should be obtained and physical examination performed, and a chest radiograph and electrocardiogram should be obtained to determine not only the degree of cardiac enlargement but also evidence of congestive heart failure or acute ischemic electrocardiographic changes. A complete blood count, chemistry profile, and urinalysis with sediment examination should be performed to assess target organ involvement. The degree of target organ involvement will have an important bearing on the selection of pharmacological agents. It is appropriate to obtain an initial plasma or urine sample for determination of catecholamines or their metabolites since a hypertensive crisis associated with pheochromocytoma is notoriously resistant to many available therapies.

The clinician must be prepared to initiate drug therapy before the results of all initial laboratory studies are available in an attempt to reduce the blood pressure to a safer level, therefore minimizing the immediate cardiovascular risks. Initial reduction in blood pressure, in a controlled fashion, to the range of 100 to 110 mmHg diastolic blood pressure or a mean arterial pressure of 120 mmHg would appear appropriate. These levels appear to represent the lower limit of the autoregulatory range of blood pressure; at lower levels cerebral blood flow may be reduced.

If this level is well tolerated, additional studies can then be undertaken should the underlying etiology of the hypertension remain in doubt. In the patient with a true emergency, controlled reduction in blood pressure to this level will be achieved with parenteral administration of an appropriate agent within one hour, while in the hypertensive urgency, gradual reduction to this level will be attained after several hours and possibly repeated dosing with a selected oral agent.

Managing the Hypertensive Urgency

Oral loading regimens have been described for a number of agents. Agents commonly used today for initial therapy in hypertensive urgencies are listed in Table 4. The availability and ease of administration of nifedipine have contributed to its frequent utilization as initial therapy in hypertensive urgencies or emergencies. The onset of action is similar with sublingual or oral administration, with peak effect observed within 60 minutes. The higher the initial blood pressure, the greater the reduction observed following nifedipine, and the initial dose-response is not controllable once the medication has been administered. Particular care should be exerted for patients in whom the status of cerebral and/

Table 4
Oral Therapy of the Hypertensive Urgency

Drug	Initial Dose (mg)	Subsequent Dose (mg)	Onset of Action (min)	Maximal Dose Effect (min)
Clonidine	0.2	0.1	30–60	90–120
Labetalol	200–400	200	60–120	90–120
Captopril	25–50	25–50	15–50	60–90
Nifedipine				
Sublingual	10	10–20	<15	60
Oral	10	10–20	15–30	60

or coronary circulation is not known since ischemic symptoms can occur with sudden, pronounced decreases in perfusion pressure. Clonidine 0.1 to 0.2 mg initially, followed by 0.1 mg hourly, has proved effective in managing the hypertensive urgency. The maximal effect of each dose will be observed within 90 to 120 minutes, and a controlled decrease in blood pressure can be achieved with repeated administrations of this central alpha-agonist agent. Preliminary clinical data suggest that clonidine may also be effective in severe hypertension when administered sublingually.

Administration of labetalol 200 to 400 mg can be associated with a prompt decline in blood pressure that can also be controlled by subsequent dosages administered at 1- to 2-hour intervals. Captopril has also been effective in the treatment of hypertensive urgencies, particularly those associated with malignant hypertension where plasma renin activity is often elevated. An initial dose of 25 to 50 mg is followed by repeated doses at 1- to 2-hour intervals. The maximal effect of a dose of captopril is observed within 60 to 90 minutes.

It is appropriate to administer a loop diuretic such as furosemide or bumetanide concomitantly, since the patient with a hypertensive urgency frequently has significant target organ dysfunction, including renal impairment, with increased sodium and volume retention. An effective diuretic will often have an additive effect with the above agents in providing prompt, stepwise reduction in blood pressure to a determined goal level. This listing does not preclude favorable responses to other available agents in the initial treatment of the hypertensive urgency, but has been limited to those agents where suitable clinical experience is available.

Managing the Hypertensive Emergency

If initial control is obtained with parenteral agents, every effort should be made to convert, as soon as feasible, to orally administered drugs. After initial reduction to the levels noted above, further, gradual titration of appropriate oral agents can be accomplished to normalize blood pressure over a period of days to several weeks, depending upon the clinical status of the patient and tolerability of selected medications.

A number of effective parenteral agents are available for treating the hypertensive emergency. I have preferred to classify these agents into two general groups: (1) vasodilating drugs that directly dilate resistance vessels, and (2) the adrenergic-inhibiting agents that interfere with sympathetic innervation of the cardiovascular system. The ideal agent should be effective regardless of the etiology of the hypertension or the severity of blood pressure elevation, reduce peripheral vascular resistance while preserving blood flow to vital organs, have a rapid onset and offset of effect, enable a smooth and controlled reduction in blood pressure, and have minimal adverse effects. A number of currently available agents share at least some of the above properties.

Vasodilating Drugs (Table 5)

Sodium nitroprusside dilates both arterioles and veins and is considered by many clinicians to be the most effective parenteral agent currently available. The rapid onset of effect and brief duration of action enables precise titration of blood pressure with a carefully monitored infusion. A variable-rate infusion pump is recommended. While effective in any hypertensive emergency, nitroprusside is particularly efficacious in hypertensive crises complicated by congestive heart failure or myocardial infarction. Fluid retention leading to tolerance is avoided by concomitant administration of furosemide or bumetanide.

Nitroprusside is converted, primarily in the liver, to thiocyanate, which is excreted by the kidneys. The risk of thiocyanate toxicity is small when renal function is adequate and as long as drug usage is limited to 24 to 48 hours. As an intermediate step, free cyanide ions are formed, but are quickly converted to thiocyanate. A few cases of cyanide intoxication have been documented in patients with advance hepatic dysfunction or severe congestive heart failure.

Nitroglycerine shares many of the advantages of sodium nitroprusside with rapid onset and offset of action, short duration of action, and can be titrated to the desired effect. It has relatively greater effect on the venous circulation and less on arterioles. Nitroglycerine also dilates collateral coronary vessels, making the drug of particular use in patients with both hypertension and coronary insufficiency. A potential advantage of nitroglycerine is the absence of significant intrapulmonary shunting and hypoxemia, which may occur with sodium nitroprusside infusions.

Nitroglycerine is not as potent an arteriolar vasodilator as nitroprusside but may be particularly useful for managing acute congestive heart failure when pretreatment blood pressure is only modestly increased. It has also been useful in patients with coronary insufficiency and in managing the acute postoperative hypertension that may follow

Table 5
Vasodilating Drugs[a]

Drug	Method of Administration			Cautions
	IM[b]	Intermittent IV[b]	Continuous IV	
Sodium nitroprusside			0.5–10 µg/kg/min	Precise control of infusion mandatory. Thiocyanate or cyanide intoxication occasional problems.
Nitroglycerin			5–200 µg/min	Special intravenous infusion equipment required. Not as potent a vasodilator as nitroprusside.
Diazoxide		50–100 mg bolus injection	15–30 mg/min until the desired effect is achieved	Reflex tachycardia and increased cardiac output. Hyperglycemia with repeated injections.
Hydralazine HCl	10–50 mg[c]	10–20 mg/20 mL[d]	100–200 mg/L	Cornary insufficiency due to reflex increase in heart rate and cardiac work.
Nifedipine	10–20 mg	Perforated capsule sublingually or orally		Rapid, uncontrolled reduction in blood pressure. May precipitate congestive heart failure in patients with aortic stenosis.
Verapamil		5–10 mg	3–25 mg/hr	Avoid in patients with cardiac conduction abnormalities. Adverse interaction with other negative inotropes.
Enalaprilat		1.25 every 6 hours		Renal failure in patients with bilateral renal artery stenosis.

[a] In most cases, a rapidly acting diuretic should be given intravenously at the beginning and at appropriate intervals throughout the treatment; [b] IM = intramuscular; IV = intravenous; [c] Start with smallest dose listed; [d] Inject from syringe at rate of 1 mg/min until the desired effect is obtained.

coronary artery bypass procedures. Headache, retching, nausea, and vomiting are the most frequent side effects observed.

Diazoxide is a potent arteriolar vasodilator that has no effect on venous capacitance vessels and therefore reduces cardiac afterload but not preload. The drug is effective in most hypertensive emergencies and offers controlled reduction in blood pressure following repeated minibolus (pulse) doses of 50 to 75 mg, repeated at 10- to 15-minute intervals until the desired effect is achieved. A gradual yet predictable reduction in blood pressure can also be obtained with continuous intravenous infusions.

Reflex tachycardia and increased cardiac output can be controlled with small intravenous doses of propranolol or esmolol. Diazoxide also causes sodium and water retention, which may result in tolerance to the hypotensive action of diazoxide. Concomitant administration of furosemide or bumetanide is recommended. Hyperglycemia regularly accompanies repeated administration of diazoxide, and use in the treatment of the hypertension associated with pre-eclampsia may lead to arrest of labor because of the drug's relaxing effect on uterine muscles.

Hydralazine reduces arterial blood pressure by direct relaxation of arteriolar smooth muscle, leading to a reduction of peripheral vascular resistance. Hydralazine has no effect on venous capacitance, and the reduction in arterial pressure is therefore associated with reflex tachycardia and increased cardiac output, which may precipitate anginal symptoms in patients with hemodynamically significant coronary artery disease.

Antihypertensive response to hydralazine is less predictable than with other parenteral agents; it is rarely used in the treatment of hypertensive emergencies today except to manage severe pre-eclampsia, where it remains the agent of choice for many obstetricians. Nausea, vomiting, tachycardia, palpitations, and dizziness are among the most common adverse effects reported. Reflex tachycardia can be prevented by beta-blockers, and the sodium and water retention by concomitant administration of a loop diuretic.

Verapamil is effective following rapid intravenous injection of 5 to 10 mg or by continuous intravenous infusion. Most experience with intravenous verapamil in the management of hypertensive emergencies comes from Europe, Brazil, and India. The observation of a heart block accompanying intravenous administration suggests the need for caution in patients with underlying cardiac conduction abnormalities or in patients being treated with other negative inotropic agents such as beta-blockers or digitalis glycosides.

Nifedipine was discussed earlier in the management of hypertensive urgencies. Because of the rapid response observed within 15 to 30 minutes of oral or sublingual administration, nifedipine has also been widely used in the management of hypertensive emergencies.

Enalaprilat is the active metabolite of the orally administered prodrug, enalapril. While onset of action may be observed within 15 minutes, full effects may not be observed for several hours, making its use in the hypertensive emergency limited. It may be particularly useful in the patient with asymptomatic hypertension when oral administration is not practical. Since plasma renin activity and plasma volumes may be variable in patients with hypertensive emergencies, the initial response to enalaprilat may be variable and difficult to predict.

Adrenergic-Inhibiting Agents (Table 6)

Labetalol is a nonselective beta-receptor blocker with selective alpha-1 antagonist activity, which produces prompt reduction of peripheral vascular resistance and blood pressure without reflex tachycardia or significant changes in cardiac output. A controlled reduction in blood pressure is achieved with repeated injections (miniboluses) of 20 to 40 mg, repeated every 10 to 15 minutes or by a continuous monitored infusion.

Usage has been extended to the treatment of hypertensive crises associated with pheochromocytoma or clonidine withdrawal, postoperative hypertension, and for acute dissection of the abdominal aorta. Since labetalol's beta-blocking properties predominate, this agent should not be used in patients with uncompensated congestive heart failure, bronchial asthma, or heart block greater than first degree. Common adverse effects include nausea, vomiting, flushing, dizziness, and tingling of the scalp or groin areas.

Trimethaphan camsylate is a ganglion-blocking agent that dilates both arterioles and veins. When given by continuous intravenous infusion, onset of effect and offset of action are rapid and cardiac output is reduced as a consequence of increased venous capacitance and decreased venous return to the heart. The therapeutic use of trimethaphan today is restricted to management of the hypertensive patient with acute aortic dissection where its acute hemodynamic effects are considered favorable.

Large doses are often required for bedridden patients and tolerance frequently develops after 24 to 48 hours. Adverse effects expected with

Table 6
Sympathetic Inhibiting Drugs

Drug	Method of Administration			Cautions
	IM[b]	Intermittent IV[b]	Continuous IV	
Labetalol		2–80 mg by intermittent injection every 10–15 min	0.5–2.0 mg/kg/min	Caution similar to those with β-adrenergic blockers. Metabolism may be diminished in hepatic insufficiency.
Trimethaphan camsylate			0.8–6 mg/min	Precise monitoring of infusion mandatory. Parasympathetic side effects with prolonged administration.
Phentolamine	5–10 mg[b]	5- to 10-mg bolus injection	0.1–100 μg/kg/min	Reflex tachycardia may induce coronary ischemia.
Esmolol		500 μg/kg bolus injection	25–200 μg/kg/min[c]	Avoid when heart block, congestive heart failure, uncontrolled asthma present

[a] In most cases, a rapidly acting diuretic should be given intravenously at the beginning and at appropriate intervals throughout the treatment.
[b] Start with smallest dose listed.
[c] Titration every 5 minutes with repeat bolus administration.

ganglionic blockade such as urinary retention, paralytic ileus, obstipation, cycloplegia, and mydriasis can pose problems during therapy.

Phentolamine is a short-acting nonselective alpha-adrenergic blocker, which generally is reserved for use in both diagnosis and initial therapy of hypertension associated with high circulating levels of catecholamines. Parenteral administration may be associated with marked tachycardia, cardiac dysrhythmias, and occasional anginal symptoms. The effect of a single injection of phentolamine is very brief, usually lasting 15 minutes or less.

Esmolol is a new ultra-short-acting, cardioselective beta-adrenergic blocker. Although largely utilized to control supraventricular tachycardias, it may be used to minimize the reflex tachycardia associated with injection or infusion of several potent vasodilating agents. There is some evidence to suggest efficacy in the treatment of blood pressure in the perioperative period.

Role of Concomitant Diuretic Therapy

Intravenous loop diuretics should be used in conjunction with parenteral antihypertensive agents to offset the sodium and water retention associated with acute blood pressure reduction. Drug pseudotolerance associated with plasma volume expansion is a well-recognized cause for apparent resistance to potent parenteral agents. Furosemide in doses of 40 to 120 mg, or bumetanide 1 to 5 mg administered intravenously and repeated as needed, will assure adequate urine flow and negate risks of volume retention. For the occasional patient with known hypersensitivity to these agents, ethacrynic acid 50 to 150 mg is a useful alternative.

Summary

The clinician has an extensive number of effective agents available for controlling blood pressure in most hypertensive patients. Truly resistant hypertension is unusual, and an intensive search for other factors should be considered.

For the patient with accelerated/malignant hypertension or a hypertensive urgency or emergency, aggressive therapy with appropriate agents will enable quick and safe control of blood pressure. The selection of appropriate agents requires a thorough knowledge of the practical clinical pharmacology of the agents considered for treatment.

Selected References

Ahmed MEK, Walker JM, Beevers DG, et al: Lack of difference between malignant and accelerated hypertension. Br Med J 292:235–237, 1986.
American Medical Association Department of Drugs, Division of Drugs and Technology: Antihypertensive agents. In: Current Drug Evaluations, Sixth Edition. Chicago, American Medical Association, 1986, pp 507–540.
Finnerty FA: Resistant hypertension. Compr Ther 8:53–59, 1982.
Garcia JY, Vidt DG: Current management of hypertensive emergencies. Drugs 34:263–278, 1987.
Gifford RW Jr: An algorithm for the management of resistant hypertension. Hypertension ll(Suppl II):II-101–II-105, 1988.
Gifford RW Jr, Tarazi RC: Resistant hypertension: diagnosis and management. Ann Intern Med 88:661–665, 1978.
Tarazi RC: Management of the patient with resistant hypertension. Hosp Prac January 16, 1981, pp 49–57.
The 1988 Report of the Joint National Committee on Detection, Evaluation, and Treatment of High Blood Pressure. Arch Intern Med 148:1023–1038, 1988.
Vandenburg MJ, Sharman VL, Drew P, et al: Quadruple therapy for resistant hypertension. Br J Clin Pract 39:17–19, 1985.
Vidt DG: Accelerated hypertension, malignant hypertension, and hypertensive emergencies. In: Messerli F (ed), Current Clinical Practice. Philadelphia, WB Saunders Co, 1986, pp 101–105.
Vidt DG: Antihypertensive agents. In: Wang RH (ed), Practical Drug Therapy. Milwaukee, Medstream Press Inc, 1987, pp 85–127.
Vidt DG: The patient with resistant hypertension: cations, volume and renal factors. Hypertension ll(Suppl II):II-76–II-83, 1988.

Chapter 18

Lipids and the Cost-Effectiveness of Antihypertensive Therapy

Katherine S. Jones and Robert J. Rubin

Introduction

Coronary heart disease is the second leading cause of death among middle aged persons (45–64 years of age) in the United States with a death rate of 269 per 100,000 in 1985. While mortality from coronary heart disease has declined, the incidence of coronary heart disease has remained fairly stable. In 1983 the incidence of coronary heart disease was 82.8 per 1,000 persons, and in 1987, the rate remained essentially the same at 82.4 per 1,000. Figure 1 shows the incidence of coronary heart disease by age group, indicating that the incidence of coronary heart disease has remained stable despite documented changes in factors contributing to risk.

Hypertension is only one of many factors contributing to the incidence of coronary heart disease. In 1979 it was estimated that only one in eight persons with hypertension was treated and controlled. This has changed dramatically, and it is now estimated that the majority of those with high blood pressure are treated. In fact, a reduction in some of the sequelae of hypertension has been observed, including reductions in renal failure, cerebrovascular accidents, and congestive heart failure. However, the expected reductions in coronary heart disease incidence have not been observed.

From Punzi HA, Flamenbaum W (eds): *Hypertension*. Mount Kisco, NY, Futura Publishing Co., Inc., © 1989.

336 • HYPERTENSION

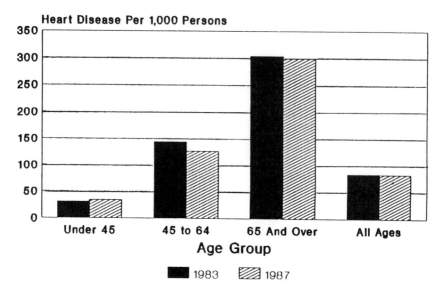

Figure 1. Incidence rates include the rate for ischemic heart disease, heart rhythm disorders, and other selected diseases of the heart. (From Vital and Health Statistics. NCHS Current Estimates from the Nation Health Interview Survey, United States 1987. Series 10, No. 166. U.S. Department of Health and Human Services.)

In treating the hypertensive patient, physicians must consider all of the various risk factors for coronary heart disease and may wish to modify the traditional step-care treatment method. In addition, they must consider issues related to compliance to the drug therapy. A drug may be useful in controlling hypertension, but if the patient does not continue on therapy, the drug will have no impact in controlling high blood pressure. Therefore, in considering the cost-effectiveness of treatment, one must consider the impact of the drug on hypertension, its influence on other risk factors, as well as compliance.

Risk Factors

Several factors, in addition to hypertension, have been identified as major risk factors for coronary heart disease (CHD). In order to be effective in reducing CHD risk, treatment for hypertension must recognize and optimize all components of risk. Factors to be considered include the blood lipid profile, glucose intolerance, fibrinogen, cigarette smoking, and level of physical activity. Some of these factors are also

Lipids and Antihypertensive Therapy • 337

related to hypertension, although for many of these factors, independent effects on CHD have been shown.

Blood Lipids

Results from the Multiple Risk Factor Intervention Trial (MRFIT) demonstrated a strong relationship between serum cholesterol level and mortality from coronary heart disease. The risk of mortality from coronary heart disease is positively correlated to serum cholesterol level (Fig. 2).

The Framingham Study followed patients over time to examine the relationship of lipid components to coronary heart disease. They reported a negative relationship between high-density lipoprotein cholesterol levels (HDL-C) and coronary heart disease and confirmed the positive relationship between total cholesterol and coronary heart disease. They concluded that the relative amount of total cholesterol carried by HDL-C was a reproducible indicator of coronary heart disease risk. Interestingly, data presented from the Framingham study demonstrate that, controlling for HDL-C levels, incidence for coronary heart disease

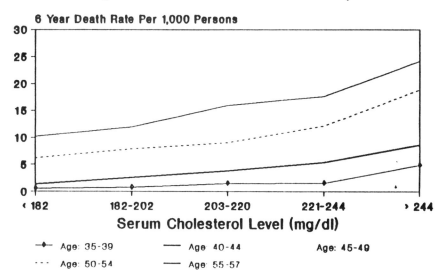

Figure 2. Six-year CHD mortality rate by age. (With permission from Kannel WB, et al: Overall and coronary heart disease mortality rates in relation to major risk factors in 325, 348 men screened for the MRFIT. Am Heart J 112:825–836, 1988.)

increases only slightly with total cholesterol. However, controlling for total cholesterol, the incidence for coronary heart disease increases dramatically as HDL-C declines.

Furthermore, several studies have now documented a decline in the incidence of coronary heart disease when total cholesterol is increased simultaneous to increasing the level of HDL-C. This is further evidence of the strong association between lipid components and coronary heart disease.

Cigarette Smoking

Cigarette smoking is associated with substantially higher risk of coronary heart disease. Data from MRFIT indicate that risk of death from CHD is 2.65 times higher for smokers than for nonsmokers. Cigarette smoking makes platelets sticky and the myocardium irritable, impairs oxygen transport, and lowers HDL-C. Similarly, data from the Framingham study indicate that smoking is a statistically significant predictor of CHD.

Glucose Intolerance

Diabetes doubles the risk of coronary heart disease for men and women in both the general and hypertensive populations. Interestingly, for women, glucose intolerance cancels out their relative advantage over men regarding risk for CHD.

Fibrinogen

Results of some recent studies suggest that hypertensive patients have higher fibrinogen values than normotensive patients, which augments their risk for coronary heart disease.

Physical Activity

A sedentary life style also increases the risk of CHD because it predisposes patients to lower levels of HDL-C, higher blood pressure, and obesity. Physical activity has been shown to reduce blood pressure and impact other factors that increase the risk of CHD.

Treatment of Hypertensive Patients

Generally a "step approach" to the treatment of hypertension has been recommended. A patient is taken through each step until blood pressure is effectively controlled.

The step approach has generally been described as: nonpharmacological treatment; first-level pharmacological treatment, which generally includes diuretics; and subsequent level pharmacological treatment, which may include other types of antihypertensives.

Nonpharmacological Therapy

In mild hypertensives (DBP 90–104 mmHg), generally nonpharmacological therapy is tried first. This includes counseling the patient to:

reduce weight level,
quit smoking
develop relaxation techniques,
exercise more frequently, and
modify diet to restrict sodium intake and reduce the level of fats in their diet.

If DBP can be controlled using these techniques, nonpharmacological approaches may be the most cost-effective therapy of hypertension.

Pharmacological Therapy

The first-line antihypertensive agent has generally been the use of a diuretic, usually a thiazide, alone. The patient is monitored to identify whether the diuretic is effective in controlling blood pressure and if a potassium supplement is required. In the past, other types of drugs have been added or tried when diuretics have failed. However, in their 1988 report, the Joint National Committee on Detection, Evaluation and Treatment of High Blood Pressure included other types of drugs in the first level of pharmacological treatment. They have suggested the use of diuretics, beta-blockers, calcium channel blockers, or angiotensin-converting enzyme (ACE) inhibitors as appropriate initial therapy for hypertension.

Selection of the Appropriate Pharmacological Control Agent

In selecting the appropriate first-line drug, several factors must be considered, including the risk factors identified above. In addition to any other factors, compliance to the drug regimen is probably the most important factor in achieving successful control of blood pressure.

There are, therefore, several important considerations in selecting the appropriate drug therapy, including: total cost of drug therapy; drug side effects and related compliance issues; and impact of the agent on risk factors. These issues are important, and in some cases, conflicting. For example, the least expensive therapy may be the one with the greatest number of side effects. Alternatively, drugs that help control hypertension and reduce total cholesterol or increase HDL-cholesterol levels may be more expensive than those that do not. Therefore, it is important to consider and weigh each of these factors.

Regardless of the efficacy of the drug, treatment will not be effective if the patient does not continue on drug therapy. Hypertensive agents have been shown to have a number of side effects that may result in lower compliance. In fact, a British survey of patients and physicians indicated that, while almost all surveyed physicians thought that hypertensive therapy was effective, only 50% of patients and virtually no relatives thought that treatment was successful. This indicates the importance of identified side effects to the patient's perception of well-being.

In addition to patient quality-of-life considerations, many of these side effects have the potential for generating additional health care costs. While it is difficult to quantify these costs, they must be considered when evaluating the total cost of therapy. Similarly, some of the drugs have secondary therapeutic effects that might be important for some patients.

The types of side effects and impact on risk factors differ by class of drug. In addition, different classes of drugs have different impacts on the risk factors discussed above. Of greatest interest in this analysis is the impact of antihypertensive agents on blood lipids. Table 1 summarizes both the potential side effects and the impact on the blood lipid profile of various classes of antihypertensive drugs.

Diuretics

Diuretics are frequently the first-line agent used to treat hypertensive patients. When used as a single agent, they are generally less ex-

Table 1
Side Effects of Antihypertensive Drugs

Drug Class	Lipid Effects	Other Side Effects
1. Diuretics/thiazides	↓ HDL ↑ LDL ↑ total cholesterol	hypokalemia; hyperuricemia; glucose intolerance; hypertriglyceridemia; sexual dysfunction; weakness
2. Beta-blockers	↑ total cholesterol ↓ HDL	bronchospasm; peripheral artery insufficiency; fatigue, insomnia; sexual dysfunction; hypertriglyceridemia; exacerbation of congestive heart failure; masking of hypoglycemia
beta-blockers with beta agonism	↑ HDL	
beta-blockers with ISA	lipid-neutral	
3. ACE inhibitors	lipid-neutral	hyperkalemia; angioneurotic edema; dysgeusia; rash; cough
4. Calcium antagonists	lipid-neutral	edema; headache; constipation; tachycardia
5. Alpha-blockers	↑ HDL ↓ total cholesterol	orthostatic hypotension; weakness; palpitations; first-dose syncope
6. Combined alpha-beta blockers	lipid-neutral	bronchospasm; peripheral vascular insufficiency; orthostatic hypotension

pensive than other drug classes (when used in combinations with potassium supplements, the cost advantage of diuretics may be diminished). There are several side effects associated with diuretics, hypokalemia being the most frequent. Other side effects include hyperuricemia, glucose intolerance, and hypertriglyceridemia. The side effects most likely to influence patient compliance include sexual dysfunction, weakness, and a general feeling of fatigue. In addition, for patients taking potassium supplements or potassium-sparing agents, hyperkalemia is a possible side effect.

Diuretics, alone or in combination with potassium supplements, have been shown to reduce HDL-C and increase total cholesterol. Therefore, while diuretics may be effective in reducing hypertension, for some population groups, they may increase the risk of coronary heart disease because of the negative effects on the patient's cholesterol profile. This may be one reason why the rate of hypertensive treatment has increased while the rate of CHD disease has not.

Beta-Blockers

Beta-blockers can cause a wide range of side effects, including bronchospasm, peripheral artery insufficiency, and hypertriglyceridemia. In addition, beta-blockers have been shown to exacerbate congestive heart failure and mask signs of hypoglycemia. Beta-blockers can also result in sexual dysfunction, fatigue, or insomnia.

Various types of beta-blockers have different effects on the lipid profile. Beta-blockers, in general, increase total serum cholesterol and reduce HDL-C. Beta-blockers with beta-agonism, however, increase HDL-C, while beta-blockers with intrinsic sympathomimetic activity (ISA) are lipid neutral.

Angiotensin-Converting Enzyme Inhibitors

Angiotensin-converting enzyme (ACE) inhibitors can cause mild hyperkalemia and may rarely result in angioneurotic edema, and dysgeusia. In addition, they may result in a rash or chronic cough. ACE inhibitors do not appear to have an adverse impact on the cholesterol profile. In fact, some studies have shown a similar positive effect on the lipid profile as observed with alpha-blockers.

Calcium Antagonists

Calcium blockers can cause edema, headache, constipation, and tachycardia. They do not appear to have any effect on the lipid profile.

Alpha-Blockers

Alpha-blockers can cause orthostatic hypotension, weakness, palpitations and can result in first-dose syncope. They increase HDL-C and reduce total cholesterol.

Combined Alpha-Beta-Blockers

Combined alpha- and beta-blockers can cause orthostatic hypotension, bronchospasm, and peripheral vascular insufficiency. They appear to be lipid-neutral.

Impact of Antihypertensive Therapy on Lipid Profile

The treatment of hypertension may have an adverse effect on the lipid profile. Studies of the adverse impact of diuretics on lipids call into question their use as a first-line agent to reduce hypertension. In fact, for some populations, they may reduce hypertension but increase the total risk for CHD by increasing total cholesterol and reducing HDL-C. Furthermore, other side effects may limit patient compliance, causing the treatment to have little effect on hypertension.

For both of these reasons, even though the cost of drug therapy might be increased, use of nondiuretic antihypertensives may increase compliance and limit the adverse impact on lipids. Therefore, treatment with more expensive agents may be cost-effective if they result in reduced risk for CHD and the associated health care costs.

Costs

The costs of various hypertensive agents differ substantially. As shown in Table 2, costs range from $28 to $582 per year, depending on the agent. While thiazides are the least expensive, when combined with a potassium supplement, their cost can be increased fourfold.

Impact on Lipids

The effect of antihypertensive agents on blood lipids was noted with early use, but not considered noteworthy until more recent research indicated the strong relationship between serum cholesterol and incidence of CHD. Several studies reported lipid changes with the use of antihypertensive agents. Some beta-blockers and thiazides were shown to increase cholesterol from 5% to 15% alone and by 20% to 30% when used in combination.

344 • HYPERTENSION

Table 2
Range of Estimated Costs of Antihypertensive Drugs

	Cost Per Year
1. Thiazides	$28–$32
2. Beta-blockers	$164–$377
3. Alpha-blockers	$277–$377
4. ACE inhibitors	$253–$325
5. Calcium channel blockers	$357–$582

Ranges presented represent the range of possible drugs in the class as well as the various dosages for a particular drug. The highest and lowest price drugs were chosen, as well as the highest and lowest recommended dosage. Annual costs reflect average wholesale prices, inflated by 10% to reflect retail markups and $2 for a dispensing fee. Average wholesale prices (AWP) are from 1989 *Red Book*, which provides AWP for all types of prescription drugs.

Recent studies have indicated that reduction in total cholesterol is linked with reduced incidence of CHD. One study comparing middle age men on a moderate cholesterol-reducing diet in which one group was given cholestyramine and another a placebo indicated that use of cholestyramine resulted in a 13.4% decrease in total cholesterol. This decrease was 8.5% greater than the group given a placebo. This reduction in total cholesterol resulted in a 24% reduction in definite CHD death and 19% reduction in nonfatal myocardial infarction. A second study compared rates of CHD in patients treated with gemfibrozil, a cholesterol-reducing agent, to patients given a placebo. In the treated group, an 11% reduction in total cholesterol resulted in a substantial change in incidence of CHD events. The group treated with gemfibrozil had a cumulative 5-year rate of cardiac events of 27.3 per thousand, compared to 41.4 per thousand in the group given the placebo.

This information suggests that, when some types of antihypertensive agents that increase cholesterol are used, the negative effects on serum cholesterol may "cancel out" the positive effect of reducing blood pressure. Therefore, traditional use of thiazides, or other agents with an adverse effect on the lipid profile, as the first treatment for hypertension may not be the most cost-effective.

Cost-Effectiveness Considerations

In considering cost-effectiveness of different types of antihypertensive drugs, some consideration must be given to risk factors other than hypertension. Clearly, one of the considerations has to be the impact of the drug on the lipid profile. It is possible that treatment with higher cost drugs can be cost-effective if the impact on lipids is sufficient to reduce the risk of CHD.

Using data from a number of different studies, it can be shown that, depending upon the cost differential of various drug types, treatment with a higher cost agent may be cost-effective. Analysis is presented here for one group, a cohort of 45-year-old males, which compares the use of a cholesterol-reducing antihypertensive to use of an agent that is assumed to be as effective in reducing blood pressure, but increases cholesterol levels. Additional analysis indicates that when lipid neutral drugs are compared to drugs that increase cholesterol, savings can also be achieved.

Assumptions

In considering the cost-effectiveness of one agent over another, data are required related to costs of the drug, incidence of hypertension, and impact of cholesterol on the risk for coronary heart disease and on the direct and indirect costs of coronary heart disease.

The data on the costs of drugs (Table 2) reflect the range of average wholesale prices for drugs in each class, marked up by 10% and including a $2.00 per prescription dispensing fee. The range of prices also reflects the range of potential dosage for each drug.

Data on the incidence of hypertension are available from a survey representative of the entire U.S. population. According to this survey, 24.2% of males age 45–54 have elevated blood pressure. Therefore, of every 100,000 males age 45, it can be estimated that 24,200 have hypertension, assuming that the rate of hypertension is the same for 45-year-old males as for the entire age group. Since the incidence of hypertension increases with age, the rate for 45-year-old males may be somewhat lower.

Data on the impact of cholesterol on coronary heart disease are also available, indicating that a reduction of 15% (from 260 mg/day) in serum cholesterol in males age 45 to 49 reduces the incidence of coronary heart disease by 270 events per 100,000 people. The estimates of changes in relative risk differ depending upon the starting cholesterol level and patient age.

Additional data provide an estimate of the distribution of coronary events by type of event (Table 3). Using these data, one can estimate

Table 3
Distribution of Coronary Events

Type of Event	Percent of Events
Sudden death	11
Fatal myocardial infarction	6
Myocardial infarction	29
Coronary insufficiency	11
Angina	43
	100

Note: Classifications used are those used in the Framingham study, see Shurtleff D: Section 30. Some characteristics related to the incidence of cardiovascular disease and death. Framingham Study, 18-year follow-up. Kannel and Gordon: The Framingham Study: An Epidemiological Investigation of Cardiovascular Disease. DHEW Pub. No. (NIH) 74-599. Bethesda, Maryland Public Health Service, 1974.

(With permission from Lewin/ICF, a division of Health and Sciences Research Incorporated, Washington, D.C.)

the type of coronary events that might be averted with a reduction in serum cholesterol.

The estimated costs of coronary events are summarized in Table 4. Costs shown in Table 4 are for 45-year-old males. Indirect costs are estimated by taking the difference in lifetime earnings between patients

Table 4
Cost Associated with Coronary Events
(Lifetime Costs for 45-Year-Old Male in 1989 Dollars)

Type of Event	Estimate Costs	
	Direct	Indirect
Sudden death	$359	$497,503
Nonsudden death	5,172	497,503
Myocardial infarction	20,448	176,633
Coronary insufficiency	21,139	154,355
Angina pectoris	15,931	147,094

(With permission from Oster G, Epstein A: Primary prevention and coronary heart disease: the economic benefits of lowering serum cholesterol. Am J Public Health 76, 1986. Inflated to 1989 using the medical care price index for direct costs and the consumer price index for indirect costs.)

with coronary heart disease and a similar group without coronary heart disease. These costs were discounted to reflect present values. Indirect cost estimates reflect work incapacity and lost earnings due to premature mortality. (There are other methods available to calculate the indirect costs associated with disease that include costs in addition to earnings. Because our analysis includes only indirect costs associated with earnings it understates indirect costs.) Direct costs are estimates of the medical care costs associated with each type of event. The figures make use of a variety of assumptions related to the types of care likely to be required, the cost of surgery where appropriate, and the cost of follow-up care, including required physician visits and costs of drug treatment, where appropriate. As shown, the direct costs associated with sudden death are much lower because it is assumed that little medical care is provided prior to death. However, the direct costs associated with coronary insufficiency are high due to the high percentage of patients that require surgery and the expected long length of hospitalization.

Analysis of Cost-Effectiveness

If these data are used, one can estimate the cost-effectiveness of using a cholesterol-reducing antihypertensive medication in one population group—45-year-old males.

For a cohort of 100,000 males age 45 years, data indicate that 24,200 will have hypertension requiring medication. If one assumes that all types of drugs can reduce blood pressure to the same level, the only differences to be considered in choosing the appropriate medication are the cost of the drug and the impact of the drug on lipids.

Table 5 shows the range of costs of medications available to treat this group of males. As shown, cost ranges from $678,000 for thiazides to $14 million for calcium channel blockers, depending on the specific drug used and dosage required. Data from previous studies indicate that diuretics increase serum cholesterol the most, while alpha-blockers decrease cholesterol the most. Therefore, we would expect alpha-blockers to provide the greatest reduction in risk for coronary heart disease associated with cholesterol, and compared with use of a thiazide, we might expect a reduction in a patient's cholesterol level of between 10%–15%. This is the result of thiazides increasing total cholesterol by 5%–8% and alpha-blockers decreasing total cholesterol by 5%–7%, resulting in a 10%–15% net reduction. One half of this reduction might occur with a change from a thiazide to a lipid-neutral agent.

Table 5
Drug Costs Associated with Treatment of 24,200 Males Age 45

Type of Drug	Costs (in 1,000s)
1. Thiazides	$ 678–$ 774
2. Beta-blockers	$3,969–$ 9,123
3. Alpha-blockers	$6,703–$ 9,123
4. ACE inhibitors	$6,123–$ 7,865
5. Calcium channel blockers	$8,639–$14,084

Ranges presented represent the range of possible drugs in the class as well as the various dosages for a particular drug. The highest and lowest price drugs were chosen, as well as the highest and lowest recommended dosage. Annual costs reflect average wholesale prices, inflated by 10% to reflect retail markups and $2 for a dispensing fee. Average wholesale prices are from 1989 *Red Book*.

As shown in Table 5 for the cohort of 45-year-old males, the additional cost of treatment with lipid-neutral antihypertensives or alpha-blockers compared to thiazides is estimated to range from $6 to $14 million on an annual basis. Use of the alpha-blocker will reduce serum cholesterol, and according to data presented earlier, may reduce the number of coronary events by 270 per 100,000 in our cohort of 45-year-old males. If one assumes that the relationship between cholesterol and coronary events is linear (as it appears to be in Fig. 2), one half of these events would be averted with the use of a lipid-neutral agent. Table 6 shows the direct and indirect cost-savings expected from averting the 270 coronary events. As shown, savings of $4.2 million in direct costs

Table 6
Estimated Savings from Averted Coronary Events

Type of Event	Events Averted	Direct Costs	Indirect Costs
Sudden death	28	10,052	13,930,084
Nonsudden death	17	87,924	8,457,551
Myocardial infarction	78	1,594,944	13,777,374
Coronary insufficiency	31	655,309	4,785,005
Angina pectoris	116	1,847,996	17,062,904
TOTAL	270	4,196,225	58,012,918

(With permission from Lewin/ICF estimates using data from Table 3.)

and $58 million in indirect costs are expected. Use of a lipid-neutral agent may achieve savings of roughly one half this amount, or $2.1 million in direct costs and $29 million in indirect costs.

If we compare these savings to the additional cost of the drugs, it is clear that use of the cholesterol-reducing or lipid-neutral antihypertensive agent is cost-effective for this population group. The additional costs cannot be justified if only direct costs-savings are considered. However, when the indirect costs associated with coronary events are considered, the additional costs can be justified.

This analysis depends upon all of the assumptions discussed earlier. It also assumes that alpha-blockers significantly reduce levels of serum cholesterol as compared to thiazides and that the change in risk for coronary heart disease that can be achieved with hypertensive patients is comparable to the general population. If these assumptions do not apply, it may significantly change the number of coronary events averted due to the use of a cholesterol-reducing agent. In addition, our analysis assumes that adverse effects on quality of life, which may effect compliance or indirect cost factors, is comparable among the various nondiuretic antihypertensive agents.

Summary

Traditional step-care treatment of hypertension suggests that thiazides may be the first pharmacological drug to be used. This is largely due to the fact that this class of drugs has been used successfully to reduce blood pressure for many years and because the drug is relatively inexpensive.

However, as do many other antihypertensive drugs, thiazides have a number of side effects. Some of these side effects can be expected to reduce the level of compliance with therapy. In addition, more recently, the negative impact of thiazides on the lipid profile has been recognized. This has been suggested as one reason why the incidence of coronary heart disease has not declined despite the fact that an increasing percentage of those with high blood pressure are being treated.

Our analysis suggests that, while treatment and control of hypertension is of paramount consideration, all other things being equal, the physician should consider a drug that either reduces lipids or is lipid-neutral. In making this decision, the physicians must evaluate the individual patient, paying particular attention to existing risk factors for coronary heart disease as well as other conditions. The example cited above makes it clear that the price of an antihypertensive may not be reflective of its true costs. The effect of an antihypertensive drug on serum cholesterol and/or HDL-C may profoundly affect a patient's risk of coronary heart disease. Therefore, treatment with a more expensive drug may result in lower costs to society as well as decreasing morbidity and even mortality among patients.

Selected References

Flamenbaum W: Hypertension, changes in high density lipoproteins, and anti hypertensive therapy: Implications for coronary heart disease risk. Am J Cardiol 63:541–571, 1989.

Frick M H, Elo O, Haapa, K, et al: Helsinki Heart Study: Primary prevention trial with gemfibrozil in middle aged men with dyslipidemia. New Engl J Med 317:1237–1245, 1987.

Grimm RH: Primary prevention trials and the rationale for treating mild hypertension. Clin Ther 9(Suppl D):20–30, 1987.

Harvard Medical School Health Letter: "High Blood Pressure: New Treatments." January 1989.

Jachuck SJ, et al: The effect of hypertensive drugs on the quality of life. J R Coll Gen Pract 32:103–105, 1982.

Kannel WB: Impact of single and multiple risk factors on coronary disease and its treatment: focus on hypertension. Clin Ther 9(Suppl D):2–19, 1987.

Kannel WB, McGee DL: Diabetes and cardiovascular disease: The Framingham Study. JAMA 241:2035–2038, 1979.

Lipid Research Clinics Program: The lipid research coronary primary prevention trial results. JAMA 251:351–364, 1987.

1988 Joint Committee: The 1988 Report of the Joint National Committee on Detection, Evaluation, and Treatment of High Blood Pressure. Arch Intern Med 148:1023–1038, 1988.

Shaw J: Antihypertensive drugs: Impact of different classes on coronary heart disease risk profiles. Clin Ther 9(Suppl D):31–36, 1987.

Stamler J: The marked decline in coronary heart disease mortality rates in the United States, 1968–1981; Summary of findings and possible explanations. Cardiology 72:11–22, 1985.

U.S. Department of Health and Human Services, Health United States 1988. Hyattsville, Maryland (March 1989 DHHS publication No. (PHS)89–1232.

Chapter 19

Renovascular Hypertension: A Radiologist's Point of View

Helen C. Redman

Introduction

Renovascular hypertension is initiated by ischemia of the renal parenchyma leading to activation of the renin-angiotensin system and then hypertension. Many radiographic techniques have been developed over the past thirty years in an attempt to define the presence of renal ischemia. Most evaluate either renal artery flow or renal size, which are indirect indicators of renal ischemia. Both decreased arterial blood flow and decreased renal size have a number of causes other than renal artery stenosis. The renal angiogram is the only unimpeachable way to demonstrate the presence of renal artery stenosis. Since the development of renal ablation techniques and percutaneous transluminal angioplasty (PTA), angiographic techniques can also be used therapeutically in some patients with renovascular hypertension.

Selection of patients for renal angiography in the evaluation of hypertension generally is done on clinical grounds. As a rule, the patients fall into one of two groups. The first group has had hypertension for some time, has not been controlled on a good medical regimen, is noncompliant with any medical regimen, or has serious side effects from an effective medical regimen. These patients are operative candidates. The second group includes patients with the documented recent onset

From Punzi HA, Flamenbaum W (eds): *Hypertension*. Mount Kisco, NY, Futura Publishing Co., Inc., © 1989.

of severe hypertension in whom the decision must be made whether to offer long-term medical control or surgical control. In general, patients who are considered for diagnostic angiography should not be older than 50 years of age. Older patients are evaluated for surgery or angioplasty only when hypertension is very severe and uncontrollable. These patients may also have declining renal function. Since children do have renovascular hypertension, there is no lower age limit for evaluation.

Preangiography Screening Tests

Concern about the complications and costs of angiography in the evaluation of hypertension frequently is voiced. It is reasonable, therefore, to consider briefly any screening tests that might help in deciding which patients should undergo angiography.

The intravenous urogram (IVU) provides an excellent evaluation of renal size and function. Congenital or acquired abnormalities of the renal parenchyma and collecting system seen with an IVU can often explain renal size discrepancies. Renal masses, primarily renal cell carcinomas and renal cysts, may also be identified. Several modifications of the standard IVU have been developed in an attempt to enhance the specificity for renal artery stenosis. The first modification (rapid sequence IVU) involves taking a series of films immediately following the rapid injection of a large bolus of contrast material. These films are generally taken at 15 seconds and then 1, 2, and 3 minutes after completion of the radiocontrast injection. A decreased nephrogram in one kidney when compared to the other kidney can be caused by decreased arterial inflow and therefore suggests the presence of a renal artery stenosis.

The second modification of the IVU is the search for delayed hyperconcentration on a late film. The theory is that the involved kidney has a diminution in renal blood and makes less urine than the normal one, so that the concentration of contrast material in the collecting system on the involved side gradually increases with time. After approximately 30 minutes, the abnormal kidney shows hyperconcentration of contrast medium in the collecting system. Urea and mannitol infusions have also been given in an attempt to enhance this finding.

Both the diminished nephrogram and delayed hyperconcentration can be difficult to detect. Bowel gas, liver overlying part or all of the right kidney, and unusual body habitus make an accurate assessment of these findings difficult. In addition, both observations depend on unilateral renal artery disease, an unrealistic expectation. In fact, the

Cooperative Study of Renovascular Hypertension found a 17% false-negative and 11.4% false-positive rate for IVU in the screening of renovascular hypertension. This error rate makes the IVU an inadequate screening technique. The "hypertensive" or rapid-sequence IVU should no longer be performed. In any specific patient with hypertension, however, a standard IVU may be indicated.

Isotopic renograms have a very low morbidity and have been used to differentiate between a normally functioning kidney and one with renal artery stenosis. The procedure relies on the decreased uptake and excretion of I131 Hippuran or, more recently, Tc-99m-DTPA in the diseased kidney when compared to the normal one. The false-positive rate (20%) and false-negative rate (14%) for the I131 Hippuran study are too great to make this procedure a satisfactory screening technique. The procedure is useful for determining renal artery and arterial graft patency, however. The Tc-99m-DTPA has fewer false-positives and false-negatives in early experience. Recently, captopril stimulation has been used to improve accuracy. While early data have been enthusiastic, use in a general or nonselective population has not been individually tried.

For some time, split renal function studies were performed during the evaluation of renovascular hypertension. This procedure required the simultaneous catheterization of both ureters with measurement of urine volume, PAH, sodium, and creatinine bilaterally. This technique was about 75% accurate in predicting surgical cure, but the complications of the procedure, including infection, obstruction, and even renal shutdown, prevented its widespread use. It is seldom performed at the present time.

Screening tests involving the renin-angiotensin system have also been used. Use of saralasin, an angiotensin II antagonist, has been described. Its limited clinical application is based on its intravenous administration. Peripheral plasma renins have actively been proposed as a screening test for renovascular hypertension. Unfortunately, as many as 20% of patients with essential hypertension have an elevated peripheral plasma renin. The test is also complicated by the fact that many of the drugs used in the therapy of hypertension either elevate or depress peripheral plasma renins. Therefore, results of such assays must be interpreted with care.

Use of selective renal venous sampling for relative renin values was proposed in the mid-1960s. It was believed that a concentration of renin one-and-a-half times that observed on the contralateral side was solid evidence of hypersecretion from an ischemic kidney. The use of a ratio assumes one normal or much more normal kidney, which may be an unrealistic assumption. Over time, the absolute renal vein renin values have assumed more importance since up to one third of patients with correctable lesions do not lateralize. Angiographically the procedure is straightforward and the morbidity is low. However, clinicians must either stop all antihypertensive drugs that modify renin secretion or be prepared to interpret the results in the light of the medication. There are a myriad of protocols for obtaining renal vein renins. The very fact that so many protocols exist makes the data received questionable. Angiotensin-converting enzyme (ACE) inhibition with captopril is currently used to accentuate the renin differences between the involved and noninvolved kidneys. When lateralization by renin ratio is greater than 1.5 to 2.0, with or without stimulation, the chances of surgical cure are markedly increased.

Doppler ultrasound, especially when color analysis is available, has developed into a noninvasive screening technique for branches of the abdominal aorta. It is very operator-dependent, and normal findings in the hands of an experienced operator are more reliable. Abnormal findings must be confirmed by angiography. Equipment for color Doppler is changing rapidly, and in the future, this technique may become the best noninvasive screening procedure for patients with renovascular hypertension.

All the tests described have real limitations as screening tests for renovascular hypertension. In any given patient one or more of these procedures may be indicated. However, renal angiography remains the only procedure that provides anatomical definition of the lesions. It is also the only procedure that the surgeon can use to determine whether surgery should be considered and what type of procedure should be undertaken.

Diagnostic Angiographic Techniques

At present there are three angiographic approaches to renovascular hypertension. These include intravenous digital subtraction angiography (IVDSA), intra-arterial digital subtraction angiography (IADSA), and standard cut-film angiography. Each procedure has its assets and drawbacks that should be clearly understood by the referring physician. Therefore, some of the important technical aspects of each approach are discussed.

IVSDA is performed by placing a catheter in the right atrium or superior vena cava and injecting 40 to 50 cc of 60% contrast medium.

Renovascular Hypertension • 355

The circulation time is taken into consideration, and filming is begun over the abdomen just before the anticipated time of arrival of the contrast medium at the renal arteries. A prolonged circulation time of any cause makes the procedure difficult since the digital filming system requires a baseline image. Information that is not on the baseline image is detected and displayed by the computer. If contrast medium has reached the field of view before the first image is obtained, the injection may be wasted. If there is too long a delay between the mask or baseline film and the arrival of contrast medium, the patient often moves when forced to breathe. Peristalsis also causes motion artifacts. The spatial resolution of all digital subtraction angiography is significantly less than that on standard cut-film angiography. Intrarenal arterial branches rarely are well evaluated by IVDSA.

Which patients should be considered for an IVDSA? Probably very few. The major advantage of IVDSA is that it is an outpatient procedure. Therefore, the patient population that can be considered is one which is fully motivated and able to remain still, even when made uncomfortable by an injection of contrast material; has no cardiac disorder and a normal circulation time; is to be evaluated only for main renal artery disease, since the branch arteries generally are not adequately seen for interpretation; and has no risk factors for large doses of intravenous contrast medium. In such patients, IVDSA is an effective screening technique, but this population is limited. The IVDSA can be used in these patients, but it remains a limited examination and, when abnormal, often must be followed by an intraarterial procedure.

IADSA minimizes many of the drawbacks of the intravenous procedure and is a more versatile examination. Outpatient studies are feasible in most patients, although bed rest for four to six hours after the procedure in a day surgery unit is necessary. In addition, these patients sometimes must have an emergency admission if hemostasis is not achieved or there is arterial injury. The procedure is performed using a 4F or 5F catheter positioned at the level of the renal arteries. The contrast medium injection is made by using 10 to 12 cc of 76% contrast medium or 40 cc to 50 cc of 25%–30% contrast medium. Timing is straightforward and not dependent on the circulation time. Motion is less of a problem since the patient needs to hold his breath for only a few seconds and frequently does not feel the injection at all. Peristalsis can still cause difficult artifacts. Because the contrast medium is injected at the level of the renal arteries, fewer opacified, but extraneous arteries hinder interpretation. Furthermore, if the digital procedure does not provide adequate information, the procedure can be changed immediately to a standard cut-film angiogram.

Which patients should have intra-arterial digital subtraction angiography? Patients with renal failure and diabetes who have an increased risk of renal problems following use of iodinated contrast medium are ideally suited for the use of this technique since the volume of contrast medium required is significantly less than that required for the other approaches. Details of the main renal arteries and their primary divisions generally are adequate with IADSA, so that many patients can have the aortic injections performed digitally and then standard cut-film angiography used for any necessary selective injections.

Standard cut-film angiography remains the "gold standard" for the angiographic evaluation of renovascular hypertension. The detail obtained is superior to digital subtraction angiography. Although the contrast medium volume is greater than that needed for IADSA, it is less than that generally needed for intravenous studies. The intrarenal detail permits visualization of branch artery involvement.

Which patients should have standard cut-film angiography in the evaluation of renovascular hypertension? All patients who need evaluation of the intrarenal branches should have at least the selective part of the angiogram performed using standard cut-film angiography. Probably all patients who are not at special risk from large doses of contrast medium are best evaluated in this fashion. When angioplasty is planned, measurements to determine balloon size are most easily and accurately made based on standard angiograms.

Angiographic Findings

The lesions that cause renovascular hypertension are most commonly atherosclerosis or medial fibroplasia. There are many other less common causes that may be encountered, including: the uncommon variants of fibromuscular hyperplasia, such as intimal fibroplasia, medial hyperplasia, and perimedial dysplasia; Takayasu's arteritis; neurofibromatosis; renal artery aneurysms; renal artery dissection; chronic perirenal hematoma; renal artery embolism; and, other unusual lesions. The majority of these lesions are best documented with angiography, and treatment planning often requires lumbar aortography as well as selective renal angiography.

Atherosclerosis increases in frequency with advancing age. Renal artery stenosis is a relatively frequent component of this aging process,

Renovascular Hypertension • 357

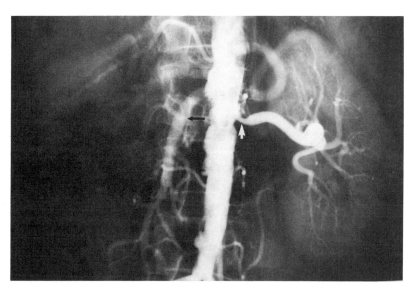

Figures 1A, B, C. Lumbar aortogram in a 60-year-old woman who had controllable hypertension for at least eight years. Her hypertension has recently become uncontrolled and kidney function has diminished. A (above). Early arterial phase. There is a moderate stenosis (⇨) of the proximal left renal artery. It appears to be renal rather than aortic in origin since the renal artery astium is not narrowed. The remainder of the left renal artery is normal. A second projection demonstrates that the possible aneurysm at the renal hilum is an arterial loop. The stenosis in the left renal artery is an appropriate one for angioplasty. The right renal artery is occluded at its origin. It reconstitutes by collaterals (→) and is seen flowing toward the right kidney. It is reasonable to postulate that occlusion of this renal artery caused the abrupt change in clinical course.

and although it may cause hypertension, it is more commonly asymptomatic or a source of increasing renal failure. The important angiographic observations in patients with renovascular hypertension caused by atherosclerosis include a determination of whether a plaque is a renal artery plaque or a plaque in the abdominal aorta encroaching on the renal artery ostium, the length and severity of the stenosis (Fig. 1); presence of collateral arterial flow (Fig. 2); and evidence of diffuse intrarenal involvement. Plaques that are aortic in origin but compromise the renal orifice may not be successfully treated by angioplasty. Diffuse intrarenal disease in addition to main renal artery involvement often makes any attempt at angioplasty or surgical repair unsuccessful. Many renal artery stenoses occur in patients who are normotensive. It is therefore a chal-

358 • HYPERTENSION

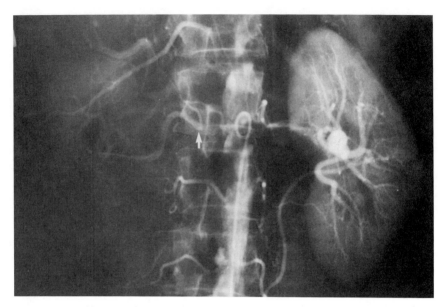

Figure 1B. Late arterial phase. The right renal artery (→) is more easily seen. Some intrarenal arteries on the right are faintly opacified.

lenge to determine which patients have renovascular hypertension. The presence of collateral circulation is evidence that the lesion is of hemodynamic significance. Evaluation of the length and degree of the stenosis will also help to determine the likelihood of success using angioplasty.

Medial fibroplasia is most frequently seen in caucasian females between 30 and 60, but may be seen in males and other racial groups. At angiography, the lesion generally spares the proximal main renal artery. In the typical case, the remainder of the main renal artery shows a series of dilatations and bands, which has been described as a "string of beads" (Fig. 3). This term is misleading since the aneurysmal outpouchings are generally not uniform and are often eccentric. The first-order segmental branches frequently are involved by the medial fibroplasia. Discrete dilations large enough to be called aneurysms occur with these lesions (Fig. 4), and these may rupture or cause arteriovenous fistulae. The disease generally is bilateral and progressive. However, the rate of progression is variable and one kidney may be far more severely involved than the other. At angiography it is important to determine the full extent of the lesion and to define the location of any associated aneu-

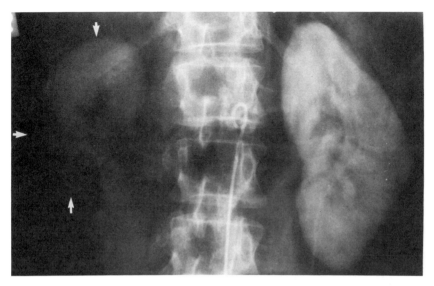

Figure 1C. Nephrogram phase. The right kidney (→) is much smaller than the left kidney, and the nephrogram is also diminished. It is sometimes possible to open an occluded renal artery using the angioplasty technique. Surgery is the other possible approach. The angiogram clearly demonstrates that the right kidney is ischemic.

rysms to determine whether angioplasty or surgery should be undertaken.

The remaining causes of renovascular hypertension are encountered relatively infrequently and will not be described in depth. Although the uncommon variants of fibromuscular hyperplasia and lesions such as Takayasu's arteritis may be amenable to angioplasty, most of the less common lesions, such as renal artery dissection (Fig. 5) or the Page kidney, require surgical intervention if medical therapy does not control the hypertension adequately. In the pediatric and adolescent hypertensive population, in particular, careful attention must be paid to the intrarenal arterial supply since branch stenoses and occlusions are relatively common in this age group. Carefully performed renal angiography is necessary in the majority of these patients.

Radiological Interventional Procedure in Renovascular Hypertension

Purposeful infarction of a kidney that has been causing malignant, uncontrollable hypertension can be offered as an alternative to surgery

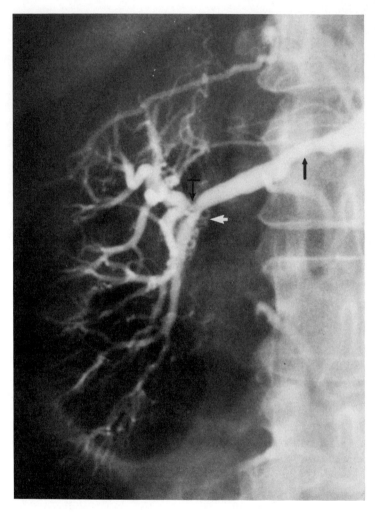

Figure 2. Selective right renal angiogram in a 21-year-old man who has had moderately well controlled hypertension for at least eight years. There is a moderate stenosis in the proximal main renal artery (→) with a slight poststenotic dilatation. This lesion is amenable to angioplasty, but further evaluation of the image demonstrates another stenosis at the bifurcation into dorsal and ventral branches (↦). Five collateral arteries are also present (⇒). Angioplasty is unlikely to be successful in treating the more distal stenosis, and surgery is the approach of choice.

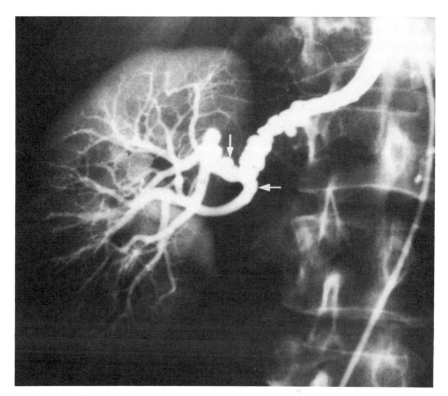

Figure 3. Medial fibroplasia in a 41-year-old woman with bad hypertension for nine years that was now becoming difficult to control. Right renal angiogram shows that the proximal right renal artery is normal. The distal two thirds shows the classical focal dilatations and bands of medial fibroplasia ("string of beads"). The lesion extends into both the dorsal and ventral branches (→). Angioplasty could be attempted in this patient, although complete dilatation of the more peripheral lesions may prove difficult or impossible.

in the very ill patient. If infarction is undertaken, the material used must be capable of occluding the fine peripheral intrarenal arteries. Occlusion of the main renal artery alone usually will cause innumerable small collateral vessels to develop, primarily from the capsular, renal pelvic, and ureteric circulations. The collaterals will result in the renal parenchyma remaining viable, but ischemia can actually worsen the hypertension. Particulate and fluid materials have been used to accomplish complete renal infarction. Currently, absolute ethanol is probably the best agent available for renal infarction. It will occlude every peripheral renal artery

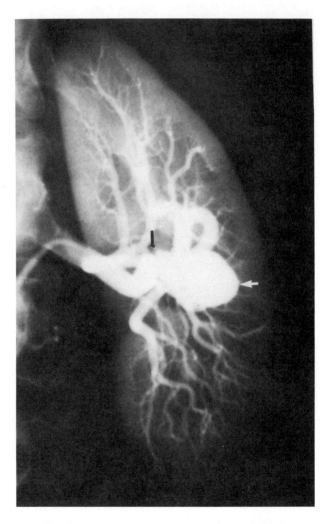

Figure 4. Medial fibroplasia and renal artery aneurysm in a 34-year-old woman with hypertension. The main renal artery is normal until near its division where some contour irregularities are seen (→). Just distal to the focus of medial fibroplasia is an aneurysm (⇒) that measures approximately 2 cm in greatest diameter. Angioplasty is not indicated since the aneurysm must be surgically treated.

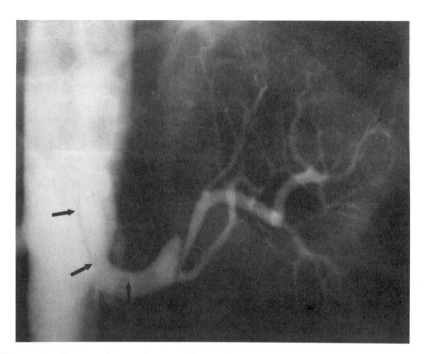

Figure 5. Traumatic renal artery dissection following a fall from scaffolding in a 54-year-old man who became acutely hypertensive during his hospitalization for other injuries. An intimal flap (→) is seen in the lumbar aorta. It extends into the renal artery severely narrowing the origins of the dorsal and ventral renal artery branches. The hypertension regressed after surgical repair.

and usually results in complete infarction. It is very neurotoxic, however, and should be injected beyond an occlusion balloon catheter to avoid any reflux into the abdominal aorta or the inferior adrenal artery. Such an infarction should be undertaken only by a seasoned angiographer with experience in embolization and the intravascular use of absolute ethanol.

Most radiological interventional procedures for renovascular hypertension are percutaneous transluminal angioplasties (PTAs). Intraoperative dilatation of medial fibroplasia has been successfully performed for many years using graduated dilators. Therefore, it is not at all surprising that renal artery PTA was begun shortly after the development of the balloon-type angioplasty catheter. The procedure has been performed in many centers since 1978 and has a significant success rate. The technique is straightforward, but should always be performed by an experienced angiographer who has had training in the angioplasty procedure.

PTA may be performed either in conjunction with the diagnostic angiogram or as a separate procedure. The individual circumstances determine which course is preferable in a specific patient. The advantage of performing both the diagnostic and therapeutic procedures at one time is that only one procedure is required. The disadvantages are the possibility of using too much contrast material, which may lead to renal failure, and the frequent need for a second arterial puncture to obtain optimum placement of the angioplasty catheter. If renal vein renin determinations are desired, this procedure must be done earlier in order to have the results available when the decision to perform an angioplasty must be made. A two-stage procedure, performing diagnostic angiography and obtaining renal vein renin samples first, and then scheduling PTA in consultation with a vascular surgeon, is the more conservative approach. The one-stage procedure, however, does have a legitimate place in the approach to renovascular hypertension.

Medial fibroplasia can be treated successfully by angioplasty in most cases where the medial fibroplasia involves only the main renal artery. The technical problems that preclude a successful dilatation in these cases are inability to traverse the lesion because of tortuosity or the use of an inappropriate balloon. When the disease involves the dorsal and ventral renal artery branches, dilatation may be contraindicated because of the danger of causing a dissection with subsequent occlusion when dilatation is performed across a bifurcation. Aneurysms found in conjunction with medial fibroplasia are also a contraindication to PTA since these, which may also lead to hypertension, commonly need to be corrected surgically.

Some of the less common causes of renovascular hypertension are amenable to angioplasty including variants of fibromuscular hyperplasia. The decision to use angioplasty in these situations must be made on a case-by-case basis. Some of these patients will have an initial incomplete response to angioplasty, but follow-up studies will show a good result. The complications of PTA are well known. Major complications, including renal artery occlusion, dissection, damage to entry site requiring surgery, and blood loss requiring transfusion, occur in less than 5% of patients with current balloons. Loss of kidney and loss of life are uncommon. Transient depressed renal function may also occur. The morbidity and mortality to correct renovascular hypertension are less than with surgery. PTA is a reasonable alternative to surgery for many patients and should be considered in each patient.

Selected References

Adler J, Einhorn R, McCarthy J, et al: Gelfoam embolization of the kidneys for treatment of malignant hypertension. Radiology 128:45–48, 1978.
Alfidi RJ, Tarar R, Fosmoe RJ, et al: Renal-splanchnic steal and hypertension. Radiology 102:545–549, 1972.
Bookstein JJ, Abrams HL, Buenger RE, et al: Radiologic aspects of renovascular hypertension. Part 2: The role of urography in unilateral renovascular disease. JAMA 220:1225–1230, 1972.
Bookstein JJ, Abrams HL, Buenger RE, et al: Radiologic aspects of renovascular hypertension. JAMA 221:368–374, 1972.
Bron KM, Redman HC: Renal arteriovenous fistula and fibromuscular hyperplasia: a new association. Ann Intern Med 68:1039–1043, 1968.
Casteneda-Zuniga W, Zollikofer C, Valdez-Davila O, et al: Giant aneurysms of the renal arteries: an unusual manifestation of fibromuscular dysplasia. Radiology 133:327–330, 1979.
Denny DF, Perlmutt LM, Bettman MA, et al: Percutaneous recanalization of an occluded renal artery and delayed ethanol ablation of the kidney resulting in control of hypertension. Radiology 151:381–382, 1984.
Ellman BA, Parkhill BJ, Marcus PB, et al: Renal ablation with absolute ethanol. Invest Radiol 19:416–423, 1984.
Ford KT, Teplick SK, Clark RE, et al: Renal artery embolism causing neonatal hypertension. Radiology 119:547–548, 1976.
Foster JH, Maxwell MH, Franklin SS, et al: Renovascular disease: results of operative treatment. JAMA 213:1043–1048, 1975.
Franklin SS, Maxwell MH: Clinical workup for renovascular hypertension. Urol. Clin North Am 2:301–310, 1975.
Fry WJ, Ernst CB, Stanley JC, et al: Renovascular hypertension in the pediatric patient. Arch Surg 107:692–698, 1973.
Gill WM, Meaney TF: Medial fibroplasia of the renal artery. Radiology 92:861–866, 1969.
Gomes AS, Sinaiko AR, Tobian L, et al: Renal vein renin sampling in essential hypertension using hydralazine and the tourniquet test. Radiology 153:619–623, 1984.
Gruenewald SM, Collins LT: Renovascular hypertension: quantitative renography as a screening test. Radiology 149:287–291, 1983.
Harper AP, Yune HY, Franken EA, et al: Spectrum of angiographically demonstrable renal pathology in young hypertensive patients. Radiology 123:141–146, 1977.
Harrington DP, Whelton PK, Mackenzie EJ, et al: Renal venous renin sampling. Radiology 138:571–575, 1981.
Havey RJ, Krumlovsky F, del Greco F, et al: Screening for renovascular hypertension. JAMA 254:388–393, 1985.
Hillman BJ, Ovih TW, Capp MP, et al: The potential impact of digital video substraction angiography on screening for renovascular hypertension. Radiology 142:577–579, 1982.
Jensen SR, Novelline RA, Brewster DC, et al: Transient renal artery stenosis produced by a pheochromocytoma. Radiology 144:767–768, 1982.

Judson WE, Helmer OM: Diagnostic and prognostic values of renal vein renin activity in renal venous plasma in renovascular hypertension. Hypertension 13:79–85, 1965.

McNeil BJ, Varady PD, Burrows BA, et al: Measures of clinical efficacy: cost-effectiveness calculations in the diagnosis and treatment of hypertensive renovascular disease. N Engl J Med 293:216–221, 1975.

Marks LS, Maxwell MH, Varady PD, et al: Renovascular hypertension: does the renal vein renin ratio predict operative results? J Urol 115:365–368, 1976.

Martin LG, Price RB, Casarella WJ, et al: Percutaneous angioplasty in clinical management of renovascular hypertension: initial and long-term results. Radiology 155:629–633, 1985.

Melman A, Donohue J, Weinberger M, et al: Improved diagnostic accuracy of renal venous renin ratio with stimulation of renin release. J Urol 117:145–148, 1977.

Mena E, Bookstein JJ, Holt JF, et al: Neurofibromatosis and renovascular hypertension in children. Am J Roentgenol 118:39–45, 1973.

Nanni GS, Hawkins IF Jr, Orak JK, et al: Control of hypertension by ethanol renal ablation. Radiology 148:51–54, 1983.

Oxman HA, Sheps SG, Bernatz PE, et al: An unusual cause of renal arteriovenous fistula—fibromuscular dysplasia of the renal arteries. Mayo Clin Proc 48:207–210, 1973.

Poutasse EF, Gonzalez-Serva L, Wendelken JR, et al: Saralasin tests as a diagnostic and prognostic aid in renovascular hypertension patients subject to renal operation. J Urol 123:306–311, 1980.

Schaeffer AJ, Stamey TA: Ureteral catheterization studies. Urol Clin North Am 2:327–340, 1975.

Scott PL, Yune HY, Weinberger MD, et al: Page Kidney: an unusual cause of hypertension. Radiology 119:547–548, 1976.

Simon N, Franklin SS, Bleifer KH, et al: Clinical characteristics of renovascular hypertension. JAMA 220:1209–1218, 1972.

Sos TA, Pickering TG, Sniderman K, et al: Percutaneous transluminal renal angioplasty in renovascular hypertension due to atheroma or fibromuscular dysplasia. N Engl J Med 309:274–279, 1983.

Srur MF, Sos TA, Saddekni S, et al: Internal fibromuscular dysplasia and Takayasu arteritis: delayed response to percutaneous transluminal renal angioplasty. Radiology 157:657–660, 1985.

Stanley JC, Fry WJ: Renovascular hypertension secondary to arterial fibrodysplasia in adults. Arch Surg 110:922–928, 1975.

Stanley P, Gyepes MT, Olson DL, et al: Renovascular hypertension in children and adults. Radiology 129:123–131, 1978.

Tegtmeyer CJ, Brown J, Ayers CA, et al: Percutaneous transluminal angioplasty for the treatment of renovascular hypertension. JAMA 246:2068–2070, 1981.

Tegtmeyer CJ, Elson J, Glass TA, et al: Percutaneous transluminal angioplasty: the treatment of choice for renovascular hypertension due to fibromuscular dysplasia. Radiology 143:631–637, 1982.

Tegtmeyer CJ, Teates CD, Crigler N, et al: Percutaneous transluminal angioplasty in patients with renal artery stenosis. Radiology 140:323–330, 1981.

Thibonnier M, Joseph A, Sassano P, et al: Improved diagnosis of unilateral renal artery lesions after captopril administration. JAMA 251:56–60, 1984.

Chapter 20

Renovascular Hypertension: An Internist's Point of View

Marc A. Pohl

Introduction

Ever since the original Goldblatt experiment in 1934 wherein experimental hypertension was produced by renal artery clamping, countless investigators and clinicians have been intrigued by the relationship between renal arterial stenosis and hypertension. In this regard, the pathophysiological role of the renin-angiotensin system has been widely discussed and much of our understanding of the role and regulation of the renin-angiotensin system has evolved from models of experimental hypertension produced by renal artery clamping. Pharmacological agents known to interfere with the activity of the renin-angiotensin system such as beta-blockers and angiotensin-converting enzyme inhibitors, fascination with numerous diagnostic screening studies designed to predict a relationship between renal artery stenosis and hypertension, controversies about surgical intervention versus medical management of renal artery stenosis, and, most recently, percutaneous transluminal renal artery angioplasty may be viewed, in one way or another, as emanating from the original Goldblatt experiment.

Under certain experimental or clinical conditions, renal artery obstruction may be the cause of hypertension. When this causality is confirmed, the term "renovascular hypertension" is used to describe this association. In a broader sense, "renovascular hypertension" may be defined as secondary elevation of the blood pressure produced by any

From Punzi HA, Flamenbaum W (eds): *Hypertension*. Mount Kisco, NY, Futura Publishing Co., Inc., © 1989.

of a variety of conditions that interfere with the arterial circulation to the kidney causing renal ischemia. Renal artery stenosis, however, is not synonymous with "renovascular hypertension." On the basis of autopsy studies and clinical-angiographic correlations, high-grade atherosclerotic renal artery stenosis without hypertension is frequent and may be observed in approximately one third to one half of normotensive patients over 60 years of age with atherosclerotic renal artery disease. In addition, not all patients with hypertension and renal artery stenosis are cured of their hypertension by operations that bypass the stenotic lesion. Thus, it is critical to distinguish between renal artery stenosis in which a stenotic lesion is present, but not necessarily causing hypertension, and renovascular hypertension, where sufficient arterial stenosis is present to produce renal tissue ischemia and initiate the sequence of pathophysiological events leading to elevated blood pressure. In the final analysis, proof that a patient has the entity of "renovascular hypertension" rests with the demonstration that the hypertension, presumed to be "renovascular," can be eliminated or substantially ameliorated following removal of the stenosis by surgical or angioplastic intervention or by removing the kidney distal to the stenosis. Thus, in its purest sense, "renovascular hypertension" is a retrospective diagnosis.

This chapter reviews the pathophysiology of renovascular hypertension, the types of renal artery stenosis frequently associated with renovascular hypertension, clinical features and diagnostic approaches to this entity, and management considerations in patients with renal artery stenosis and presumed renovascular hypertension. Although the thrust of this chapter will be devoted to renovascular hypertension, evolving concepts regarding the issue of renal artery stenosis as a threat to renal function are presented.

Pathogenesis

Figure 1 is a schematic representation of renovascular hypertension. This diagram shows the classic model of "Goldblatt hypertension," two kidney-one clip (2K,1C), in which one renal artery is constricted and the contralateral kidney is left intact. In the presence of hemodynamically sufficient unilateral renal artery stenosis in the 2K,1C model, the kidney distal to the stenosis is rendered ischemic, activating the renin-angiotensin system, and producing high levels of angiotensin II, which presumably cause a "vasoconstrictor" type of hypertension. Numerous studies have established the causal relationship between angiotensin II-

Renovascular Hypertension

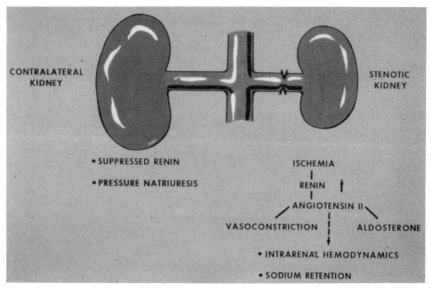

Figure 1. Schematic representation of renovascular hypertension.

mediated vasoconstriction and hypertension in the early phase of renovascular hypertension. In addition, the high levels of angiotensin II stimulate the adrenal cortex to elaborate larger amounts of aldosterone such that the involved kidney demonstrates sodium retention. Mild or moderate degrees of renal artery stenosis do not initiate the above-described sequence of events; the degree of renal artery stenosis necessary to produce hemodynamically significant reductions in perfusion, triggering renal ischemia and activating the renin-angiotensin system, generally does not occur until there is reduction of 80% or more of both diameter and cross-sectional area of the renal artery.

The model of two kidney-one clip Goldblatt hypertension implies that the contralateral (nonaffected) kidney is present and that it's renal artery is not hemodynamically significantly narrowed. As indicated in Figure 1, the contralateral kidney demonstrates a suppressed renin and a pressure natriuresis. Why do these phenomena occur in the contralateral kidney? Recall that angiotensin II-induced vasoconstriction generated due to the stenotic kidney and angiotensin II-induced increases in aldosterone result in vasoconstriction and sodium retention, leading to systemic elevation of blood pressure. This elevation in systemic pressure results in suppression of renin release and enhanced excretion of sodium (pressure natriuresis) by the contralateral kidney.

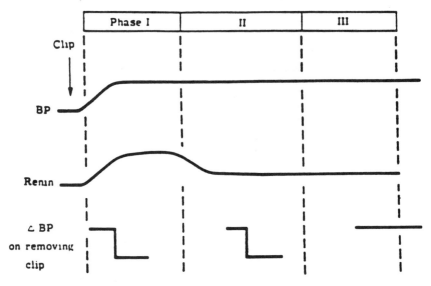

Figure 2. Sequential phases reproduced in 2K,1C hypertension. Effect on blood pressure and renin secretion. After the clip is put on one main renal artery, with the contralateral kidney left untouched, blood pressure and renin secretion increase. In Phase II, the blood pressure remains high but renin secretion falls. In Phase III, the blood pressure remains elevated despite removal of the clip, presumably reflecting vascular damage in the contralateral kidney. (With permission from Brown JJ, Davies DL, Morton JJ, et al: Mechanisms of renal hypertension. Lancet i:1219, 1976.)

The pathophysiological schema of renovascular hypertension as depicted in Figure 1 is an oversimplification. In fact, the course of experimental two kidney-one clip hypertension may be divided into three sequential phases (Fig. 2). In phase I, renal ischemia and activation of the renin-angiotensin system is of fundamental importance and, in this early phase of experimental hypertension, the blood pressure elevation is renin-dependent . Acute administration of angiotensin II antagonists, administration of angiotensin-converting enzyme inhibitors, removal of the renal artery stenosis (i.e., removal of the clip in the experimental animal), or removal of the "stenotic kidney" will promptly normalize the blood pressure. However, several days after renal artery clamping, renin levels fall, but blood pressure remains elevated. This second phase of 2K,1C hypertension may be viewed as a pathophysiological transition phase that, depending upon the experimental model and species, may last from a few days to several weeks. During this transition phase

(Phase II), salt and water retention are observed as a consequence of the effects of hypoperfusion of the stenotic kidney; augmented proximal renal tubular reabsorption of sodium and water and angiotensin II-induced stimulation of aldosterone secretion (secondary aldosteronism) contribute to this sodium and water retention. In addition, the high levels of angiotensin II stimulate thirst, which further contributes to an expansion of the extracellular fluid volume. The expanded extracellular fluid volume results in a progressive suppression of peripheral renin activity as depicted in Figure 2. During this transition phase, the hypertension is still responsive to removal of the unilateral renal artery stenosis, to angiotensin II blockade, or unilateral nephrectomy, although these maneuvers do not normalize the blood pressure as promptly and consistently as in the acute phase.

After several days to several weeks, this evolves into a chronic phase (Phase III) where removal of the stenosis (or unclipping the renal artery in the experimental animal) does not lower the blood pressure. Most likely, this failure of "unclipping" to lower the blood pressure in the chronic phase of 2K,1C hypertension is due to widespread arteriolar damage to the contralateral kidney consequent to prolonged exposure to high blood pressure and high levels of angiotensin II. In this chronic phase of 2K,1C, renovascular hypertension, extracellular fluid volume expansion and systemic vasoconstriction are the main pathophysiological abnormalities. The blood pressure remains elevated despite the fact that the plasma renin activity has returned to a normal level. The pressure natriuresis of the contralateral kidney blunts the extracellular fluid volume expansion caused by the "stenotic kidney" (Fig. 1), but as the contralateral kidney suffers vascular damage from prolonged exposure to the increased blood pressure, its excretory function diminishes and extracellular fluid volume expansion persists. In Phase III of 2K,1C hypertension, acute blockade of the renin-angiotensin system fails to lower the blood pressure. Sodium depletion may ameliorate the hypertension but does not normalize it.

Systemic vasoconstriction also contributes to the elevated blood pressure, despite normalization of renin, in Phase III of two kidney-one clip hypertension. Whether the peripheral renin level is elevated or not, this phase of renovascular hypertension is associated with increased sensitivity to angiotensin II, increased levels of vasopressin, and increased peripheral and central sympathetic nervous system activity. Some authors have postulated a renin-angiotensin system localized in vascular tissues, possibly contributing to the generation of vasoconstriction by acting through adrenergic nerves on vascular smooth muscle.

Hypertension-induced structural changes in the vascular wall may also contribute to the maintenance of hypertension in this chronic phase of 2K,1C hypertension. Thus, although in the early phase of two kidney-one clip hypertension the basis of the hypertension appears to be predominantly renin-dependent and the hypertension ameliorated by interference with the renin-angiotensin system, revascularization, or nephrectomy, the pathogenesis of blood pressure elevation in the chronic phase is multifactorial and less clearly defined. Extrapolating these observations to patients, one might presume that the sooner an arterial lesion causing "renovascular hypertension" is removed, the more likely the chance for relief of the hypertension. Admittedly, this clinical suggestion, based on a complexity of experimental observations, may be stretching the experimental observations too far. Nevertheless, clinical experience indicates that corrective surgery for unilateral renal artery stenosis as the presumptive cause for hypertension is far more successful in patients with a brief history of hypertension (e.g., less than five years) in contrast to patients with a longer duration of hypertension.

The above discussion of the pathophysiology of renovascular hypertension has focused on the two kidney-one clip model of renovascular hypertension ("two kidney hypertension"); where the contralateral nonaffected kidney is present. The most common clinical counterpart to this type of hypertension is unilateral renal artery stenosis. It should be appreciated, however, that several other clinical circumstances might be associated with this type of hypertension including, unilateral renal artery aneurysm, arterial embolus, congenital and traumatic arteriovenous fistula, segmental arterial occlusion, pheochromocytoma compressing a renal artery, and metastatic tumor compressing either the renal artery or renal parenchyma. Unilateral renal trauma with development of a calcified fibrous capsule surrounding the injured kidney, causing compression of the renal parenchyma may produce "renovascular hypertension." This clinical situation is analogous to the experimental Page kidney wherein cellophane wrapping of one of two kidneys causes hypertension, which is relieved by removal of the wrapped kidney.

There is another type of "renovascular hypertension," known as one kidney-one clip hypertension ("one kidney hypertension") that should be distinguished from two kidney-one clip hypertension ("two kidney hypertension"). In experimental one kidney-one clip (1K,1C) hypertension, one renal artery is constricted and the contralateral kidney is removed. Clinical counterparts of one kidney-one clip hypertension include renal artery stenosis in a solitary functioning kidney, bilateral

Renovascular Hypertension • 373

renal arterial stenosis, coarctation of the aorta, vasculitides such as polyarteritis nodosa and Takayasu's arteritis, atheroembolic renal artery disease, and renal artery stenosis in a transplanted kidney. In experimental one kidney-one clip hypertension, initial increase in renin release is responsible for the early rise in blood pressure, as in the two kidney-one clip model of renovascular hypertension. However, in the absence of an unclipped contralateral kidney, sodium retention from angiotensin II-induced secondary aldosteronism becomes extremely important early in the course of the one clip-one kidney model. Thus, extracellular fluid volume expansion is a prime feature of "one kidney hypertension," and the pathophysiological features described for the chronic phase of 2K,1C hypertension develop more quickly. In this situation, there is no contralateral kidney to offset the developing rise in systemic blood pressure and sodium retention. Renal perfusion pressures reach levels sufficient to suppress renin to normal levels at the price of high blood pressure sustained mainly by salt and water retention. Accordingly, one might expect plasma renin levels to be normal and the blood pressure elevation to be independent of circulating angiotensin II. Although these expectations are basically correct in the volume expanded state, the role of angiotensin II may be unmasked under conditions of salt depletion, resulting in systemic vasoconstriction and maintenance of elevated blood pressure.

Types of Renal Artery Stenosis

Since the most common clinical circumstance producing the syndrome of renovascular hypertension is renal arterial stenosis, it is important to describe the main renal arterial lesions associated with this type of hypertension. Fibromuscular dysplasia and atherosclerosis of the renal artery are by far the most common causes of significant renal artery stenosis. Other relatively rare causes, such as Takayasu's arteritis, renal artery aneurysm, and arteriovenous fistula have been previously mentioned. The remainder of this chapter describes the two major types of renal arterial disease, fibromuscular dysplasia, and atherosclerosis.

Fibrous Renal Artery Disease

Fibrous dysplasia of the renal artery is estimated to account for 30%–40% of renal artery lesions. There are five different types of fibrous renal

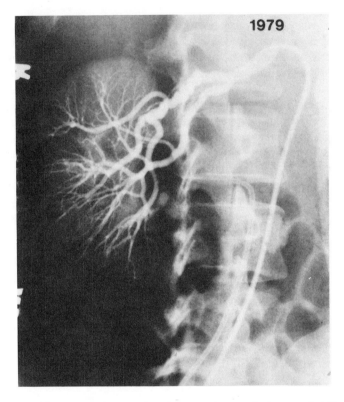

Figure 3. Selective right renal arteriogram demonstrates medial fibroplasia involving the distal renal artery. (With permission from Schreiber MJ, Pohl MA, Novick AC: The natural history of atherosclerotic and fibrous renal artery disease. Urol Clin North Am 11:383–392, 1984.)

artery disease: medial fibroplasia, perimedial fibroplasia, medial hyperplasia, intimal fibroplasia, and periarterial fibroplasia. Although the true incidence of these specific types of fibrous renal artery disease is not clearly defined, medial fibroplasia is the most common and estimated to account for 60% to 70% of fibrous renal artery disease. The lesion of medial fibroplasia characteristically affects the distal half of the main renal artery, frequently extending into the major branches, is often bilateral, and angiographically gives an appearance of multiple aneurysms ("string of beads") because the diameter of the aneurysms is wider than the apparently unaffected portion of the renal artery (Fig. 3). The majority of cases of medial fibroplasia are diagnosed between the ages of 30–50 years and it is more common in women. Although medial fibroplasia progresses to higher degrees of stenosis in about one third of cases, complete arterial occlusion or ischemic atrophy of the involved kidney are rare. The stenotic lesions in medial fibroplasia are secondary to thickened fibromuscular ridges replacing the normal structure of the intima and media of the artery. These areas alternate with thinned areas that do not have an internal elastic membrane and may become aneurysmal.

Perimedial fibroplasia is the second most common of the fibrous dysplasias, accounting for 15%–25% of fibrous renal artery lesions. This lesion also occurs predominantly in women between the ages of 15 and 30 and angiographically is often characterized by a small string of beads, with the beads being of similar width or less wide in diameter than the diameter of the apparently unaffected portion of the renal artery (Fig. 4). This lesion typically affects the distal half of the main renal artery, is frequently bilateral, highly stenotic, and may progress to total occlusion. Collateral blood vessels and renal atrophy on the involved side are frequently observed. Pathologically, the outer layer of the media varies in thickness and is densely fibrotic with very little smooth muscle, producing a severely stenosing lesion that is often irregular. Mural aneurysms occasionally may be associated with perimedial fibroplasia although less commonly than with medial fibroplasia.

Medial hyperplasia and intimal fibroplasia are not common, estimated to make up only about 5% of fibrous renal artery lesions. Intimal fibroplasia (Fig. 5) occurs primarily in children and adolescents and angiographically gives the appearance of a localized, highly stenotic, smooth lesion, with post stenotic dilatation. It may occur in the proximal portion of the renal artery, is progressive, and is occasionally associated with dissection or renal infarction. Pathologically, idiopathic intimal fibroplasia is due to a proliferation of the intimal lining of the arterial wall. Intimal fibroplasia of the renal artery may also occur as an event secondary to atherosclerosis or as a reactive intimal fibroplasia consequent to an inciting event such as prior endarterectomy. Medial hyperplasia is found predominantly in adolescents and angiographically also appears a smooth linear stenosis that may extend into the primary renal artery branches. There is great difficulty in the arteriographic differentiation between intimal fibroplasia and medial hyperplasia and, in the literature, these two types of fibrous renal artery disease may be grouped together. Periarterial fibroplasia is the least common of the fibrous lesions and is characterized by dense collagen replacing the adventitia and extending into the periarterial fibro-fatty tissues. This lesion, usually occurring in children and adolescents is extremely rare.

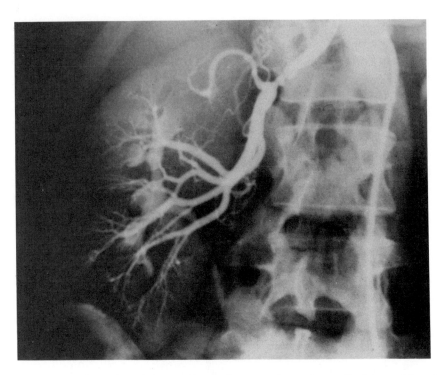

Figure 4. Selective right renal arteriogram shows a small string of bead appearance typical of perimedial fibroplasia. Note that the beads are of smaller diameter than the unaffected portion of the renal artery. Note also the presence of collateral vessels typically seen with perimedial fibroplasia. (With permission from Pohl MA, Novick AC: Natural history of atherosclerotic and fibrous renal artery disease: clinical implications. Am J Kidney Dis 5:A120-A130, 1985.)

An appreciation of the distinct types of fibrous renal artery disease has important clinical implications. Medial fibroplasia may demonstrate progressive stenosis angiographically but rarely progresses to total occlusion. Accordingly, the risk of losing renal function over time due to progressive medial fibroplasia is small and renal revascularization or percutaneous transluminal angioplasty need not be considered because of fear of losing kidney function. These modalities of treatment should be utilized for patients with hypertension refractory to medical therapy in whom clinical evaluation strongly suggests that the hypertension is "renovascular." On the other hand, patients with perimedial fibroplasia,

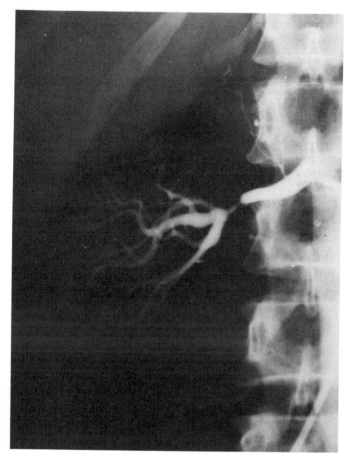

Figure 5. Selective right renal arteriogram demonstrating intimal fibroplasia of the distal renal artery. Note the localized, highly stenotic, smooth lesion.

medial hyperplasia, and intimal fibroplasia are at substantial risk for developing high-grade renal artery stenosis, which might threaten long-term renal function. In addition, these patients not infrequently have hypertension resistant to drug therapy. Since these patients are generally quite young, have more severe hypertension, and are at greater risk for losing kidney function, renal revascularization is usually recommended for these patients in order to avoid life long antihypertensive therapy and to prevent renal atrophy.

Atherosclerotic Renal Artery Disease

Atherosclerotic renal artery disease (ASO-RAD) is estimated to account for 60%–70% of all renal artery lesions. This lesion predominately affects men in the fifth to seventh decades of life, but is not uncommon in women of similar ages or in younger adults. Renal artery atherosclerosis is very common in older patients with or without hypertension simply as a consequence of generalized atherosclerosis obliterans. Renal arteriograms performed in patients presenting with various forms of peripheral vascular disease indicate that one third to one half have significant degrees of renal artery obstruction due to atherosclerosis. Correlations of hypercholesterolemia and cigarette smoking with renal artery atherosclerosis are not unequivocally clear, but one might presume that they represent risk factors for renal artery atherosclerosis just as they represent risk factors for atherosclerosis in other vascular beds.

Atherosclerotic renal artery disease is typically associated with atherosclerotic changes of the abdominal aorta. Anatomically, the majority of these patients demonstrate atherosclerotic plaques located in the proximal third of the main renal artery. In the majority of cases (70%–80%), the obstructing lesion is an aortic plaque invading the renal artery ostium. Twenty to thirty percent of patients with ASO-RAD demonstrate the atherosclerotic narrowing 1–3 cm beyond the take-off of the renal artery, i.e., nonostial lesions. Patients with unilateral renal atrophy where the atrophy is due to large vessel atherosclerotic occlusive disease may be expected to have significant obstruction of the renal artery supplying the contralateral normal sized kidney in anywhere from one third to one half of cases (Fig. 6).

Although carefully acquired prospective information on the natural history of ASO-RAD is lacking, retrospective studies suggest that ASO-RAD is a progressive disorder. In a large series from the Cleveland Clinic, serial renal arteriograms obtained in nonoperated patients indicated progression of renal artery obstruction in 44% of patients. Progression to total occlusion was not uncommon. Renal artery atherosclerotic lesions with more than 75% stenosis on the initial renal arteriogram seemed to be at highest risk for progression to more severe occlusion. Further, patients with progressive atherosclerotic renal artery disease had a significantly higher frequency of clinically detectable loss of renal function as indicated by rising serum creatinine levels and reduction in ipsilateral renal size in contrast to patients with nonprogressive (angiographically) atherosclerotic renal artery disease.

Taken together, important clinical clues to the presence of signifi-

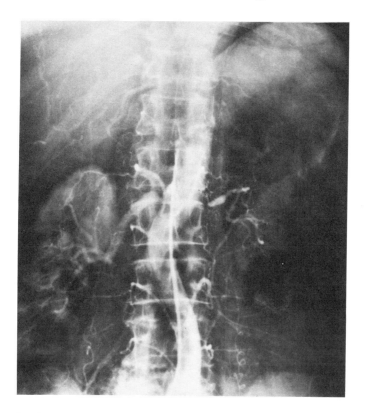

Figure 6. Aortogram in a 62-year-old woman demonstrating bilateral atherosclerotic renal artery stenosis. Note the total occlusion of the left renal artery and high-grade stenosis of the proximal right renal artery with a normal-sized right kidney. (With permission from Pohl MA, Novick AC: Natural history of atherosclerotic and fibrous renal artery disease: clinical implications. Am J Kidney Dis 5:A120-A130, 1985.)

cant atherosclerotic renal artery disease, which is often bilateral, include the following: (1) patients with generalized atherosclerosis obliterans; (2) hypertension, often presumed to be renovascular hypertension; (3) a unilateral small kidney; (4) mild to moderate azotemia; (5) deterioration in renal function with blood pressure lowering, particularly with the use of angiotensin-converting enzyme inhibitor drugs. These clinical clues strengthen the indications for angiographic study to define the degree of renal artery stenosis, which is potentially instrumental in the pathogenesis of hypertension and in identifying patients for whom the risk of renal functional impairment from progressive arterial occlusion is greatest.

In summary, patients with fibrous renal artery disease are predominantly women, between the ages of 15 and 40 years. ASO-RAD occurs predominantly in men more than 45–50 years of age and with other risk factors for generalized atherosclerosis. Although many of these patients have hypertension, and some certainly turn out to have renovascular hypertension, the majority of patients with ASO-RAD probably have two mutually exclusive disorders, essential hypertension and generalized atherosclerosis obliterans. Although the differences between patients with ASO-RAD and fibrous renal artery disease have been emphasized, both forms of renal artery disease have a propensity to cause hypertension, are much less frequent in blacks, and occur bilaterally in 30%–50% of patients.

Clinical Characteristics of Renovascular Hypertension

Prevalence estimates of renovascular hypertension range from 2%–30%, depending upon the population of hypertensive patients studied. The prevalence of renovascular hypertension reported by tertiary care medical centers may be as high as 20%–30%. In contrast, prevalence figures of renovascular hypertension generated from the hypertensive population at large suggests a prevalence of no more than 2%. When patients with severe or accelerated hypertension are considered, the yield of finding renovascular hypertension may be as high as 15%–20%. Since the great majority of hypertensive patients have mild or moderate degrees of blood pressure elevation, with only about 10% of hypertensives having "severe" hypertension (diastolic blood pressure greater than 120 mmHg), a prevalence estimate of 2%–3% for renovascular hypertension seems most reasonable. The special appeal of diagnosing renovascular hypertension centers around the observation that this form of hypertension is the most common type of potentially curable hypertension with the possible exception of hypertension induced by oral contraceptives or excessive alcohol intake.

The medical history and physical examination provide important clues suggesting renovascular hypertension. In contrast to essential hypertension, renovascular hypertension should be suspected if the family history is negative for hypertension. However, one quarter to one third of patients with proven renovascular hypertension have a positive family history for hypertension. The abrupt onset of moderate to severe hypertension at any age, particularly if the patient is less than 20 years or greater than 45 years of age, suggests renovascular hypertension. Caucasian children and young adults with a history of abrupt onset of moderate to severe hypertension are strong candidates for fibrous renal artery disease as the cause of the hypertension. Adults over 45 years of age, particularly if Caucasian and with a history of cigarette smoking, are strong candidates for ASO-RAD as the cause of the hypertension.

The severity of the hypertension is another clinical clue that the blood pressure elevation may be renovascular in origin. Patients with persistent diastolic hypertension >110 mmHg, which is resistant to a rational triple drug regimen, are strong candidates for renovascular hypertension. Acceleration of previously stable and well-controlled blood pressure is another important clue to renovascular hypertension. An excellent antihypertensive response to converting-enzyme inhibitor drugs, such as captopril, enalapril, or lisinopril, therapeutic agents that block the renin-angiotensin system most effectively, suggests renovascular hypertension. The history of acute flank pain with or without hematuria, followed by the onset of hypertension, also suggests renovascular hypertension.

Clues to renovascular hypertension from the physical examination include advance hypertensive retinopathy such as retinal hemorrhages and exudates with or without papilledema. In one series, nearly 40% of patients with these characteristics on fundus examination (group III or IV retinopathy) turned out to have renovascular hypertension. Evidence of atherosclerotic occlusive disease characterized by carotid bruits and/or claudication, in conjunction with the historical clues mentioned above, suggests atherosclerotic disease of the renal artery. A systolic/diastolic bruit in the epigastrium, particularly in a young, white woman, suggests fibrous renal artery disease as a potential cause for the hypertension. A systolic bruit without a diastolic component is much less specific and is frequently heard in elderly patients who do not have renal artery stenosis. There are no clear-cut historical or physical findings that discriminate with certainty patients with renovascular hypertension from the larger pool of patients with essential hypertension, with the possible exception of a systolic/diastolic bruit in the epigastrium of a young Caucasian woman. Nevertheless, when several of the above-described historical or physical examination clues are present, renovascular hypertension should be considered.

Having suspected renovascular hypertension from the history and physical examination, there are a number of diagnostic or screening tests

Table 1
Diagnostic Tests for Presumed Renovascular Hypertension

Hypokalemia

Rapid-Sequence ("hypertensive") IVP

Radionuclide Scan
  Conventional
  Pre- and postcaptopril

Peripheral Renin Activity (PRA)

Captopril PRA (Captopril Test)

IV-DSA

Renal Arteriography
  Conventional
  IA-DSA

Renal Vein Renin Ratio

---

that might enhance the clinician's ability to predict renovascular hypertension. These screening tests are summarized in Table 1. Hypokalemia in the untreated state or in response to a thiazide diuretic is a frequent clue to renovascular hypertension since the pathophysiology of this disorder is associated with secondary aldosteronism. Activation of the renin-angiotensin system with subsequent increased aldosterone levels tend to reduce the serum potassium level. Thiazide diuretics accentuate this phenomenon in renovascular hypertension.

The rapid sequence ("hypertensive") intravenous pyelogram (IVP) holds a time-honored place in evaluating patients for renovascular hypertension. Although the rapid sequence IVP is utilized less frequently now than in the past, it remains an excellent screening test for renovascular hypertension particularly if one wishes to gain other additional information about the anatomy of the urinary tract, e.g., a patient with moderately severe hypertension and a history of kidney stones or urinary tract infection. Features of the rapid sequence IVP that suggest unilateral renal artery stenosis include: (1) a disparity in kidney size of 1.5 cm or more (recall that the left kidney is 0.5 cm greater than the right kidney); (2) delayed nephrogram on the early minute films; (3) a disparity in appearance time of contrast medium in the collecting system; (4) a persistent nephrogram of the kidney on the side of the presumed arterial stenosis. Unfortunately, with the hypertensive IVP, there is a 15%–20% false-negative rate and a 10%–13% false-positive rate in surgically proven unilateral renovascular hypertension. Numerous studies have indicated that the sensitivity of an IVP in detecting unilateral renovascular hypertension is relatively poor (about 75%) and the overall sensitivity in detecting patients with bilateral renal artery disease is only about 60%. These shortcomings of the IVP, in addition to the potential risk of contrast media-induced acute renal failure, are the major reasons for the decreased popularity of this procedure as a screening test for presumed renovascular hypertension. However, since renovascular hypertension has a low prevalence in the general population (between 2% and 4%), when one applies Bayh's theorem to the utility of the rapid sequence IVP as a screening test for renovascular hypertension, a negative intravenous pyelogram provides strong evidence (98%–99% certainty) against renovascular hypertension.

Dynamic renal flow scans with technetium-99m diethylenetri-aminepentaacetic acid (DTPA) is a less invasive, less risky, screening test for presumed renovascular hypertension. Decreased uptake of isotope on the involved side should, theoretically, correlate fairly well with ipsilateral renal artery stenosis. However, this diagnostic test has a lower specificity than the rapid sequence IVP, and false-positive rates in the range of 25% have been reported. Attempts to enhance the sensitivity and specificity of nuclear imaging techniques by comparing the radionuclide scan before and after administration of captopril are under active investigation.

The casual measurement of peripheral plasma renin activity (PRA) is of little value as a diagnostic screening test for renovascular hypertension. The notion that patients with high PRA, even in the face of high urinary sodium excretion, will turn out to have renovascular hypertension is not supported by numerous clinical observations. Indeed, approximately one fourth of patients with essential hypertension have high peripheral plasma renin activity. However, the short-term (60–90 minute) response of blood pressure and PRA to an oral dose (25–50 mg) of captopril (captopril provocation test) has gained recent popularity as a screening test for presumed renovascular hypertension. The patient is prepared by remaining off all antihypertensive drugs from one to two weeks and is subsequently studied in a sodium replete state. A baseline blood pressure and PRA are obtained after which 25–50 mg of captopril crushed (to facilitate absorption) is administered. Sixty minutes after captopril administration, a "post-captopril" peripheral renin level is obtained along with repeat measurements of the blood pressure. Renin criteria that distinguish patients with proven renovascular hypertension from those with essential hypertension are the following: (1) a stimulated PRA of 12 ng/mL/hour or more and; (2) an absolute increase in PRA of 10 ng/mL/hour or more and; (3) an increase in PRA of 150% if the baseline PRA is greater than 3 ng/mL/hour or an increase of PRA of 400% if baseline PRA was less than 3 ng/mL/hour. Early reports with this test indicate an extremely high sensitivity and specificity (95%–100%) in identifying renovascular hypertension if all three of the above described renin criteria are met. Equally important is the observation that a post-captopril PRA of less than 3 ng/mL/hour virtually excludes the possibility of renovascular hypertension, assuming that the patient is not taking drugs known to suppress PRA (e.g., beta-blockers).

Intravenous digital subtraction angiography (IV-DSA) is a technique of imaging blood vessels whereby the background of bone and soft tissues of the body are subtracted from images made with iodinated contrast medium in the blood vessels. The final images reveal only the contrast medium outlining the lumen of the blood vessels. Accordingly, IV-DSA is less invasive than a formal renal arteriogram or intra-arterial DSA, which requires direct arterial puncture. However, the required dosage of contrast medium is relatively high, and visualization of the main renal arteries does not compare with that of either standard arteriography or intra-arterial DSA. Nevertheless, IV-DSA has become a popular diagnostic modality for diagnosing renal artery stenosis mainly because this procedure can be readily employed in an outpatient setting and does not require arterial cannulation. Unfortunately, the false-negative rate of IV-DSA approximates that of the rapid sequence IVP, and one large review of IV-DSA studies indicated that 7%–10% of these studies are considered uninterpretable due to motion artifact, overlying bowel gas, mesenteric vessels, and dependence on adequacy of cardiac output. Although many centers have done away with the rapid sequence IVP in favor of IV-DSA, the precision of this technique currently provides an inadequate basis for the interventional radiologist or vascular surgeon to intervene on the basis of an IV-DSA study alone. This technique frequently misses orificial atherosclerotic lesions as well as branch lesions and does not allow adequate evaluation of intrarenal vasculature. For patients at risk from contrast media acute renal failure (e.g., elderly patients and those with azotemia or proteinuria), the risks are similar for IV-DSA and conventional IVP.

Formal renal arteriography remains the gold standard for making the anatomical diagnosis of renal artery stenosis due either to atherosclerotic or fibrous renal artery disease. A complete arteriographic study of the renal arterial tree usually includes oblique and lateral views to better visualize the origin of the renal arteries as well as the origin of the celiac artery. Selective renal arteriograms help identify branch stenoses. If significant atherosclerotic stenosis is present at the orifice of the main renal artery, selective renal arteriography generally should be avoided because of the risk of dissecting or occluding the renal artery or of generating atheroemboli to the renovascular bed. Intra-arterial digital subtraction angiography (IA-DSA) is based on the same principle described for IV-DSA. Many centers are routinely utilizing IA-DSA rather than conventional arteriography since IA-DSA requires smaller volumes of contrast medium than conventional arteriography and the main renal artery vasculature is visualized just as well. Experienced radiologists obtain oblique and lateral views with the IA-DSA technique.

The presence of a stenotic lesion on a formal renal arteriogram or IA-DSA obviously confirms the diagnosis of renal artery stenosis but does not necessarily confirm that the stenotic lesion is instrumental in the pathogenesis of the hypertension. For approximately 25 years, determination of renal vein renin (RVR) ratios (ipsilateral divided by contralateral) have been utilized to help assess the functional significance of angiographically documented renal artery stenosis. A comparison of renin activity from the effluent venous blood of the suspected ischemic kidney to that of the contralateral nonstenotic kidney has been used to predict improvement in hypertension following an interventive procedure. Lateralization of renal vein renin to the side of the stenotic kidney predicts benefit from surgery in approximately 90% of patients. That is, lateralizing renal vein renins have a very high predictive value (90%–93%) for surgic success. However, there is an extremely high false-negative rate in that approximately 50% of patients with nonlateralizing renal vein renin ratios will benefit from surgery.

As indicated in Figure 1, 2K,1C Goldblatt hypertension is characterized by increased renin levels from the stenotic kidney (SK) and a suppressed renin from the contralateral kidney (CK). Accordingly, a renal vein renin ratio equal to or greater than 1.5—2.0 (SK/CK) predicts a beneficial response to surgery. However, in predicting a beneficial response to surgery or angioplasty (the final proof that the patient has renovascular hypertension), one should also observe a suppressed renin from the contralateral noninvolved kidney (CK). For example, if renal vein renin values in a patient with high-grade left renal artery stenosis measured 10 ng/mL/hour from the left renal vein and the renin level from the right renal vein measured 5 ng/mL/hour, this RVR ratio of 2.0 would seem to indicate a beneficial response to an interventive procedure on the left renal artery. However, if the renin level in the low inferior vena cava, below the renal veins, (reflecting a peripheral renin activity measurement) measured 2 ng/mL/hour, then clearly both kidneys are making renin and renin production from the unaffected right kidney is not suppressed. In contrast, if the renin value from the low inferior vena cava measured 5 or 6 ng/mL/hour, such data would indicate not only a 2:1 RVR ratio (left/right), but also that renin production from the contralateral right kidney is suppressed. The beneficial effect of the interventive maneuvers in patients with presumed renovascular hypertension due to unilateral renal artery stenosis is significantly enhanced by observing a lateralizing renal vein renin ratio in conjunction with suppressed renin from the contralateral side. Unfortunately, the utility of renal vein renin measurements in patients with bilateral renal artery stenosis is notoriously unreliable. In many cases, renin production is high in both kidneys and the RVR ratio loses its predictive value. In such situations, a higher renal vein renin on one side in comparison to the other, in conjunction with the appearance of the lesion on the angiogram may be useful in assisting the surgeon or interventional radiologist in determining which side to act upon.

One might argue that if strong historical clues are present to suggest renovascular hypertension, that one might proceed directly to formal renal arteriography or IA-DSA with concomitant measurement of the renal vein renin ratio. This approach would bypass other less invasive tests such as intravenous pyelography, radionuclide scan with or without captopril, and the captopril provocation test. For patients without a strong history to support a diagnosis of renovascular hypertension and particularly if such patients require several drugs to control the blood pressure, then additional diagnostic screening studies may be useful in influencing the physician to proceed with the more invasive IA-DSA or formal renal arteriogram. Most importantly, as cure or amelioration of the hypertension following renal revascularization, angioplasty, or nephrectomy is the ultimate criterion for the diagnosis of renovascular hypertension, the physician and patient should agree to one of these interventive maneuvers before expending considerable energy and expense with diagnostic screening tests.

Treatment of Renovascular Hypertension

The main goals in the treatment of renovascular hypertension are to control the blood pressure, prevent target organ complications, and to avoid the loss of renal function. Although the issue of renal function may be viewed as mutually exclusive from the issue of controlling the blood pressure, there is increasing concern that even in the presence of excellent blood pressure control, progressive arterial stenosis might worsen renal ischemia and promote renal atrophy and fibrosis. Thus, for many patients where the hypertension is presumed to be renovascular, concerns regarding overall renal function may affect the clinician's judgment regarding treatment options for the hypertension.

Therapeutic options include pharmacological antihypertensive therapy, percutaneous transluminal angioplasty (PCTA), and surgery. Surgical procedures consist primarily of revascularization of the kidney. Occasionally, ablative procedures such as total or partial nephrectomy are utilized. All of these therapeutic options have been found to be effective to varying degrees, and the indications for one treatment modality versus the other depends on several important factors. Among these factors are the accuracy of the diagnosis of renovascular hypertension, the likelihood of patient compliance with antihypertensive drug regimens, the presence of concurrent disorders, the risk-to-benefit ratio associated with the available treatment modalities, the severity of the hypertension, the threat to renal function, the medical condition of the patient and potential morbidity of surgical therapy, and the results of surgical therapy or angioplasty at a given medical center. The type of renal artery disease responsible for the elevated blood pressure should also be considered.

Prior to the early 1970s, the medical management of presumed renovascular hypertension was empirical and similar to that of essential hypertension. With the availability of beta-adrenergic blocking drugs and the angiotensin-converting enzyme inhibitors (ACEI), drugs that interfere with the renin-angiotensin system, the medical treatment of these patients is rarely truly resistant to pharmacological drugs. The administration of a beta-blocker, especially when combined with a diuretic, and the use of angiotensin-converting enzyme inhibitors when used alone, or in conjunction with diuretics and/or a beta-blocker are effective drug regimens for renovascular hypertension. Medical therapy is often the treatment of choice for some patients, including those with advanced age, disseminated atherosclerotic vascular disease who pose high surgical risks, and in situations where renal revascularization is thought to be infeasible due to technical difficulties of the potential surgery or irreversible atrophy of the kidney. However, relative contraindications to medical treatment of presumed renovascular hypertension include the inability to control the blood pressure pharmacologically,

Table 2
Relative Efficacy of Revascularization Versus PCTA for Renal Artery Disease

Lesion	% Success PCTA	% Success Revascularization
Atherosclerotic		
Nonostial (20%)	80–90	90
Ostial (80%)	25–30	90
Fibrous Dysplasia		
Main (50%)	80–90	90
Branch (50%)	Not Available	90

progressive atrophy of the kidney distal to the stenosis, and drug side effects that interfere with patient compliance or patient well-being. Surgical therapy for renovascular hypertension should be considered when the hypertension is refractory to medical management, for younger patients, for patients who are good surgical risks, and when the specific type of renal artery disease poses a threat to renal function from progressive arterial stenosis.

Considerable controversy exists over the issue of medical management versus surgery versus percutaneous transluminal angioplasty for renovascular hypertension. To date, no prospective randomized trials have been published addressing the long-term benefits, risks, and success of these three treatment modalities. Nevertheless, the bulk of the literature supports an interventional approach (i.e., surgery or angioplasty) when the clinical evaluation of the patient suggests that the patient will turn out to have renovascular hypertension. As shown in Table 2, abundant experience indicates that a high percentage of patients (at least 90%) will be successfully revascularized with improvement in blood pressure control for both fibrous and renal artery disease. However, the success rate for transluminal angioplasty with atherosclerotic ostial lesions of the renal artery and for patients with branch stenoses due to fibrous renal artery disease is less encouraging than if similar patients are treated surgically.

Medical management, although avoiding the risks of vascular surgery, is associated with several problems: the long-term metabolic side effects of drug therapy; problems of patient compliance; the potential deleterious effects of uninterrupted renal artery stenosis on renal function; the potential for blood pressure lowering below a critical renal perfusion pressure to impair overall glomerular filtration rate; and the potential for ACEI-induced acute renal failure. Approximately 10% of patients with high-grade bilateral renal artery stenosis will develop impaired renal function while on ACE inhibitor drugs. Fortunately, this complication is usually completely reversible upon discontinuance of these agents.

With regards to the surgical management of patients with presumed renovascular hypertension, unilateral nephrectomy rarely is indicated. In situations wherein a hyperreninemic atrophic kidney (e.g., less than 7–8 cm in height by laminography) is present, and especially if the blood pressure cannot be controlled medically, a simple nephrectomy by the posterior approach technique may be recommended and is a low-morbidity procedure. A variety of bypass procedures using autologous or synthetic grafts are the most common methodology for renal revascularization of atherosclerotic and fibrous renal artery diseases. A detailed review of the pros and cons of one surgical technique over the other is beyond the scope of this chapter. However, there appears to be a changing approach to surgical intervention in some centers in that alternative bypass procedures such as splenorenal, hepatorenal, and iliorenal bypass are being utilized in order to avoid operation on a badly diseased aorta. These surgical techniques have been associated with improved overall morbidity and mortality. For patients suspected of having generalized atherosclerosis, more favorable surgical results may be obtained by the preoperative screening and correction of coexisting coronary or carotid artery disease prior to undertaking elective renal revascularization. If co-existing generalized atherosclerosis is widespread, medical management or PCTA may be the treatments of choice.

Morbidity and mortality following surgical treatment of atherosclerotic renal artery disease ranges from 2% to 10%, depending upon the particular surgical series, with risk factors including coexisting coronary artery disease, bilateral renovascular disease, impaired renal function, and the magnitude of the operation. An operative mortality rate of 2% in patients with atherosclerotic renovascular disease has been achieved in some centers by paying careful attention to co-existing vascular disease, avoidance of operation on a severely diseased aorta, and by undertaking unilateral renal revascularization in patients with bilateral renovascular disease. The incidence of postoperative renal artery thrombosis or stenosis has been reported to be as low as 4%–5%.

Over the past several years, PCTA has surfaced as a popular interventional modality for the treatment of patients with presumed renovascular hypertension. Although PCTA provides a nonsurgical treatment option, it is an invasive procedure and not without complications. The technical success rates of PCTA as summarized in Table 2 are encouraging. In patients with fibrous renal artery disease, approximately 60% of patients are cured of their hypertension or demonstrate marked improvement in blood pressure control following successful dilatation. For patients with unilateral, nonostial atheromatous lesions, the "cure rate" of the hypertension is much lower, approximately 30%. Unfortunately, large numbers of patients presenting to physicians for evaluation and treatment for presume renovascular hypertension have high-grade bilateral atherosclerotic renal artery disease with either totally occluded renal arteries, or ostial lesions. For these patients, the technical success rates of PCTA are low, and the complication rates are high. These complications include: contrast-induced acute renal failure, atheroembolic renal failure, rupture or dissection of the renal artery, thrombotic occlusion of the renal artery, and occlusion of a branch renal artery. One rarely encounters balloon malfunction or balloon rupture. Although the long-term patency rates of successfully dilated stenoses is not entirely clear, available data suggest that stenosis recurs in about 15% to 20% of fibrous renal artery lesions, 30% to 50% of nonstial atherosclerotic lesions, and 50% to 70% of ostial atherosclerotic lesions at one to two years of follow-up. In comparison to renovascular surgery, PCTA has the advantages of substantially lower morbidity and mortality, diminished rate of nephrectomy, markedly lower cost, and the ease of repeating this procedure if the first attempt is unsuccessful. Further, a patient failing with PCTA therapy can always opt for surgery. Despite these potential advantages of PCTA, the potential complications should be taken seriously and PCTA should be viewed as an interventive maneuver that requires considerable angiographic expertise.

Summary

The management of patients with renovascular hypertension is a challenging one, requiring the cooperation and experience of the internist, nephrologist, radiologist, and vascular surgeon. The crucial step in approaching these patients is determining the likelihood that the patient has renovascular hypertension. Subsequently, the advantages and disadvantages of the various therapeutic options should be carefully considered for each individual patient, this decision making to include the experience and expertise of the treating physicians. As we enter the decade of the 1990s, there will be more efficacious and better-tolerated pharmacological agents for the medical management of these patients, and more experience with PCTA should establish this procedure as effective treatment for many. The development of better methods of surgical revascularization (e.g.. for patients with branch renal artery disease, and severely atherosclerotic aortas), and the improved safety and efficacy of surgical revascularization, particularly in elderly patients, will be forthcoming. Finally, as we learn more about the potential for atherosclerotic renal artery disease to affect kidney function, future efforts to diagnose renal artery disease may be initiated with a view toward preservation of overall renal function, rather than for relief of hypertension.

Selected References

Canzanello VJ, Millan VG, Spiegel JE, et al: Percutaneous transluminal renal angioplasty in management of atherosclerotic renovascular hypertension: results in 100 patients. Hypertension 13:163–172, 1989.

Chrysant SG, Dunn M, Marples D: Severe reversible azotemia from captopril therapy. Arch Intern Med 143:437–441, 1983.

Dean RH, Kieffer RW, Smith BM, et al: Renovascular hypertension: anatomic and functional changes during drug therapy. Arch Surg 116:1408–1415, 1981.

Dunnick NR, Svetkey LP, Cohan RH, et al: Intravenous digital subtraction renal angiography: use in screening for renovascular hypertension. Radiology 171:219–222, 1989.

Dustan HP, Humphries AW, de Wolfe VG, et al: Normal arterial pressure in patients with renal arterial stenosis. JAMA 187:1128–1129, 1964.

Foster JH, Maxwell MH, Franklin SS, et al: Renovascular occlusive disease: results of operative treatment. JAMA 231:1043–1048, 1975.

Gifford RW Jr: Evaluation for renovascular hypertension and selection of patients for surgical treatment. In: Novick AC, Straffon RA (eds), Vascular Problems in Urologic Surgery. Philadelphia, WB Saunders, 1982, pp 139–154.

Gifford RW Jr, McCormack LJ, Poutasse EF: The atrophic kidney: its role in hypertension. Mayo Clin Proc 40:834–852, 1965.

Goldblatt H, Lynch J, Hanzal RF, et al: Studies on experimental hypertension. I. The production of persistent elevation of systolic blood pressure by means of renal ischemia. J Exp Med 59:347, 1934.

Goncharenko V, Gerlock AJ, Shaff MI, et al: Progression of renal artery fibromuscular dysplasia in 42 patients as seen on angiography. Radiology 139:45–51, 1981.

Gruntzig A, Kuhlman U, Vetter W, et al: Treatment of renovascular hypertension with percutaneous transluminal dilatation of a renal artery stenosis. Lancet 1:801–802, 1978.

Hughes JS, Dove HG, Gifford RW Jr, et al: Duration of hypertension: a predictor of surgical cure for renovascular hypertension. Am Heart J 101:408, 1981.

Hunt JC, Sheps SG, Harrison EG Jr, et al: Renal and renovascular hypertension: a reasoned approach to diagnosis and management. Arch Intern Med 133:988–999, 1974.

Hussain RA, Gifford RW Jr, Stewart BH, et al: Differential renal venous renin activity in diagnosis of renovascular hypertension. Review of 29 cases. Am J Cardiol 32:707–715, 1973.

Jacobson HR: Ischemic renal disease: an overlooked clinical entity? Kidney Int 34:729–743, 1988.

Kaplan NM: Renal vascular hypertension. In: Kaplan NM (ed), Clinical Hypertension. Baltimore, Williams and Wilkins, 1986, pp 317–344.

Klinge J, Mali WPTM, Puijlaert CBAJ, et al: Percutaneous transluminal renal angioplasty: initial and long-term results. Radiology 171:501–506, 1989.

Madias NE: Renovascular hypertension. American Kidney Foundation Nephrology Letter 4:27–42, 1986.

Maxwell MH, Lupu AN: Excretory urogram in renal arterial hypertension. J Urol 100:395–406, 1968.

McCormack LJ, Poutasse EF, Meaney TF, et al: A pathologic arteriographic correlation of renal arterial disease. Am Heart J 72:188–198, 1966.

Muller FB, Sealey JE, Case DB, et al: The captopril test for identifying renovascular disease in hypertensive patients. Am J Med 80:633–644, 1986.

Nally JV Jr, Gupta BK, Clarke HS, et al: Captopril renography for the detection of renovascular hypertension. Cleve Clin J Med 55:311–318, 1988.

Novick AC (ed): The Urologic Clinics of North America, Volume 11, Number 3. Philadelphia, W.B. Saunders, 1984.

Novick AC, Pohl MA, Schreiber MJ, et al: Revascularization for preservation of renal function in patients with atherosclerotic renovascular disease. J Urol 129:907–912, 1983.

Novick AC, Straffon RA, Stewart BH, et al: Diminished operative morbidity and mortality in renal revascularization. JAMA 246:749–753, 1981.

Novick AC, Ziegelbaum M, Vidt DG, et al: Trends in surgical revascularization for renal artery disease. Ten years' experience. JAMA 257:498–501, 1987.

Parrot TS, Woodard JR, Trulock TS, et al: Segmental renal vein renins and partial nephrectomy for hypertension. J Urol 131:736–739, 1984.

Pickering TG, Laragh JH, Sos TA: Renovascular hypertension. In: Schrier RW, Gottschalk CW (eds), Diseases of the Kidney, Fourth Edition. Boston, Little, Brown and Company, 1988, pp 1597–1622.

Pickering TG, Sos TA, Vaughan ED Jr, et al: Predictive value and changes of renin secretion in hypertensive patients with unilateral renovascular disease undergoing successful renal angioplasty. Am J Med 76:398–404, 1984.

Pohl MA, Novick AC: Natural history of atherosclerotic and fibrous renal artery disease: clinical implications. Am J Kidney Dis 5:A120-A130, 1985.

Ratliff NB: Renal vascular disease: pathology of large blood vessel disease. Am J Kidney Dis 5:893, 1985.

Renovascular Hypertension • 393

Reiss MD, Bookstein JJ, Bleifer KH: Radiologic aspects of renovascular hypertension: IV arteriographic complications. JAMA 221:374–378, 1972.

Schreiber MJ, Pohl MA, Novick AC: The natural history of atherosclerotic and fibrous renal artery disease. Urol Clin North Am 11:383–392, 1984.

Smith MC, Dunn MJ: Renovascular and renal parenchymal hypertension. In: Brenner BM, Rector FC Jr (eds), The Kidney, Third Edition. Philadelphia, W.B. Saunders, 1986, pp 1221–1251.

Sos TA, Pickering G, Sniderman K, et al: Percutaneous transluminal renal angioplasty in renovascular hypertension due to atheroma or fibromuscular dysplasia. N Engl J Med 309:274–279, 1983.

Stewart BH: Renovascular hypertension: surgical treatment. Monographs in Urology 5:3–36, 1981.

Textor SC, Novick AC, Tarazi RC, et al: Critical perfusion pressure for renal function in patients with bilateral atherosclerotic renal vascular disease. Ann Intern Med 102:308–314, 1985.

Thibonnier M, Joseph A, Sassano P, et al: Improved diagnosis of unilateral renal artery lesions after captopril administration. JAMA 251:56–60, 1984.

Vaughan ED Jr, Carey RM, Ayers CR, et al : A physiologic definition of blood pressure response to renal revascularization in patients with renovascular hypertension. Kidney Int 15:S83, 1979.

Vaughan ED Jr, Sos TA, Sniderman KW, et al: Renal vein renin secretory patterns before and after transluminal angioplasty in patients before and after transluminal angioplasty in patients with renovascular hypertension: verification of analytic criteria. In: Laragh JH (ed), Frontiers in Hypertension Research. New York, Springer-Verlag, 1981.

Williams GH: Converting-enzyme inhibitors in the treatment of hypertension. N Engl J Med 319:1517–1525, 1988.

Wollenweber J, Sheps SG, David DG: Clinical course of atherosclerotic renovascular disease. Am J Cardiol 21:60–71, 1968.

Working Group on Renovascular Hypertension: Detection, evaluation, and treatment of renovascular hypertension. Final report. Arch Intern Med 147:820–829, 1987.

Ying CY, Tifft CP, Gavras H, et al: Renal revascularization in the azotemic hypertensive patient resistant to therapy. N Engl J Med 311:1070–1075, 1984.

Chapter 21

The Future

Henry A. Punzi and Walter Flamenbaum

The future of clinical hypertension will, as has been true to date, parallel the course of medicine in general. Regardless of the etiology of essential or primary hypertension, we will continue to focus on improved methods of diagnosis and therapy. Basic research will continue to dissect away the roles of inheritance, volume homeostasis, and the various neurogenic and/or hormonal mechanisms controlling vascular tone. Separate efforts will continue to elucidate the interaction of blood pressure and altered "core" organ function. The relevance of changes in intrarenal hemodynamics with regard to the occurrence or progression of renal disease may be followed by similar understandings with regard to cerebral or cardiac function.

The future, in the near term, will see some increasing efforts to refine our diagnostic and prognostic techniques. There is already an increasing emphasis on the accuracy and appropriateness of our diagnosis of hypertension. Improvements in methodology will almost certainly place a greater reliance on techniques such as ambulatory blood pressure monitoring for diagnostic purposes. As we continue to dissect out the relative and relevant changes in systemic blood pressure, the relationship between shear forces and rates of rise in systemic pressure to the need for treatment, the rapidity of therapy, and the long-term implications of therapy will almost certainly evolve. In this regard, we will very likely see the fruits of the current trend in selecting agents that are vasodilators *because* increased total peripheral resistance is the common physiological denominator of the hypertensive disease state.

From a therapeutic viewpoint we see a tendency to continue with

From Punzi HA, Flamenbaum W (eds): *Hypertension*. Mount Kisco, NY, Futura Publishing Co., Inc., © 1989.

the current trends. We believe that the influence of the "J-curve"—that is, the potential negative impact of a relative excessive lowering of blood pressure on morbidity and mortality—will require long-term study prior to being settled. For the present, most physicians will use prudent clinical judgment with the possibility of a persistence in the trend to undertreat and, therefore, undercontrol of the blood pressure of patients with hypertension.

In the short term, there will be an increase in various vasodilatory agents—both those that act through converting enzyme inhibition, as well as those functioning as calcium (or other ionic) channel blockers. We very likely have not seen the last of agents such as atrial natriuretic peptide. Agents that can simultaneously vasodilate and promote a natriuresis are very attractive, as is evident from some of the considerations surrounding certain calcium channel blockers. We should not be deterred by the current necessity to inject such compounds; especially if we remember the parenteral predecessors of the converting enzyme inhibitors.

We almost certainly will see continued growth in the availability of specific agents interfering with the actions of the renin-angiotensin system axis. These "renin inhibitors" will be therapeutically specific and dramatic in their antihypertensive effects. Similarly, there will be greater therapeutic control over prostanoid vasodilators and vasoconstrictors. The net effect will be to lower blood pressure and reduce vasculotoxic events important in the sequelae of hypertension and the pathogenesis of atherosclerosis.

The interaction of hypertension with other risk factors and the interaction among the various antihypertensive agents will have a larger impact on the provision of health care to hypertensive patients. We will gain reasonable perspective about the interaction of blood pressure per se and altered lipid profiles in the genesis of cardiovascular disease. Certainly altered lipid profiles will not outweigh the prognostic import of the absolute reductions achieved in systemic blood pressure; *but*, all things being equal, we opt for less disturbance in lipid profile. Therapeutic agents that will safely and effectively normalize lipid profile will be used intelligently with antihypertensive agents.

The recrudescence of interest in combination therapy will result, in part, from our concerns about long-term side effect issues and in part from the consideration of "quality-of-life" issues. Side effects are perceived as being dose-related. The nature of studies resulting in the FDA approval process has resulted in higher than necessary doses being utilized for the therapy of hypertension. These two factors together will result in our using lower doses of therapeutic agents and leaning towards the earlier use of nonfixed- and fixed-dose combination therapies.

The events of the future would suggest an overall improvement of the care provided to patients with hypertension. The earlier and more accurate diagnosis of hypertension should result in a greater reduction in the overall morbidity and mortality associated with the disease. Improved pharmacotherapy—newer agents, the better and more appropriate use of all agents—will result in a larger percentage of patients achieving better control of their ambulatory blood pressures. The commingling of therapeutic goals—reduction in blood pressure, avoidance of side effects, maintenance of quality of life, and considerations of cofactor interaction for the pathogenesis of cardiovascular disease—are on the horizon. Thirty to forty years ago the therapy of hypertension was moving from the empiric to the specific; the next chapter shall not take as long in the coming.

Index

ACE inhibitors *see* Enzyme inhibitors
Acute ischemic stroke, 71–72
Adrenergic blockers, 71
Age, 2–4
Alcohol, 99–100
Aldosteronism, 36–38
Allergic reactions, 125
Alpha blockers, 321–322, 342–343
Ambulatory monitoring, 43–55
   accuracy, 45–46
   data analysis, 50–51
   instrumentation, 44–45
   physiological relevance, 47–50
   use in research, 54–55
   use in treatment, 53–54
Angiography, 354–359
Angiotensin II, 88–90
Antihypertensive agents
   centrally acting, 207–218, 310–311
   effect on cerebral blood flow, 70–71
   and pregnancy, 310–311
   see also specific drugs
Arrhythmias, 254–255
Arthritis, 264–265
Atherosclerotic renal artery disease, 378–380
Atrial natriuretic factor, 18–19

Baroreceptors, 178
Beta-adrenergic blockade, 143–144, 167–179, 342
   alpha-adrenergic activity, 171–172
   and alpha blockers, 321–322, 343
   cardiovascular effects, 175–179
   ISA, 171
   MSA, 170, 178
   pharmacodynamic properties, 167–172
   pharmacokinetic properties, 172–175
   potency, 168
   selectivity, 170–171
Binswanger's disease, 73
Blood lipids *see* Lipids

Blood pressure
   and beta-adrenergic blockade, 175–179
   classification of readings, 29
   cuff size, 25–26
   follow-up criteria for first measurements, 30
   home measurements, 27–29
   measurement of, 24–25
   pseudohypertension, 26–27
   role of ambulatory monitoring, 43–55
Borderline hypertension, 2–3
Brain, 9
   baroceptor reflexes, 68, 70
   cerebral autoregulation, 65–68, 69
Breast feeding, 311–312

Calcium, 20, 106–107
Calcium antagonists, 71, 131–150, 311, 322, 342
   as antihypertensive agents, 137–138
   antihypertensive therapy with accompanying diseases, 140–142
   and beta blockers, 144
   combination therapy, 142–144
   demographic considerations, 139–140
   differences among, 133
   discontinuation syndrome, 146
   dosage, 147–148
   drug interactions, 149
   metabolic effects, 146–147
   and other vasodilators, 135–136
   pharmacokinetics, 133–135
   pharmacology, 138–139
   side effects, 144–146
   see also specific channel blockers
Calcium metabolism, 124–125
Carbohydrates, 112–113
Central nervous system, 175–176
Cerebral autoregulation, 65–68, 69
Cerebral blood flow, 65–71, 286–287
Cerebral vascular disease, 71–74

Chloride, 110
Cholesterol, 36, 147
   see also Lipids
Chronic obstructive pulmonary
   disease, 264
Chronotropic effects, 175
Cigarette smoking, 338
Clonidine, 208, 212–215
Congestive heart failure, 252–254, 255
Coronary heart disease, 251–252, 253, 335–338
   blood lipids, 337–338
   risk factors, 336–337

Demographics, 10, 139–140
Diabetes, 257–261, 263
Diazoxide, 196–197, 329, 330
Diet, 104–113
Dihydralazine, 70–71
Dilevalol, 321
Diltiazem, 133–134, 145–146
Diuretics, 117–130, 333, 339, 340–342
   and elderly, 274–275
   loop-blocking, 126–128
   potassium-sparing, 128–130
   and pregnancy, 307–308
   thiazide, 118–126
Drugs, 339–340
   antihypertensive, 70–71, 207–218, 310–311
   beta blockers, 143–144, 167–179, 342
   calcium antagonists, 71, 131–150, 311, 322, 342
   diuretics, 117–130, 307–308, 333, 339, 340–342
   see also specific drugs

Echocardiography, 57–63
Elderly, 4, 269–279
   diuretics, 274–275
   sympatholytics, 275–276
   therapy, 273–274
   vasodilators, 276–279
Electrocardiogram (ECG), 36
Emergencies, 202, 323–326, 327–328
Enalaprilat, 329, 331
Enzyme inhibitors, 155–165, 311, 323, 342
   currently available, 159–160
   guidelines for use, 160–164
   pharmacological basis for antihypertensive action, 157–158
   renal effects of, 90–92
Esmolol, 332, 333
Essential hypertension, 1–21, 296–297
Exercise, 101–103, 338

Fat, 111–112
Fiber, 112
Fibrinogen, 338
Fibrous renal artery disease, 373–377

Ganglionic blockers, 71
Gender, 10
Glucose, 147, 338
Guanabenz, 215
Guanafacine, 216

Heart, 5–6
   congestive failure, 252–254, 255
   functional changes in hypertensive, 59–60
   structural changes in hypertensive, 57–59
   surgery, 289–290
   see also Coronary heart disease
Hydralazine, 192–194, 201–202, 310, 329, 330
Hyperglycemia, 125–126
Hyperlipoproteinemia, 123
Hypertension
   accelerated, 318–321
   beta-adrenergic blockade in systemic, 167–179
   borderline, 2–4
   and calcium antagonists, 131–150
   and concomitant diseases, 247–266
   converting enzyme inhibitors, 155–165
   core organ effects, 57–92
   diagnosis and evaluation of, 23–41, 52–53, 60–61
   and echocardiography, 57–63
   in elderly, 4, 269–279
   essential, 1–21, 296–297

Hypertension (cont.)
  malignant, 319–321
  monitoring in hospitalized patient, 39
  new patient currently receiving treatment, 40–41
  nondrug therapy, 97–114
  and obesity, 11–16, 98–99
  pathophysiological and pathogenic aspects of essential, 1–21
  in perioperative period, 283–292
  and pregnancy, 293–312
  quality of life for patients, 221–241
  renovascular, 351–391
  resistant, 316–321
  secondary, 203
  treatment for, 339
  urgent, emergent, and refractory, 315–334
  and vasodilators, 190–192, 201–203
  see also Blood pressure
Hyperuricemia, 125
Hypochloremic metabolic alkalosis, 122–123
Hypokalemia, 121–122
Hyponatremia, 121

Inotropic effects, 175
Intubation, 285

Kidneys, 6, 8–9
  chronic renal disease, 297–298
  intrarenal effects of angiotensin II, 88–90
  pathophysiology of essential hypertensive, 83–87
  renal effects of ACE inhibitors, 90–92
  renal impairment, 256–257, 258
  therapeutic considerations, 87–88
  see also Renovascular hypertension

Labetalol, 321, 331, 332
Laboratory tests, 35–38
Lacunar infarcts, 72–73
Large arteries, 190
Left ventricular hypertrophy, 191, 250–251
Lipids, 335–350

and antihypertensive therapy, 343–349
  cost effectiveness of drugs, 344–345, 347–349
Loop-blocking diuretics, 126–128

Magnesium, 109–110
Medical history, 31–32
Methyldopa, 207–212, 310–311
Minoxidil, 194–196, 202
MSA see Quinidine effect
Myocardial infarction, 287–288

Nervous system, central see Central nervous system
Nervous system, sympathetic see Sympathetic nervous system
Nicardipine, 134–135, 145, 322
Nifedipine, 133–134, 135, 145, 322, 329, 331
Nitroglycerin, 199–200, 328, 329
Nitroprusside see Sodium nitroprusside

Obesity, 11–16, 98–99
Osler's maneuver, 27

Perioperative period, 283–292
Peripheral blood flow, 177
Peripheral vascular disease, 256
Phentolamine, 332, 333
Pheochromocytoma, 38–39
Phosphorus, 110–111
Phototoxicity, 123
Physical examination, 32–35
Pinacidil, 200–201
Plasma renin, 176–177
Postcerebral infarction, 73–74
Potassium, 107–109, 147
Potassium-sparing diuretics, 128–129
Pre-eclampsia, 298–302, 309–310
  clinical features of, 301–302
  differential diagnosis, 302
  pathophysiology of, 299–301
Pregnancy
  antihypertensive therapy, 302–309
  breast feeding, 311–312
  chronic renal disease, 297–298
  and hypertension, 293–312
  pre-eclampsia, 298–302, 309–310

402 • HYPERTENSION

Prejunctional beta-receptors, 178–179
Protein, 112
Pseudohypertension, 26–27
Pulmonary disease, chronic obstructive, 264

Quality of life, 221–241
Quinidine effect (MSA), 170, 178

Race, 10
Renal artery stenosis, 373–380
Renal blood flow, 287
Renal system see Kidneys; Renovascular hypertension
Renin-angiotensin system, 17–18
Renovascular hypertension, 351–391
 angiographic findings, 356–359
 clinical characteristics, 380386
 diagnostic angiographic techniques, 354–356
 internist's view, 367–391
 pathogenesis, 368–373
 preangiography screening, 352–354
 radiological interventional procedure, 359–364
 radiologist's view, 351–364
 treatment of, 386–390
Research, 54–55
Reserpine, 216–218

Sexual dysfunction, 124
Smoking, 338
Sodium, 104–106, 317
Sodium nitroprusside, 71, 197–199, 328, 329
Stress, 103–104
Stroke
 acute ischemic, 71–72
 prevention of, 74–78
 primary prevention, 74–76
 secondary prevention, 76–78
Surgery
 cardiac, 289–290
 factors predicting cardiovascular risk, 288
 hemodynamic changes during, 284–288
 increased risk in hypertensive patients, 283–284
 intubation, 285
 perioperative myocardial infarction, 287–288
 recovery, 287
Sympathetic nervous system, 16–20
Sympatholytics, 275–276

Target organ disease, 5–9
Thiazide diuretics, 118–126
Tobacco, 100–101
Transient ischemic attacks, 72
Trimethaphan camsylate, 331, 332

Uric acid, 147
Uric acid metabolism, 261–262, 264

Vascular disease, peripheral, 256
Vascular factors, local, 19–20
Vascular resistance, 177
Vascular smooth muscle tone, 184–185
Vasodilators, 183–203, 328–331
 compensatory responses to, 189–190
 control of vascular smooth muscle tone, 184–185
 differences between calcium antagonists and others, 135–136
 effect on large arteries, 190
 and elderly, 274–275
 mode and site of action of, 185–187
 and pregnancy, 310
 and structural alterations in hypertension, 190–192
 uses in hypertension, 201–203
 see also specific vasodilators
Venous tone, 177
Verapamil, 133, 145–146, 329, 330